DIABETES
TECHNOLOGY
SCIENCE AND PRACTICE

Edited by Boris Draznin, MD, PhD

Associate Editors:
Steven Edelman, MD
Irl B. Hirsch, MD
David C. Klonoff, MD

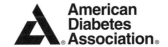

American Diabetes Association

Associate Publisher, Books, Abe Ogden; *Director, Book Operations,* Victor Van Beuren; *Managing Editor, Books,* John Clark; *Associate Director, Book Marketing,* Annette Reape; *Acquisitions Editor,* Jaclyn Konich; *Senior Manager, Book Editing,* Lauren Wilson; *Editorial Services,* Cenveo Publisher Services; *Composition,* Cenveo Publisher Services; *Cover Design,* Vis-a-Vis Creative; *Printer,* Lightning Source®.

Printed in the United States of America
1 3 5 7 9 10 8 6 4 2

The suggestions and information contained in this publication are generally consistent with the *Standards of Medical Care in Diabetes* and other policies of the American Diabetes Association, but they do not represent the policy or position of the Association or any of its boards or committees. Reasonable steps have been taken to ensure the accuracy of the information presented. However, the American Diabetes Association cannot ensure the safety or efficacy of any product or service described in this publication. Individuals are advised to consult a physician or other appropriate healthcare professional before undertaking any diet or exercise program or taking any medication referred to in this publication. Professionals must use and apply their own professional judgment, experience, and training and should not rely solely on the information contained in this publication before prescribing any diet, exercise, or medication. The American Diabetes Association—its officers, directors, employees, volunteers, and members—assumes no responsibility or liability for personal or other injury, loss, or damage that may result from the suggestions or information in this publication.

Dr. Barry Ginsberg conducted the internal review of this book to ensure that it meets American Diabetes Association guidelines.

⊗ The paper in this publication meets the requirements of the ANSI Standard Z39.48-1992 (permanence of paper).

ADA titles may be purchased for business or promotional use or for special sales. To purchase more than 50 copies of this book at a discount, or for custom editions of this book with your logo, contact the American Diabetes Association at the address below or at booksales@diabetes.org.

American Diabetes Association
2451 Crystal Drive, Suite 900
Arlington, VA 22202

DOI: 10.2337/9781580406932

Library of Congress Cataloging-in-Publication Data

Names: Draznin, Boris, editor.

Title: Diabetes technology : science and practice / Boris Draznin (editor).
Description: Arlington : American Diabetes Association, [2019] | Includes bibliographical references and index.
Identifiers: LCCN 2018056277 | ISBN 9781580406932 (softcover : alk. paper)
Subjects: | MESH: Diabetes Mellitus—therapy | Blood Glucose Self-Monitoring | Insulin Infusion Systems | Equipment and Supplies
Classification: LCC RC660 | NLM WK 815 | DDC 616.4/62—dc23
LC record available at https://lccn.loc.gov/2018056277

Contents

Preface

Diabetes is anything but a simple disease. In addition to having the potential to affect every organ and every system of the body, it influences every day of a person's life, every single thing one does. And it never goes away. Diabetes affects more than 10% of the U.S. population, and close to 1.5 million people in this country live with type 1 diabetes, many of whom enjoy otherwise healthy and productive lives while managing their diabetes.

Advances in technology and the application of this technology to healthcare in general, and diabetes in particular, have added tremendous benefits to patients with diabetes, but not without a trade-off: The complexity and cost of diabetes technology quickly became factual and undeniable obstacles in its widespread utilization.

Despite the newly added complexity, diabetes technology is improving diabetes management: so much so that many patients and their healthcare providers can no longer imagine life without it.

Yet, only a fraction of patients with diabetes use diabetes technology to its full capacity. Putting the cost of diabetes technology aside (which is, unfortunately, impossible to do in real life), we still have to deal with the fact that most physicians simply lack the knowledge of this critical aspect of contemporary diabetes management to guide their patients through the complexity of these new devices and apps.

Patients, too, must be educated about what is available on the market today to help them manage their disease and advised about how to use rapidly improving technology for the daily self-management of diabetes.

Notwithstanding this difficulty, the editors and contributors to this volume realize that the future of diabetes technology is even more interesting and exciting than what is unfolding today. This technology will continue to transform the lives of patients with diabetes until the inevitable day when diabetes is cured.

We hope that our book, which may well be somewhat obsolete at the time of publication, offers practical guidelines to today's diabetes technology for healthcare providers. We present real-life cases to illustrate how the use of diabetes technology has helped patients control their disease under a variety of circumstances. Finally, leading diabetes specialists, who themselves live with type 1 diabetes, share their personal and inspiring life stories, including their experiences with, and thoughts about, the benefits of diabetes technology.

Boris Draznin, MD, PhD
Steven Edelman, MD
Irl B. Hirsch, MD
David C. Klonoff, MD

Introduction

Diabetes technology evolved rather rapidly in the past decade, showing significant improvements every year. Interestingly, and somewhat paradoxically, one could argue that advances in technology also have increased the burden of managing diabetes, defined by *1)* increased complexity of monitoring and therapy, *2)* commitment and knowledge on behalf of patients and their healthcare providers, *3)* intricacy of the structure of the clinics caring for patients who utilize diabetes technology, and *4)* expenditure of financial resources.

Despite these barriers, the number of patients and providers who are embracing diabetes technology continues to grow as technology clearly improves treatment outcomes and the lives of our patients. A fully automated artificial pancreas the size of a pager or a cellphone is no longer a dream but rather is a rapidly approaching reality.

Integrating information and communication technology into the overall diabetes-related technology expands advances in management and offers huge potential for improving healthcare in general and diabetes care in particular. Mobile apps and text messaging already have been shown to improve glycemic management along with other crucial components of diabetes self-management, such as meal planning, dietary interventions, and activity tracking, as well as education and motivation.

Digital health for continuous glucose monitoring and insulin delivery is ready to explode, bringing to the market new avenues for therapy of both type 1 and type 2 diabetes. Social media undoubtedly will prove to be extremely useful for diabetes management.

These exciting developments also bring significant challenges to diabetes care. With publication of this book, we seek to bring practical solutions and guidelines to many physicians and their patients in this country and around the world, offering expert opinion as to how to overcome many real and perceived obstacles in successful and expanded use of diabetes technology.

Part 1 of this book is written by leaders in this field, and each chapter attempts to integrate seamlessly the data and experience with diabetes technology available to us today with the clinical decision-making process most physicians face in their daily practice. Every author contributing chapters to this book is open to answer any questions the readers might have. Nothing would compliment us more than knowing that this book is helping others to better manage diabetes by involving diabetes technology into therapeutic armamentarium.

Part 2 of this book presents clinical examples of how certified diabetes educators (CDEs) use the latest diabetes technology to manage their patients, addressing the most complex and frequently urgent problems. We hope their experiences would introduce invaluable examples to other CDEs, endocrinologists, and primary care providers and entice them to fully embrace diabetes technology in their practice.

Finally, Part 3 of this book represents the most unique contribution of physicians who have the most intimate, first-hand experience with type 1 diabetes and diabetes technology. These doctors have lived, breathed, and endured diabetes every day and every minute of their lives for decades. They describe their journey into the realm of diabetes technology, their acceptance of this technology, and their successes in managing their own disease and in their professional and family lives. They are true heroes of our time, inspiration to many of us, and role models not only for future generations of doctors and patients but also for humanity. We are so grateful to all of them for sharing their stories with us.

Chapter 1
The History and Future of Diabetes Technology

David C. Klonoff, MD, FACP, FRCP (Edin), Fellow AIMBE[1]

INTRODUCTION

Diabetes technology refers to the application of scientific principles or the use of practical experience to create tools for people with diabetes and to develop products to fight this disease. Diabetes technology spans the spectrum of technologic applications derived from the physical sciences, which can be used to treat, monitor, diagnose, or prevent diabetes. Diabetes technology is a new approach. Traditional approaches to diabetes seek to improve the physiological capabilities of patients to produce more insulin or survive better with existing production of insulin. A bioengineered approach does not seek to cure the disease, but rather it seeks to provide sensor data and effector capabilities to allow patients to take steps or to automatically take steps to compensate for the physiological deficits present in this disease.[1] Two goals of the discipline of diabetes technology are to promote the development and use of technology; therefore, advances in this discipline come both from scientists who are developing tools and from clinicians who are using these tools on patients. The first medical journal to focus on the field of diabetes technology and whose name included the first mention of the term diabetes technology was *Diabetes Technology & Therapeutics*, which was launched in 1999. This journal was followed by the second journal to cover this field: *Journal of Diabetes Science and Technology*, which was launched in 2007. Both were quickly accepted into PubMed and between them today they cover the spectrum of topics related to diabetes technology. The Artificial Pancreas Center at Thomas Jefferson University was founded in 1998 by Dr. Jeffrey Joseph to address a key element of the field of diabetes technology. The University of Virginia established the Center for Diabetes Technology (CDT) in 2010 to advance the use of technology, including analytics, to allow improved management, monitoring, and therapies for patients with type 1 diabetes (T1D).

WIDELY USED DIABETES TOOLS

Self-Monitoring of Blood Glucose

During the first two-thirds of the 20th century, diabetes patients could measure their blood glucose levels only by measuring the concentration of glucose in

[1]Medical Director, Diabetes Research Institute, Mills-Peninsula Medical Center, San Mateo, CA; Clinical Professor of Medicine, University of California, San Francisco, San Francisco, CA.

urine and then attempting to estimate the corresponding blood glucose level. This approach was inaccurate because of the threshold for the appearance of glucose in urine (the blood glucose level had to be at least 180 mg/dL) and because of the time lag between a rise in the blood glucose concentration above the threshold and the appearance of glucose in the urine.

Dry regent test strips for blood glucose were introduced in the 1960s and, for the next 20 years, patients could have a blood glucose tested at a physician's office or even test their own glucose level with a strip that would change color according to the glucose concentration. A color wheel could be used to determine a semi-quantitative glucose level. The color wheels were crude and color separation was difficult to visualize, so it was difficult to obtain an exact reading. In the 1970s, tabletop reflectance photometry glucose monitors reading strips became available for physician's offices and hospitals. These devices required training and regular calibration and were not suitable for home use.

In the 1980s, portable battery-powered reflectance meters for measuring strips became widely available. Over this decade, these products became smaller, faster, and more accurate. Many of them had a data storage capability. In 1987, the first electrochemical glucose monitor was developed. This product allowed blood to be added to a strip that was already inserted into the meter. No washing, wiping, or blotting of strips was needed with this type of product. By the mid-1990s, self-monitoring of blood glucose (SMBG) had become established as a mainstream part of care in part because this method was used in two major studies of this period, the Diabetes Control and Complications Trial and the *U.K. Prospective Diabetes Study* (UKPDS) Trial and, in part, because operator dependent sources of error were being engineered out of the products.[2]

On the basis of patient preferences for ease of testing and physician preferences for lack of interference from oxygen, during the first decade of the 21st century, glucose oxidase systems were being replaced gradually by glucose dehydrogenase systems. These systems used the coenzyme pyrroloquinoline quinone (PQQ) as a cofactor. Although these products were becoming widely used, two types of pharmaceutical products also were coming onto the market that contained glucose-derived substances that interfered as false positive substances. Peritoneal dialysis fluid contained glucose polymers (icodextrin) or glucose disaccharides (maltose) and parenteral immunoglobulin preparations used maltose as an excipient to stabilize the protein in the solution. In the first decade of the 2000s, several cases of falsely elevated glucose readings followed by inappropriately high doses of insulin resulting in death were reported.[3] At that point, manufacturers of electrochemistry blood glucose monitors (BGMs), which used PQQ as a cofactor, switched from PQQ to other coenzymes with which icodextrin and maltose did not interfere.

In the 21st century, SMBG was widely established as a tool for recognizing real-time blood glucose levels, so that either treatments can be made in response to blood glucose levels or as an educational and inexpensive tool so patients can understand what happens to their blood glucose levels when they experience a particular dietary or lifestyle event.

Continuous glucose monitors (CGMs) are now emerging as a popular tool for obtaining real-time glucose results, which for some products are so accurate that no calibration of the sensor by SMBG testing is required and no confirmatory testing with SMBG before taking an action in response to the glucose reading is mandated by the product label. Even for users of these products, SMBG still may be indicated if the CGM is suspected to be inaccurate, such as if low- or high-glycemic symptoms do not match the CGM glucose value or during periods of rapid changing glucose when changes in the CGM readings might be lagging behind changing blood glucose values.

Assisted Monitoring of Blood Glucose

The concept of assisted monitoring of blood glucose (AMBG) was first reported following a collaboration between Centers for Disease and Prevention (CDC) and Diabetes Technology Society (DTS), which culminated in a meeting in 2010 called Sticking with Safety: Eliminating Bloodborne Pathogen Risks during Blood Glucose Monitoring. Later that year, the two organizations coined the term AMBG.[4] AMBG is similar to self monitoring of blood glucor (SMBG), but unlike SMBG for which patients perform the monitoring, a healthcare provider or other caregiver performs AMBG for the patient with diabetes. AMBG and SMBG both have had long traditions in practice, but it is important that AMBG be recognized more broadly as a distinct concept to address safety concerns. In many instances, the equipment and processes that are appropriate for an individual performing SMBG are not appropriate in an AMBG setting. The primary reason for this is the ever-present risk of transmitting bloodborne viruses between individuals who are having capillary blood sampled and tested. This risk is heightened when finger-stick lancing devices, blood glucose meters, or other equipment are used for multiple patients.

Settings in which AMBG is practiced include hospitals, nursing homes, assisted living facilities, health fairs, schools, prisons, medical practitioners' offices or clinics, and children's camps. The differences between SMBG and AMBG relate to the risk of transmitting bloodborne viruses, such as hepatitis B, hepatitis C, or HIV, between individuals who are undergoing capillary blood sampling and testing. This risk is heightened when finger-stick lancing devices, BGM systems, or other paraphernalia are used for multiple patients.

Documented outbreaks of hepatitis B (but not hepatitis C or HIV to date) have occurred in hospitals, nursing homes, and other long-term care facilities. In the U.S., the Centers for Disease Control and Prevention (CDC) monitors these outbreaks. The CDC recommends that *1)* finger-stick devices should never be used for more than one person; and *2)* whenever possible, blood glucose meters should not be shared, but if they must be shared, then the device should be cleaned and disinfected after every use, per the manufacturer's instructions. Furthermore, if the manufacturer does not specify how the device should be cleaned and disinfected, then it should not be shared.

Finger-stick devices, also called lancing devices, are devices that are used to prick the skin and obtain drops of blood for testing. There are two main types of finger-stick devices: *1)* those that are disposable and for single-use; and *2)* those that are designed for reuse. Because of difficulties with cleaning and disinfection after use, failures to change disposable components, and their link to multiple hepatitis B infection outbreaks, the CDC recommends that the reusable devices never be used for more than one person. If these devices are to be used, then they should be used only by people using these devices for SMBG. Likewise, in their most recent draft guidance for accuracy of BGMs in 2018 the U.S. Food and Drug Administration (FDA) separated the requirements into two guidance documents—one for Self-Monitoring Blood Glucose Test Systems for Over-the-Counter Use (which is for SMBG[5]) and one for Blood Glucose Monitoring Test Systems for Prescription Point-of-Care Use (which is for AMBG[6]). This bifurcation was performed in part to emphasize that the latter class of BGMs cannot be operated with reusable lancing devices and that systems for AMBG must have validated cleaning and disinfection procedures.

It is not adequate to disinfect multiuser lancing devices with 70% isopropyl alcohol, even with disposable lancets. Poor access to a tight channel surrounding the lancet impedes sufficient contact with blood. Furthermore, rapid evaporation makes prolonged contact with a lancing device difficult, and alcohol often damages devices that contain shellac, plastic, or rubber.

Noninvasive Optical Glucose Monitoring

Many patients hope that an optical noninvasive glucose monitor can be developed to avoid needle sticks as well as the need for any subcutaneous or implanted glucose-monitoring device. Although noninvasive glucose monitors have been approved with a Conformité Européenne (CE) mark indicating safety, the FDA has not approved a noninvasive glucose monitor for outpatients. This fact indicates that no product has demonstrated a sufficient amount of both effectiveness and safety to satisfy this scientifically rigorous agency.

In 2003, the Pendragon Medical noninvasive glucose monitoring device became the first such device ever to receive clearance. The system was based on a measuring system called impedance spectroscopy. It was cleared for use in Europe with a CE mark. Unfortunately, the product's accuracy was poor, and the Swiss manufacturer soon went out of business. In 2012, the second noninvasive glucose monitor, the C8 Optical Glucose Monitoring System, received its CE mark. The system was based on Raman spectroscopy. Unfortunately, this product's accuracy was also poor and the U.S. manufacturer soon went out of business. In 2013, the Israeli company Integrity received a CE mark for its noninvasive glucose monitor, the GlucoTrack DF-F. It uses three simultaneous measuring technologies: ultrasound, electromagnetic, and thermal technologies to obtain blood glucose readings. In 2017, the Israeli company CNOGA received a CE mark for its noninvasive glucose monitor. This system uses a mathematical approach to predict glucose concentrations based on multiple optical signals and a neural brain network. Another method for noninvasive glucose monitoring has used biocompatible nanosensing polymers implanted under the skin, like a tattoo. They can fluorescence proportionate to the glucose concentration in the surrounding *interstitial fluid* (ISF) when interrogated by a laser beam.[7] Other investigators and companies have attempted to measure glucose in tear fluid using a sensor embedded in a contact lens.[8]

Continuous Glucose Monitoring

The concept of automatic, accurate, around-the-clock measurement of glucose has captivated patients and healthcare professionals for 20 years. The field has seen developments in such products, which are becoming increasingly accurate and easy to use. The goal for many patients is to be able to use any one of these systems as the sole measurement tool. Early products were cleared for adjunctive use only, which meant that, in some cases, a patient had to test more often with one of these devices (to be allowed to act on the data) than they were testing before using an automatic measurement system. In the late 2010s, we have seen products that are so accurate that the FDA is clearing them for nonadjunctive use, which means that patients do not need to confirm a CGM reading with a blood glucose reading. In 2018 the FDA created a new category for continuous glucose monitors called iCGM for products that could be integrated for use with compatible devices.

The first CGM was cleared by the FDA in 1999. It was not intended to provide real-time readings, but instead the data were collected, downloaded, and analyzed by a physician. It was a sensor based on reverse iontophoresis. The device was shaped like a wristwatch and applied a current to the wrist skin. This led to a flux of electrolytes and glucose out from the skin. A sensor on the back of the watch measured captured tissue fluid and measured tissue glucose every 15 min. This device provided novel insights into glycemia (especially overnight), but the product's accuracy eventually was deemed inadequately accurate; its 3-h warm-up period was considered inconvenient and, in some patients, it caused local skin irritation and pain. The manufacturer was acquired in 2004 and, in 2007, the product went out of production. In 2008, manufacturer support for the product was terminated.

Over the past nearly 20 years, three international companies came to dominate the field of continuous glucose monitoring. All of them produce a subcutaneous sensor containing glucose oxidase, which uses electrochemistry to measure electric current, which is proportionate to the ISF glucose concentration. Eventually, new enzymes are expected to replace glucose oxidase, which can suffer from interference by hypoxemia. A fourth company recently launched a long-term implanted glucose sensor that has been approved for 90 days in the U.S. and 180 days in Europe. It uses an optical technology to measure fluorescence, which is proportionate to the ISF glucose concentration.

Over this period, these products have become increasingly more accurate and their permitted dwell times have gradually increased. The longest-functioning needle sensor CGMs now may be used for 14 days before they have to be replaced. Over this period, there has been a shift in popularity from retrospective (or so-called professional or physician-owned) systems to real time (or so-called patient-owned) systems both because *1*) this is what most patients and physicians want and *2*) these manufacturers have been able to build such systems and get them cleared by the FDA. The most recent hurdle that has been overcome by two products is the development of real-time CGMs that do not require calibration and that have been cleared by the FDA for a nonadjunctive indication. The glucose results may be available in real time either automatically without user intervention or intermittently with user intervention.

In the second half of the 2010s, a series of landmark clinical trials of real-time CGM products demonstrated improved A1C levels, improved time-in-range, and decreased hypoglycemia. The opportunity to use a CGM that does not require calibration or confirmatory testing means that patients who use these products and future similar ones will not necessarily have to perform any SMBG testing whatsoever, unless their CGM is not functioning properly.[9]

With greater use of CGMs, the realization that A1C is not the only robust biomarker for mean glycemia has increased. The concentration of this substance in the blood is affected by various factors that influence hemoglobin synthesis and that are unrelated to glycemia. Various metrics that can be derived from CGM and appear to be better correlated than A1C with development of complications, include mean glycemia, time within a target glycemic range, glycemic variability, the incidence of hypoglycemia, and the incidence of hyperglycemia.[10] The use of CGM to generate these metrics to assess overall control is now being investigated.

Insulin Pumps

An insulin pump is a battery-powered, programmable effector device that delivers rapid-acting insulin in small doses into the subcutaneous space to mimic the pattern of natural insulin released by the pancreas. By dosing rapid-acting insulin in a more controlled manner, the user often has improved blood glucose, increased flexibility, and improved quality of life.

The use of a pump for controlled subcutaneous insulin infusion was first reported in 1978.[11] During the1980s, many large heavy insulin pump products were on the market, but none was widely used and most lacked features that are now considered important, such as safety alarms, flexibility in dosing, and soft (nonmetallic) infusion sets. Infections and occlusions were common. By the 1990s, the quality of insulin pumps had improved and most had greater flexibility in dosing with fewer occlusions, and robust alarms for occlusions did occur. In the 2000s, flexible infusion sets became popular and bolus calculator software became a standard feature in insulin pumps.[12] In the middle of the decade, the first and only pod pump was released, which allowed patients to not have to disconnect their infusion set when they did not want to be encumbered with tubing. At the end of the first decade, the FDA cleared the first patch pump and it had a smaller form factor than the pod pump. Since then, a variety of these patch pumps have been cleared, and the difference between a pod and a patch has blurred. In the 2010s, all types of pumps (both traditional catheter type and pod type) have been shown to provide similarly good control.[13]

Current pump manufacturers want to deliver more concentrated insulins than the standard U100, so that their reservoirs will contain a longer number of days' worth of insulin. In addition, current insulin manufacturers are looking to develop faster-acting insulins in the hope that such products will be particularly well suited for insulin pump users who want to get insulin into their systems with or even slightly before a meal. As of 2019, one ultra-rapid-acting subcutaneous insulin was on the market and other ultra-rapid-acting subcutaneous insulins were in the pipeline. In the 2010s, pump manufacturers have shown interest in using various types of patch pumps for controlled insulin delivery in patients with type 2 diabetes.

Smart Insulin

Smart insulins or glucose-responsive insulins, which self-regulate their release in response to ambient glycemic levels, are being designed to break apart only when insulin is needed and to remain fully assembled when they are not. In this paradigm, a pool of insulin would respond quickly to an elevation in the blood glucose level, but during falling glucose levels, it would shut off release to prevent insulin over-dose. To prevent insulin overdose and immediate hypoglycemia, these systems have to not allow burst release. The strategies for incorporating glucose sensing into formulations can be broadly categorized into three subsets: enzymatic sensing, natural glucose-binding proteins, and synthetic molecular recognition.

The smart insulin concept has been written about since the turn of this century. This is when continuous glucose monitoring became feasible as an enabling technology for automatic abiotic closed-loop insulin release; several glucose-responsive insulin models have been developed. All the systems were reported in vitro until 2015, at which point several in vivo systems have been reported to control blood glucose in mice very effectively, including after meals. Currently, several universities, startup companies, and large pharmaceutical com-panies are working to commercialize a smart insulin product.[14]

Closed-Loop Control

The idea of closed-loop control dates back to of the middle of the 20th cen-tury. Until around the turn of the 21st century, the problem seemed impractical to solve for outpatients to use accurate wearable devices. The Artificial Pancreas Meeting under the leadership of Jeffrey Joseph and Marc Torjman began in 1999 and in 2001 this meeting absorbed by the DTS. Three issues that have been dis-cussed at this annual meeting include interoperability of devices from different manufacturers, a sense of whether the three main components of such a system (e.g., sensor, infusion pump, and algorithm) were adequately precise for the neces-sary job, and whether off-the-shelf glucagon could be used in solution for a two-hormone system. The Society eventually determined that the hardware could be made interoperable, as seen with other mechanical and electronic systems. In 2018, the FDA created a new category of CGM authorization called an integrated CGM system (iCGM) for a continuous glucose monitoring system that could be used as part of an integrated system with other compatible medical devices and electronic interfaces. These devices may include automated insulin dosing sys-tems, insulin pumps, blood glucose meters, or other electronic devices used for diabetes management.[15] In 2019, the FDA created a new category of insulin pump called alternate controller enabled (ACE) for products that can be used with dif-ferent components that make up a diabetes therapy system. A regulatory pathway for software to automatically control a closed-loop automated insulin delivery (AID) system is under development at the FDA.

By the end of the first decade of the 2000s, the three main components of closed-loop systems were already adequate and, throughout the 2010s, they have continued to improve each year. We are also on the cusp of having access to ultra-rapid insulin for artificial pancreas systems, which is ideal for a hybrid closed-loop system or a fully closed-loop system. When blood glucose begins to rise following food ingestion, it is imperative to get insulin into the blood stream as quickly as possible to match the glycemic rise. Whether a patient must trigger a mealtime bolus (which is the definition of a hybrid closed-loop system) or the system itself triggers the bolus delivery (which is the definition of a fully closed-loop system), the faster the insulin is absorbed, the more natural its effect will be.

In the 1980s, hospitals had access to a closed-loop system called the Biostator. Inpatients could be hooked up to three intravenous lines (two of which are merged into a double lumen catheter). The patient was connected to the Biostator by way of a blood withdrawal line in one arm and a Y infusion line, which was used to administer the insulin or glucose, in the other arm. The system contained a pump for continuous withdrawal and mixing of blood, a blood glucose analyzer for continuous analysis of the glucose concentration, a computer programmed with algorithms to determine the amount of insulin or glucose to be infused according to the blood glucose level, an infusion pump for insulin or glucose delivery, and a printer to display continuous glucose readings every minute.[16] These devices were expensive and labor intensive and are no longer being manufactured; as a result, they are rarely used other than in a few research centers. A next-generation glucose clamping system is CE marked and used in Germany and a similar system is used in Japan (REF); however, neither system has been cleared by the FDA.

The first product with any automatic insulin delivery functionality or closed-loop control was a CGM-pump-algorithm system from a single manufacturer that had a threshold low-glucose suspend feature.[17] Similar versions of the same product were approved in Europe in 2009 and in the U.S. in 2013. The most notable difference between the U.S. system and the European system was the threshold for triggering suspension of insulin: 60–90 mg/dL in the U.S. and 40–110 mg/dL in Europe. This system was followed by a series of similar systems over the next 4 years with a more accurate predictive low-glucose suspend feature. In 2017, the first product that the manufacturer considered to be a closed-loop system was approved. This hybrid closed-loop system requires the user to manually deliver a bolus dose at mealtime.[18] Meanwhile, several insulin pump companies, several CGM companies, and several algorithm companies are working on their own closed-loop systems. By 2020, one or more of these so-called plug-and-play systems with components worthy of being designated as integrated, from multiple manufacturers, are expected to apply to the FDA for clearance.

Digital Health

A modern paradigm for providing information and decision support advice is digital health. The combination of a wearable, carried, or implanted glucose sensor (which can all be part of the Internet of Things) and software (known as mobile applications) allows data to be collected and sent wirelessly to a smartphone. Data then can be analyzed and returned to the patient in the form of processed information or else as decision support. Furthermore, data can be automatically uploaded to the cloud for storage and more intensive analysis.[19] Until the 2010s, virtually all sensors and effectors did not communicate wirelessly, were manually controlled, and did not connect to anything else. SMBG data usually were messy and disorganized, lacked accurate time stamping, and were not amenable to storage in a digital database. There was no such thing as digital health. With the new Internet of Things paradigm, these devices are now mostly connected to each other and to the cloud. We will increasingly see smart sensors linked to effectors for automatic control and maintenance of physiologic homeostasis for various perturbations, which is how an artificial pancreas works.[20]

Some insulin pens, known as smart pens, can now connect wirelessly to the cloud. These pens transmit important information about the actual doses and timing of insulin therapy that patients are using. This information can help a physician rationally adjust insulin dosing by knowing exactly how much insulin patients actually are treating themselves with.[21] The combination of a smart pen, a CGM, and insulin-dosing software can enable a patient using basal insulin to have the dose of this medication automatically and safely titrated using software that accounts for whether the patient needs more or less insulin than the dose that the patient is actually using. This approach can be considered to be a future type of closed-loop control for patients who are not using controlled insulin infusion with a pump, but who instead are using basal once-daily injections. The idea of closed-loop control for patients on injectable insulin would be inconceivable without the recent technologies of smart pens, CGMs, and decision support software.

With the use of sensors and software, mobile health can be personalized and made scalable. For many accountable healthcare organizations, this communication tool offers the potential of communicating information, reminders (known as nudges), and suggestions for lifestyle modifications with a goal of improving adherence to treatment.

Although more than 2,000 diabetes apps are available at app stores or are described in the medical literature, only a tiny percentage of these are associated with published outcomes data in the medical literature or are FDA approved or CE marked. As of 2017, only 18 diabetes apps had been cleared or approved by the FDA.[22] Many mobile apps are poorly written, embody poor usability, or are dangerous.[23]

In 2018, the FDA announced a Digital Health Innovation Action Plan that would: *1)* issue new implementation guidance (in response to recent legislation) regarding medical software and decision support software; *2)* revise its approach to digital health product oversight by looking first at the software developer or digital health technology developer, not the product; and *3)* hire new staff for its Digital Health Program, as supported by additional user fee funding. In 2018, additional details were released about how the FDA would treat medical software, which they designate as Software as a Medical Device (SaMD) and by which they mean "software intended to be used for one or more medical purposes that perform these purposes without being part of a hardware medical device." This type of software is in contrast to two other types of medical device software, including software that is integral to a medical device (also known as software in a medical device) and software used in the manufacture or maintenance of a medical device.[24]

Cybersecurity

The dark side of digital health is the risk of a data breach by an unauthorized agent into the digital health ecosystem. Threats to the accurate flow of diabetes sensor and effector information and device commands may compromise the function of these devices and put their users at risk of health complications. Sound cybersecurity of connected diabetes devices is needed to maintain confidentiality, integrity, and availability of their data and commands.[25] Security is needed to protect the following: *1)* safety (which is generally an engineering issue); and *2)* privacy (which is generally a legal issue). Medical device safety is in the purview of the FDA. Medical device privacy is in the purview of the U.S. Department of Health and Human Services Office for Civil Rights.

In 2016, DTS led a coalition of cybersecurity, information technology, and diabetes experts for government, professional organizations, industry, and academia to develop the DTS Cybersecurity Standard for Connected Diabetes Devices (DTSec). This is a cybersecurity standard whose goal is to raise confidence in the security of network-connected diabetes devices through independent expert security evaluation. This standard initially targets networked life-critical devices, such as insulin pump controllers, but inherently it could be used in any medical product or component contributing to the protection of high-value assets. This standard will provide the foundation for effective cybersecurity standards across other connected devices and the broader Internet of Things. DTSec-approved labs evaluate the products applying for certification to ensure they meet their claimed security requirements. Successfully evaluated products are then publicly listed for the world to see.

In 2018, DTS developed the DTS Platform Controlling a Diabetes Device Security and Safety Standard (DTMoSt). This is a consensus cybersecurity guidance, which complements DTSec, and whose goal it is to provide assurance that consumer mobile phones can safely control diabetes devices. DTMoSt aims to ensure that sufficient security measures are taken to protect the privacy, integrity, and availability of data for patients who will entrust precious medical information and control of medical devices to their smartphones. DTMoSt identifies such threats to mobile phone–controlled diabetes devices, such as battery depletion, loss of wireless communication, and insufficient central processing unit time. The DTMoSt Guidance is the first standard with both performance requirements and assurance requirements for manufacturers of connected medical devices controlled by a mobile platform. DTMoSt was built upon the principles of DTSec. In 2018, both DTSec and DTMoSt were turned over to a consortium of Underwriters Lab and Institute of Electrical and Electronics Engineers to become a use case standard for the cybersecurity of diabetes devices and a potential model standard for the cybersecurity of devices used for other diseases. This will be the first standard that these two standard development organizations have ever co-managed.

THE FUTURE OF DIABETES TECHNOLOGY

Diabetes technology has become a science of data. Two current issues for diabetes data are as follows: *1*) how the data are collected and *2*) how the data are protected. Many new types of wearable and implanted sensors are being developed, and they will provide a rich multimodal picture of our behavior and our phenotype. With artificial intelligence, relationships based on this sensor data will become increasingly clear as part of the paradigm of precision medicine. The predictive power of these new sensors and analytics tools will be astounding and likely positive. At the same time, this tsunami of data—both stored ("data at rest") and transmitted from sensors to physicians and hospitals ("data in motion")—is at risk of being hacked. In 2017, hospital security reported 477 breaches, affecting 5.6 million patients. There is increasing concern that data must be protected. For the healthcare industry to move into the modern world like other segments of the economy, such as finance, energy, and transportation, it will be necessary for health data to be protected. Standards and guidance, such as that provided by DTSec and DTMoSt, are a start in that process. Eventually, it is likely that devices for other diseases will adopt similar standards and guidance. In the past 20 years, diabetes technology has gone from initially emphasizing hardware, to just 5 years ago covering software, to now covering data. Leaders in the field of diabetes technology must be prepared to promote effective use as well as safe protection of this flood of data.

As technology becomes increasingly pervasive in the monitoring and treatment of diabetes, data and artificial intelligence will become widespread tools for treatment decisions. These decisions will be based on both structured information about patients collected from sensors and surveys, as well as unstructured information collected from social media and video. Eventually, we might not see any data input from physicians into the electronic medical record. There will remain, however, a need for human judgment and for empathy to treat and motivate patients with diabetes. The increasing digitalization of diabetes care and healthcare, in general, will not replace the human touch. The nonlinear qualities needed for physicians to treat diabetes and other diseases, which include judgment, compassion, and context, will not be available from computers for the foreseeable future.

REFERENCES

1. Klonoff DC, Friedl CKE, Grodsky GM, Heinemann L. *J Diabetes Sci Technol Diabetes Technol Community*. (Online) 2007;1:1–2

2. Clarke SF, Foster JR. A history of blood glucose meters and their role in self-monitoring of diabetes mellitus. *Br J Biomed Sci* 2012;69:83–93

3. Frias JP, Lim CG, Ellison JM, Montandon CM. Review of adverse events associated with false glucose readings measured by GDH-PQQ-based glucose test strips in the presence of interfering sugars. *Diabetes Care* 2010; 33:728–729

4. Klonoff DC, Perz JF. Assisted monitoring of blood glucose: special safety needs for a new paradigm in testing glucose. *J Diabetes Sci Technol* 2010;4: 1027–1031

5. U.S. Department of Health and Human Services FaDA. Self-monitoring blood glucose test systems for over-the-counter use: guidance for industry and Food and Drug Administration staff. Washington, D.C., U.S. Department of Health and Human Services, 11 October 2016

6. U.S. Department of Health and Human Services FaDA. blood glucose monitoring test systems for prescription point-of-care use: guidance for industry and Food and Drug Administration staff. Washington, D.C., U.S. Department of Health and Human Services, 11 October 2016

7. Thomas A, Heinemann L, Ramirez A, Zehe A. Options for the development of noninvasive glucose monitoring: is nanotechnology an option to break the boundaries? *J Diabetes Sci Technol* 2016;10:782–789

8. Lin CE, Ito Y, Deng A, et al. A disposable tear glucose biosensor-part 5: improvements in reagents and tear sampling component. *J Diabetes Sci Technol* 2018;12:842–846

9. Klonoff DC, Ahn D, Drincic A. Continuous glucose monitoring: a review of the technology and clinical use. *Diabetes Res Clin Pract* 2017;133:178–192

10. Wright LA, Hirsch IB. Metrics beyond hemoglobin A1C in diabetes management: time in range, hypoglycemia, and other parameters. *Diabetes Technol Ther* 2017;19:S16–S26

11. Pickup JC, Keen H, Parsons JA, Alberti KG. Continuous subcutaneous insulin infusion: an approach to achieving normoglycaemia. *Br Med J* 1978;1: 204–207

12. Gross TM, Kayne D, King A, Rother C, Juth S. A bolus calculator is an effective means of controlling postprandial glycemia in patients on insulin pump therapy. *Diabetes Technol Ther* 2003;5:365–369

13. Leelarathna L, Roberts SA, Hindle A, et al. Comparison of different insulin pump makes under routine care conditions in adults with type 1 diabetes. *Diabet Med* 2017;34:1372–1379

14. Chen G, Yu J, Gu Z. Glucose-responsive microneedle patches for diabetes treatment. *J Diabetes Sci Technol* 2019;13(1):41–48

15. U.S. Department of Health and Human Services FaDA. FDA authorizes first fully interoperable continuous glucose monitoring system, streamlines review pathway for similar devices. Washington, D.C., U.S. Department of Health and Human Services, 27 March 2018

16. Gin H, Catargi B, Rigalleau V, et al. Experience with the Biostator for diagnosis and assisted surgery of 21 insulinomas. *Eur J Endocrinol* 1998; 139:371–377

17. Bergenstal RM, Klonoff DC, Garg SK, et al. Threshold-based insulin-pump interruption for reduction of hypoglycemia. *N Engl J Med* 2013;369:224–232

18. Bergenstal RM, Garg S, Weinzimer SA, et al. Safety of a hybrid closed-loop insulin delivery system in patients with type 1 diabetes. *JAMA* 2016; 316:1407–1408

19. Klonoff DC, Kerr D. Overcoming barriers to adoption of digital health tools for diabetes. *J Diabetes Sci Technol* 2018;12:3–6

20. Klonoff DC. Smart sensors for maintaining physiologic homeostasis. *J Diabetes Sci Technol* 2011;5:470–475

21. Klonoff DC, Kerr D. Smart pens will improve insulin therapy. *J Diabetes Sci Technol* 2018;12:551–553

22. U.S. Department of Health and Human Services FaDA. Examples of pre-market submissions that include MMAs cleared or approved by FDA. Washington, D.C., U.S. Department of Health and Human Services, 21 January 2017

23. Drincic A, Prahalad P, Greenwood D, Klonoff DC. Evidence-based mobile medical applications in diabetes. *Endocrinol Metab Clin North Am* 2016;45: 943–965

24. U.S. Department of Health and Human Services FaDA. Software as a medical device (SaMD). Washington, D.C., U.S. Department of Health and Human Services, 26 March 2018

25. Klonoff DC. Cybersecurity for connected diabetes devices. *J Diabetes Sci Technol* 2015;9:1143–1147

Chapter 2

Infrastructure of Diabetes Clinics and Centers to Support Diabetes Technology

Boris Draznin, MD, PhD,[1] and Michael McDermott, MD[1]

W e live in a century of technological revolution and have witnessed the birth and maturity of artificial intelligence. Technological advances of the past few decades have not only transformed biomedical sciences, but also have profoundly changed clinical medicine.[1–4] Like every other sphere of our life, diabetes-related technology is moving forward at lightning speed. Technological innovations and bioengineering have produced increased capacity for accurate continuous glucose monitoring (CGM), more physiological insulin delivery, and direct communication between glucose monitoring devices and insulin delivery systems.[5] This information also can be easily communicated to patients' designated family members and their healthcare providers. Diabetes-related technology has already changed diabetes therapeutic capabilities significantly and will continue to provide advances in our ability to manage diabetes and to improve the lives of people who struggle daily with this chronic, challenging disease.[5,6]

CGM systems, continuous subcutaneous insulin infusion devices (CSII or insulin pumps), and feedback-regulated insulin delivery systems (hybrid closed-loop systems) currently provide dramatically improved methods of reducing hemoglobin A_{1c} (A1C) levels, decreasing glucose variability, and preventing hypoglycemia.[7,8] These devices have gained sophistication and acceptance as reliable methods of glycemic measurements and insulin delivery, providing enhanced accuracy and flexibility.

The problem is that technology is moving ahead much faster than we, physicians and other healthcare professionals, can incorporate these advances into our practices. Both physicians and patients often feel left hopelessly behind, much like parents and grandparents trail their children and grandchildren in using ever-evolving technology. Furthermore, the organization and structure of healthcare systems also lags significantly behind. It is true that progress in technology is reshaping the healthcare workplace,[9,10] but the rate of healthcare change is much slower than the prolific technological advances. For the sake of the health of millions of patients, we must keep pace with the technology curve and help steer the enormous ship of healthcare bureaucracy to incorporate medical technology seamlessly into the daily practice of medicine.

Remarkable advances in the function and utility of CGM devices, insulin pumps, smart insulin pens, and feedback-regulated insulin delivery systems

[1]Division of Endocrinology, Diabetes, and Metabolism, University of Colorado Anschutz Medical Campus, Aurora, CO.

(hybrid closed-loop and, eventually, fully closed-loop systems) demand equally significant improvements in the structure and organization of diabetes centers, clinics, and practices. Successful translation of technological advances into clinical practice poses challenges and opportunities for providers, patients with diabetes, and healthcare administrators. For providers who are familiar with and promote diabetes-related technology to incorporate these tools into their daily practices, the infrastructure of such innovative practices must be fully supportive of their efforts.[11]

DIABETES CENTERS OF EXCELLENCE

The challenges of successfully translating technological advances into clinical practice are best met in the setting of Diabetes Centers of Excellence (DCOE), where trained and dedicated teams of providers and support staff have first-hand knowledge of and experience with all aspects of diabetes-related technology.[11] DCOEs should implement comprehensive education for motivated patients; have the manpower and dedicated time to solve the complex and frequently urgent issues that patients using technology commonly encounter; and have the structure to deal with preauthorizations, delays, denials, and other problems posed by the many layers of health insurance and coverage for medications and durable medical equipment. The DCOEs must have the readily available expertise that is necessary to guide patients, troubleshoot a multitude of essential issues, and make ongoing therapy adjustments.

We realize that not all diabetes programs, diabetes clinics, diabetes practices, or even diabetes centers would qualify to be named "centers of excellence." Nevertheless, to ensure successful integration of diabetes technology into clinical practice, certain elements must be in place. Even though diabetes management, like management of many other chronic diseases, relies heavily on the self-management skills of individual patients, it is impossible to obtain the full benefits of diabetes-related technology without DCOEs that have experience in CGM, insulin pump, and hybrid closed-loop system data interpretation; the expertise necessary to make proper and timely adjustments of treatment plans; and the ability to troubleshoot a multitude of emerging issues.

This expertise is not trivial and not inexpensive. It is best concentrated in highly specialized centers and programs that can utilize the economy of scale to advance proficiency in diabetes technology to obtain optimal glycemic control for a wide range of patients.

Recently, primarily for the sake of discussion, many authors have divided the diabetes technology subject into two groups: proximal and distal technology.[12] Proximal technology refers to the devices and applications in immediate proximity to the patients, such as glucose meters, CGM devices, and insulin delivery systems. In contrast, distal technology encompasses capabilities and services provided remotely, such as telehealth, mobile health (mHealth), patient portals, and social platforms. In many instances, successful use of proximal technology may rely on distal technology, such as when data downloads from meters, CGMs, and insulin delivery systems need to be analyzed remotely. Thus, the optimal DCOE must have expertise in both proximal and distal technologies to provide optimal care for patients with diabetes.

DIABETES MANAGEMENT SOFTWARE

Needless to say, the ability to download glucose meters, CGM devices, insulin pumps, and feedback-regulated insulin delivery systems presents a minimal requirement for a comprehensive diabetes center or program.[13] The on-site software must be able to create an interface with multiple products produced by various manufacturers. The emergence of mobile devices demands a user-friendly interface of diabetes management programs with mobile applications as well. The manufacturers of the diabetes management software and the end users must have appropriate concerns and safeguards about the integrity of patient data and their privacy.

Diabetes management software must be able to efficiently organize data downloads into easily readable and understandable graphs, charts, and summaries. These downloads must be capable of being printed, imported from various sources, archived in electronic health records (EHR), and shared, as needed, by fax, e-mail, or online. They must enable rapid visualization of trends and patterns to facilitate adjustments in insulin regimens. This information, presented in various formats to include plots, piecharts, daily views, and basal and bolus insulin delivery patterns, must be available quickly for detailed analyses of glycemic data and insulin use patterns so that accurate and timely therapy adjustments can be readily made. Thus, the availability of adaptable diabetes management software is a critical prerequisite for successful integration of diabetes technology into clinical practice.

No data downloads can be useful unless patients and providers have adequate knowledge and training in organizing and interpreting data from the various available devices. This is likely the single most important reason why patients with type 1 diabetes (T1D) as well as those with type 2 diabetes (T2D) who are using diabetes technology, should be followed in specialized centers and programs. Frequently, even the best primary care providers lack sufficient knowledge and time to deal with these issues. It is not uncommon to meet patients with diabetes who are much more knowledgeable about diabetes technology than their providers. Invariably, this leads to diminished returns in terms of clinical benefit for these patients.

PERSONNEL

Putting patient-related issues aside for this chapter, the main obstacle for diabetes centers, programs, and clinics is the absence of a sustainable business model. Essential personnel for a diabetes specialty center should include medical doctors and doctors of osteopathic medicine (MD/DO), advanced practice providers (APP), and certified diabetes educators (CDE). MD/DOs must have extensive knowledge of all aspects of diabetes management and a passion for caring patients with this disease. APP (e.g., certified nurse specialists, nurse practitioners, physician assistants) must have a special interest and training in diabetes management, and CDEs must have a background in clinical nutrition or nursing and must receive extensive, diabetes-focused training to be certified or eligible for certification through the CDE examination administered by the American Association of Diabetes Educators (AADE).[14–16] Whenever possible, the centers and programs must have at least one dedicated social worker and clinical pharmacist to assist with the myriad socioeconomic and clinical-administrative issues that frequently arise and that represent roadblocks for the delivery of optimal diabetes care. It is also highly desirable for a diabetes specialty center to employ a patient care coordinator to provide their patients with timely and convenient access to affiliated specialties, such as ophthalmology, nephrology, neurology, podiatry, and cardiology.

DIABETES CARE PROVIDERS: MD, DO, OR APP

An unresolved question is what the optimal staffing level and mix should be for a successful diabetes program. On the basis of our own experience and a national survey,[17–19] we assume that a diabetologist (MD/DO, APP) sees between 10 and 15 complex patients a day. Assuming that these providers see their patients every 3 or 4 months, this would create a 600–800 patient panel for each provider, generating 2,400 to 3,200 patient visits per year. Going beyond this number of patients would reduce significantly the time that could be allotted for each visit and thereby would impair the quality of care provided.

We believe an initial visit to a diabetes specialist should last no less than 1 h, and the return visits should be no less than 30 min long. It is impossible to assess a patient's medical and psychological status, collect and discuss lifestyle history and problems, perform the necessary physical examination, interrogate their technology devices, interpret the data, and recommend insulin delivery adjustments and other medication management in shorter periods of time.

Patients who use diabetes technology have been documented to achieve better control and to spend more time within target glucose ranges, but at the same time, they are more susceptible to developing acute complications, such as diabetic ketoacidosis or hypoglycemia, if and when their devices malfunction for any reason.[20,21] These patients may have urgent questions about ever-changing life situations (such as nondiabetic medications, dietary habits, exercise patterns, night shifts, concurrent illnesses, upcoming elective procedures or hospitalizations, air travel) so that quality time spent communicating with their healthcare provider is often of paramount importance. To answer their concerns in a sensitive and understandable manner is not a trivial task. The clinics and centers must also have well-informed, dedicated staff available to answer patient and family phone calls, texts, e-mails, and other forms of communication in between clinic visits.

Furthermore, instant availability of distal technology allowing patients with urgent questions to transmit their data to knowledgeable on-call professionals is of great importance to provide accurate and proper advice based on the real-time data.

CDEs

The optimal number of CDEs is also difficult to approximate, but one CDE for every two or three providers is a good starting estimate for a center devoted to the expert utilization of diabetes technology. One full-time CDE usually sees five to seven patients per day in one-to-one sessions lasting up to 1 h per patient and often teaches one or more classes for groups of patients with diabetes and their families each week. This would generate at least 1,100 to 1,500 patient visits per year.

Reimbursement for CDE services is another critical issue. Federal insurance payers (Medicare, Medicaid, Tricare) and many commercial insurance plans do not reimburse for the services provided by a CDE unless their program has undertaken the rigorous and extensive application process for recognition by the American Diabetes Association (the Association) that ensures adequate oversight, quality, and documentation by the CDE program.[15] Without this official Association recognition, CDE services generally are not reimbursed, leaving the costs of employing and resourcing a CDE team to be absorbed as overhead for the diabetes specialty center. This underscores the importance not only of employing skilled and dedicated CDEs but also of pursuing and obtaining Association recognition so that their services are adequately compensated.

PROFESSIONAL EDUCATION

Training of endocrinologists, diabetologists, and APPs to ensure that they have the expertise to initiate, download, and interpret the data available from diabetes technology is an absolute necessity. Practical first-hand knowledge of glucose meters, CGM devices, insulin pumps, and the various emerging feedback-regulated insulin delivery systems is indispensable for a successful diabetes practice.

CDEs and registered nurses who work with patients who have diabetes in diabetes specialty centers must be thoroughly trained in starting and using these devices, analyzing the downloaded data they provide, answering the myriad questions that come from patients via phone or e-mail, and facilitating interactions with pharmacies and insurance companies. They must also have the experience, dedicated time, and rapid access to current, accurate coverage and copay information to enable them to efficiently and effectively complete the high volume of paper and electronic forms that is required for approval and renewal of the various diabetes devices, supplies, and protective footwear.

PATIENT VISITS AND EDUCATION

Of all attempts to influence patient motivation, knowledge of self-management, and adherence to therapeutic regimens, frequent face-face meetings are arguably, but certainly in our opinion, the most beneficial method. Maintaining this pattern of practice is particularly important when taking care of patients participating in intensive diabetes management programs and utilizing diabetes technology. Although the original meaning of "face-to-face" may be yielding to telemedicine and mHealth, the underlying importance of frequent communication remains the same. Patients must be seen every 3–4 months (and sometimes more often when acute needs arise); their glycemic data must be analyzed with constant periodicity; their questions must be answered expeditiously; and adjustments in lifestyle, medications, and device settings must be made in a timely manner. The contemporary diabetes center or clinic must be well equipped to handle regularly scheduled visits and all aspects of distal diabetes-related technology.

The devices and applications presented by diabetes technology to the community of patients and their healthcare providers are not only accurate and helpful but also sophisticated. They require a certain level of knowledge, insight, and learning capacity on the part of the user.

Patient education is a lifelong learning process as self-management skills must be constantly refined and updated. Experience teaches us that new, unpredictable, and unforeseen circumstances arise frequently and baffle even the most proficient and educated patients. Thus, any diabetes center or program dealing with diabetes technology must be organized to provide both initial training in diabetes-related technology as well as continuous support for refining user skills.

CONCLUSION

Patients using diabetes-related technology are best served when their care is concentrated in specialized diabetes centers and programs. Such centers and programs should be adequately staffed to allow for sufficient time to be allocated for patient visits. Staff working at these centers and programs should be well trained and experienced with all forms of proximal and distal technology and be equipped with appropriate software to download and analyze patient data. Both clinical decision support systems and training programs for healthcare providers and their patients must seamlessly integrate technologies into daily clinical workflow. These centers and programs must have a sufficient number of CDEs and their educational programs must be accredited by the Association. Finally, these centers and programs should be able to respond promptly to patients' urgent questions and concerns 24/7, 365 days a year.

REFERENCES

1. Walton A, Nahum-Shani B, Crosby L, Klasnja P, Murphy S. Optimizing digital integrated care via micro-randomized trials. *Clin Pharmacol Ther* 2018; doi:10.1002/cpt.1079

2. Banova, B. The impact of technology on healthcare, 24 April 2018. American Institute of Medical Sciences and Education. Available from www.aimseducation.edu/blog/the-impact-of-technology-on-healthcare. Accessed 17 May 2018

3. New opportunities, new challenges: the changing nature of biomedical science. Available from www.ncbi.nlm.nih.gov/books/NBK43496. Accessed 17 May 2018

4. Topol E. Digital medicine: empowering both patients and clinicians. *Lancet* 2016;388:740–741

5. Klonoff DC, Ahn D, Drincic A. Continuous glucose monitoring: a review of the technology and clinical use. *Diabetes Res Clin Pract* 2017;133:178–192

6. Fatehi F, Menon A, Bird D. Diabetes care in the digital era: a synoptic overview. *Curr Diabetes Rep* 2018;18:38

7. Garg SK, Weinzimer SA, Tamborlane WV, Buckingham BA, Bode BW, Bailey TS, Brazg RL, Ilany J, Slover RH, Anderson SM, Bergenstal RM,

Grosman B, Roy A, Cordero TL, Shin J, Lee SW, Kaufman FR. Glucose outcomes with the in-home use of a hybrid closed-loop insulin delivery system in adolescents and adults with type 1 diabetes. *Diabetes Technol Ther* 2017;19:155–163

8. Fonseca VA, Grunberger G, Anhalt H, Bailey TS, Blevins T, Garg SK, Handelsman Y, Hirsch IB, Orzeck EA, Roberts VL, Tamborlane W; Consensus Conference Writing Committee. Continuous glucose monitoring: A consensus conference of the American Association of Clinical Endocrinologists and American College of Endocrinology. *Endocr Pract* 2016;22:1008–1021

9. Carbo A, Gupta M, Tamariz L, Palacio A, Levis S, Nemeth Z, Dang S. Mobile technologies for managing heart failure: a systematic review and meta-analysis. *Telemed J E Health* 2018; doi:10.1089/tmj.2017.0269

10. Mikk KA, Sleeper HA, Topol EJ. The pathway to patient data ownership and better health. *JAMA* 2017;318:1433–1434

11. Draznin B, Kahn PA, Wagner N, Hirsch IB, Korytkowski M, Harlan DM, McDonnell MF, Gabbay RA. Clinical diabetes centers of excellence: a model for future adult diabetes care. *J Clin Endocrinol Metab* 2018;103:809–812

12. Duke DC, Barry S, Wagner DV, Speight J, Choudhary P, Harris MA. Digital technologies and type 1 diabetes management. *Lancet Diabetes Endocrinol* 2018;6:143–156

13. Allepo G, Laffel LM, Ahman AJ, Hirsch IB, Kruger DF, Peters A, Weinstock RS, Harris DR. A practical approach to using trend arrows on the Dexcom G5 CGM system for the management of adults with diabetes. *J Endocr Soc* 2017;1:1445–1460

14. Facing today's challenges in diabetes education, 2008. *Endocrine Today*. Available from www.healio.com/endocrinology/diabetes/news/print/endocrine-today/%7B4a5f80f6-0a86-402b-b463-a8743f4af033%7D/facing-todays-challenges-in-diabetes-education. Accessed 17 May 2018

15. Benefits of education recognition. American Diabetes Association. Available from https://professional.diabetes.org/content-page/benefits-education-recognition. Accessed 17 May 2018

16. Rinker J, Dickinson JK, Litchman ML, Williams AS, Kolb LE, Cox C, Lipman RD. The 2017 diabetes educator and the diabetes self-management education national practice survey. *Diabetes Educator* 2018; doi: 10.1177/0145721718765446

17. Vigersky RA, Fish L, Hogan P, Stewart A, Kutler S, Ladenson PW, McDermott M, Hupart KH. The clinical endocrinology workforce: current status and future projections of supply and demand. *J Clin Endocrinol Metab* 2014;99:3112–3121

18. Endocrinology: Growing need, but shrinking workforce. Available from www.medscape.com/viewarticle/881849. Accessed 17 May 2018

19. Endocrine clinical workforce: supply and demand projections, 2014. Endocrine Society. Available from www.endocrine.org/-/media/endosociety/files/

advacacy-and-outreach/other-documents/2014-06-white-paper--endocri-nology-workforce.pdf?la = en. Accessed 17 May 2018

20. Pease A, Lo C, Earnest A, Liew D, Zoungas S. Evaluating optimal utilization of technology in type 1 diabetes mellitus from a clinical and health economic perspective: protocol for a systematic review. *Systematic Rev* 2018;7:44–50

21. Karges B, Schwandt A, Heidtmann B, Kordonouri O, Binder E, Schiertoh U, Boettcher C, Kapellen T, Rosenbauer J, Holl RW. Association of insu-lin pump therapy vs insulin injection therapy with severe hypoglycemia, ketoacidosis, and glycemic control among children, adolescents, and young adults with type 1 diabetes. *JAMA* 2017;318:1358–1366

Chapter 3
Insulin Pumps

Eda Cengiz, MD, MHS[1]

The late 1970s marked the integration of insulin pump therapy, commonly referred to as the continuous subcutaneous insulin infusion (CSII), into diabetes management. The CSII has become a key milestone for incorporating technology into diabetes treatment and ignited the decades-long mission to mimic physiologic insulin secretion and blood glucose control using technological devices. The CSII introduced a new insulin basal-bolus treatment concept that was different from the insulin injection method and has emerged as an ideal tool to intensify insulin treatment while minimizing hypoglycemia.[1,2] The idea behind the insulin pump treatment was to infuse insulin continuously through a transcutaneous catheter with a tip in the subcutaneous tissue to deliver basal insulin 24 h/day and bolus insulin doses to cover for carbohydrate intake or to correct hyperglycemia.[3] The first external insulin pump systems have evolved over the course of several years and were replaced by modern high-technology insulin pump devices (Figure 3.1).

One of CSII's most remarkable contributions to insulin treatment has been the ease and flexibility of insulin treatment with respect to meal and snack timing. Most modern pumps have preprogrammed, adjustable multiple basal rate and bolus ratio functions to mimic the needs of each person. Consequently, clinicians can titrate insulin basal doses hourly as well as implement multiple different correction and insulin to carbohydrate ratios at different times of the day to account for changes in insulin glycemic response and their patients' age, sex, daily activities, and other factors that might affect their response to insulin. CSII use has been particularly advantageous in certain conditions; CSII treatment has been used to manage patients with severe or recurring hypoglycemia because of the more physiologic insulin replacement by insulin infusion.[4] Notably, CSII has been successfully used in pediatric subjects.[5] Better dosing precision and accuracy than injection therapy in small insulin doses and the small insulin infusion rate function that accommodates for low insulin dose requirements make the CSII an appealing treatment choice for management of toddlers and young children with diabetes.[6] The immediate or extended insulin bolus options adjust the insulin delivery rate, amount, and duration to match the rate of absorption of meals, such as high-fat-content meals that are slowly absorbed from the gastrointestinal tract or for patients with gastroparesis. CSII treatment offers numerous benefits to

---

[1]Associate Professor, Yale School of Medicine, New Haven, CT; Visiting Professor, Bahçeşehir University Faculty of Medicine, Istanbul, Turkey.

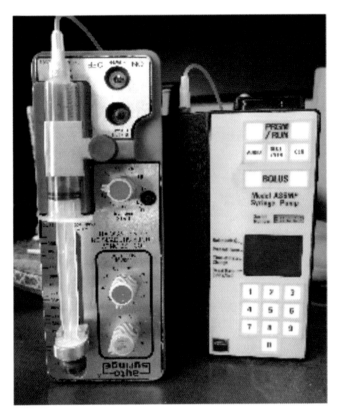

Figure 3.1. First- and second-generation insulin pumps.

accommodate an active lifestyle, particularly for people with diabetes at high risk for exercise-related hypoglycemia. People with diabetes can disconnect the pump during exercise for an extended period of time or adjust the insulin delivery rate during and after exercise to mitigate exercise-related hypoglycemia. Overall, carbohydrate counting coupled with CSII offers greater flexibility and satisfaction for patients.

Rapid-acting, short-acting insulins and, more recently, a faster-acting insulin analog have been shown to be compatible with insulin pumps.[7,8] Lower HbA$_{1c}$ levels (0.26%) among users of rapid-acting insulin (RAI) analog compared with short-acting insulin have been reported in adult patients with type 1 diabetes (T1D), which is suggestive of superior glycemic control when RAI is used in the CSII compared with regular insulin.[9] In general, the total daily insulin requirement is decreased by 10–20% while transitioning patients from the multiple daily injection (MDI) to the CSII. This could be partly due to the more even insulin absorption resulting from the insulin depo in the catheter infusion site. Evidence suggests that the insulin absorption from an insulin infusion site is enhanced after few days of insertion.[10,11] CSII could be used to infuse diluted or concentrated insulin.

Diluted rapid-acting insulin (U50, U10) has been used in pumps to treat infants and young children[12] and concentrated insulin infusion has been typically used for insulin-resistant patients.[13]

INSULIN PUMP TYPES

Most insulin pumps have three major components: the pump itself (which is a programmable electronic device that includes a user interface, electronic processor, worm-screw to control dosing, and batteries); a disposable reservoir that stores the insulin; and a disposable infusion set (which is the tubing that connects to the reservoir and which terminates in a cannula or needle through which the insulin is infused). The cannula is inserted under the skin with a small needle that is removed after it is in place, and the insulin pump itself is externally worn. (See examples of different pump types in Figure 3.2.)

The interior of the insulin pump consists of a device that contains a large syringe-like cartridge or reservoir to hold several days' worth of insulin (180–300 units). The syringe-like cylindrical insulin reservoir is connected to a mechanical screw and a plunger at one end and attached to tubing on the other end. Small gears inside the pump rotate and slowly turn the mechanical screw that pushes the plunger slightly to deliver a measured amount of insulin from the reservoir to the flexible tubing with a catheter at the end. The catheter is inserted in the subcutaneous tissue to infuse insulin and is secured to the skin with an adhesive patch. The insulin flows from the reservoir into the tubing and is infused into the subcutaneous tissue through the catheter. The electronic processor in the pump controls the mechanical system that dispenses the insulin in an amount that is programmed into the system. The entire unit of tubing and catheter is called the infusion set and must be compatible with the specific insulin pump.

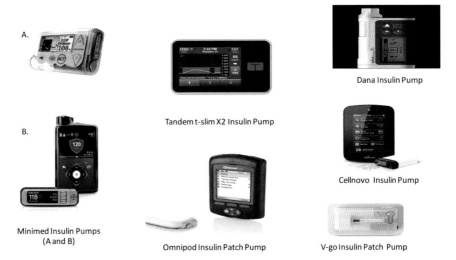

Figure 3.2. Tethered and patch insulin pump types.

The display screen and buttons on the pump are used to program insulin settings and delivery to inform the user of the insulin delivery status. Safety and user features may include programmable bolus profiles, customizable reminders, alerts for missed bolus dose or missed glucose measurement, and alarms in the event of a blockage that prevents the continuous infusion of the insulin through the pump. Insulin delivery data, alerts, alarms, blood glucose data (if entered in to the pump via Bluetooth link or manual entry), and CGM data (if the pump has an interface with the CGM) could be accessed from the insulin pump memory.

Insulin patch pumps introduced a slightly different design with a disposable pod containing the insulin reservoir and the delivery mechanism that sits on the skin (Figure 3.3). A catheter at the bottom of the pod is inserted directly into the subcutaneous tissue without tubing. Typically, patch pumps require that a handheld device be connected to the pod via a wireless link to enable adjustments in insulin dosing and settings. Patch pumps offer a combination of basal-bolus insulin delivery.

Despite the differences in design, both pump types have similar features and functions to infuse insulin. Major differentiating characteristics of different insulin pump models are summarized in Table 3.1.

The Digital Insulin Pump Technology

Pump technology has continued to evolve throughout the years, and the major shift in insulin pump technology occurred during the digital age. Modern pump designs have incorporated sophisticated pumping mechanisms, touchscreen features, Bluetooth connectivity, and digitally enhanced systems into the CSII. Insulin pumps have become more advanced with multiple features and an interface with glucose meters, continuous glucose monitors (CGM), and potentially other relevant devices. Initially, insulin pumps were linked with glucometers; they were later paired with the CGM, which eased some of the diabetes treatment burden by reducing the need to manually enter blood glucose data. CGM augmented insulin pump systems; commonly referred to as sensor-augmented pump treatment has become the tipping point for interconnected diabetes management ecosystems. The traditional stand-alone insulin pumps have been gradually replaced by interconnected systems with smart insulin pumps that are equipped with insulin delivery decision-making algorithms augmented by CGM trends. First-generation sensor-augmented pumps improved safety by suspending infusion during hypoglycemia.[14] A large multicenter randomized control trial (RCT) demonstrated the benefits of a low-glucose suspend system in hypoglycemia-prone subjects age 16 years and older. New-generation sensor-augmented insulin pumps have taken this feature a step further by regulating insulin delivery based on predicted sensor glucose values, thus enabling detection of glucose values that are anticipated to fall outside the lower limit of the target range.[15,16] Similar to many other things in our lives that are handled by technology, the next logical steps are to leverage technology to improve diabetes care and to create technology-driven systems in which the devices and digital systems do all the tracking, observation, estimating, and planning both automatically and passively. As a matter of fact, the idea of improving diabetes management with an automated insulin system has been around for a long time, almost since the beginning of insulin pump therapy. The artificial pancreas system research project was mothered by this necessity and gave significant momentum to the development of interconnected, automated

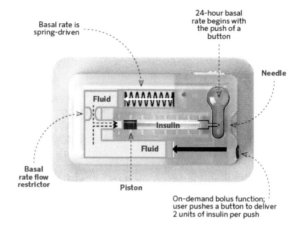

Basal rate is
spring-driven

24-hour basal
rate begins with
the push of a
button

Needle

Fluid

Insulin

Fluid

Basal
rate flow
restrictor

Piston

On-demand bolus function;
user pushes a button to deliver
2 units of insulin per push

V-Go Insulin Pump
Schematic [1]

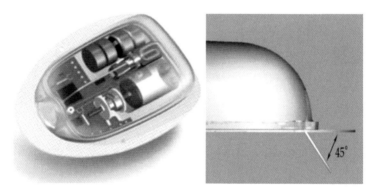

Omnipod patch insulin pump internal components and the catheter
view demonstrating 45-degree angle and 6.5 mm vertical depth[2]

1. Available at http://www.diabetesforecast.org/2014/09-sep/how-insulin-pumps-work.html.
2. Republished with permission of Springer Science and Business Media, from "The OmniPod Insulin Management System: the latest innovation in insulin pump therapy," Howard C. Zisser, from Diabetes Therapy, Volume 1, Issue 1, 2010, p. 10–24; permission conveyed through Copyright Clearance Center, Inc.

Figure 3.3. Internal structure of insulin patch pumps.

diabetes management systems. The artificial pancreas system research subsequently has generated interest in diabetes data collection and relevant software design. The ability to upload insulin delivery and CGM data onto shared platforms, such as the cloud or various smartphone applications, has become a mainstay of diabetes management and has enabled further advancements within diabetes data analytics.

Table 3.1. Insulin Pump Models and Their Technical Features

Insulin pump brand name, model	Pump size and technical specifications	Pump features, reservoir and infusion set	Basal insulin delivery	Bolus insulin delivery	Other features
MiniMed 530G System	3.7 × 2 × 0.82 in. 3.7 oz. with battery and full reservoir 1 AAA battery Monochromatic screen without a touchscreen feature	The MiniMed 530G combo pump–CGM uses SmartGuard technology to stop insulin delivery for up to 2 h if the glucose level reaches a preset low limit and the user doesn't react to a low-glucose alarm. 300-unit reservoir Compatible with Medtronic infusion sets only	Minimum insulin delivery: 0.025 units/h Maximum insulin delivery: 35 units/h Insulin delivery in 0.025-unit increments for up to 0.975 units. Increments of 0.05 units for between 1 and 9.95 units. Increments of 0.1 units for 10 units or more.	Minimum insulin delivery: 0.025 units. Maximum insulin delivery: 25 units. Insulin delivery in increments of 0.1 units.	Pump is not waterproof and needs to be disconnected from the body before bathing, swimming, and doing other water activities. Continuous Glucose Monitor (CGM): Communicates only with the Medtronic CGM Pump and CGM data could be uploaded using Carelink software, Glooko and Tidepool data-management systems.
MiniMed 630G System	2.1 × 3.78 × 0.96 in. 3.7 oz. without battery and with empty reservoir a full-color screen without touchscreen features 1 AA battery	The MiniMed 630G combo pump–CGM uses SmartGuard technology to stop insulin delivery for up to 2 h if the glucose level reaches a preset low limit and the user doesn't react to a low-glucose alarm. 300-unit reservoir Compatible with Medtronic infusion sets only	Minimum insulin delivery: 0.025 units/h Maximum insulin delivery: 35 units/h Insulin delivery in 0.025-unit increments for up to 0.975 units. Increments of 0.05 units for between 1 and 9.95 units. Increments of 0.1 units for 10 units or more.	Minimum insulin delivery: 0.025 units. Maximum insulin delivery: 25 units. Insulin delivery in increments of 0.025 units.	Pump is waterproof for 12 feet deep for up to 24 h and features. Pump has limited remote bolus functionality via the Contour Next Link 2.4 meter. CGM: Communicates only with the Medtronic CGM Pump and CGM data could be uploaded using Carelink software, Glooko and Tidepool data-management systems.

(continued)

Device	Physical specifications	Description	Basal insulin delivery	Bolus insulin delivery	Additional features
Minimed 640G System	2.1 × 3.78 × 0.96 in. MMT-1512: 85 × 53 × 24 mm MMT-1712: 96 × 53 × 24 mm 3.7 oz. without battery and with empty reservoir a full-color screen without touch-screen features 1.5 V AA lithium (FR6) battery or 1.5 V AA alkaline (LR6) battery	The MiniMed 640G with SmartGuard technology monitors glucose levels and suspends basal insulin delivery if a glucose level below preset threshold is predicted to occur in the next 30 minutes. Basal insulin delivery restarts automatically once the glucose is above the preset threshold and is rising. Model MMT-1512: 180unit reservoir MMT-1712: 300unit reservoir	Minimum insulin delivery: 0.025 units/h Maximum insulin delivery: 35 units/h Insulin delivery in increments of 0.025 units for basal amounts in the range of 0.025 to 0.975 units. Increments 0.05 units for basal amounts in the range of 1 to 9.95 units Increments of 0.1 units for basal amounts of 10.0 units or larger	Minimum insulin delivery: 0.025 units. Maximum insulin delivery: 35 units. Insulin delivery in increments of 0.025, 0.05, and 0.1 unit.	The pump would cease delivering insulin if blood sugar levels became low Pump has limited remote bolus functionality via the Contour Next Link 2.4 meter. Pump is waterproof to a depth of up to 3.6 meters (12 feet) for up to 24 h CGM: Communicates only with the Medtronic CGM
MiniMed 670G System	2.1 × 3.78 × 0.96 in. 3.7 oz. without battery and with empty reservoir 1 AA battery Pump has a full-color screen without touchscreen features	The MiniMed 670G, a hybrid closed-loop pump, uses SmartGuard technology to adjust background insulin delivery based on an insulin delivery decision making algorithm. The levels of insulin delivery automation varies depending the selected mode. The auto-mode feature automatically adjusts basal insulin delivery based on the user's CGM sensor glucose readings and recent insulin delivery. Users are required to announce their meals/snacks by manually entering the carbohydrate count of their meals and confirm the insulin bolus delivery. The predicted low-glucose sensor mode (PLGS) stops insulin delivery for up to 2 h if the glucose level reaches a preset low limit and the user doesn't react to a low-glucose alarm. 300-unit reservoir Compatible with Medtronic infusion sets only	Minimum insulin delivery: 0.025 units/h Maximum insulin delivery: 35 units/h Insulin delivery in increments of 0.025 units for basal amounts in the range of 0.025 to 0.975 units. Increments 0.05 units for basal amounts in the range of 1 to 9.95 units. Increments of 0.1 units for basal amounts of 10.0 units or larger.	Minimum insulin delivery: 0.025 units. Maximum insulin delivery: 25 units. Insulin delivery in increments of 0.025, 0.05, and 0.1 units.	Approved for use by adults and children 7 years and over with T1D. Pump is waterproof for 12 feet deep for up to 24 h and features. Pump has remote bolus functionality via the Contour Next Link 2.4 meter. CGM: Communicates only with the Medtronic CGM The system could be uploaded using Carelink software, Glooko and Tidepool data-management systems.

(continued)

Table 3.1. Insulin Pump Models and Their Technical Features (*continued*)

Insulin pump brand name, model	Pump size and technical specifications	Pump features, reservoir and infusion set	Basal insulin delivery	Bolus insulin delivery	Other features
MiniMed Paradigm Revel	3.7 × 2 × 0.84 in. 3.5 oz. with battery and full reservoir 1 AAA battery	300-unit reservoir Compatible with Medtronic infusion sets only	Minimum insulin delivery: 0.025 units/h Maximum insulin delivery: 35 units/h Insulin delivery in increments of 0.025 units for basal amounts in the range of 0.025 to 0.975 units. Increments of 0.05 units for between 1 and 9.95 units. Increments of 0.1 units for 10 units or more.	Minimum insulin delivery: 0.025 units. Maximum insulin delivery: 35 units. Insulin delivery in increments of 0.025 to 25 units.	The MiniMed Paradigm Revel is a stand-alone pump with optional CGM capabilities. Pump is not water-proof and needs to be disconnected from the body before bathing, swimming, or other water activities. Continuous Glucose Monitor (CGM): Communicates only with the Medtronic CGM. The system could be uploaded using Carelink software, Glooko and Tidepool data-management systems. Pump also works with MiniMed Connect, which allows data to be displayed via Apple or Android smart devices. MiniMed Connect can text updates to family and friends.

(continued)

Tandem T:slim X2	3.13 × 2 × 0.6 in. 3.95 oz. with battery and full reservoir Flat reservoir design and micro-delivery technology allow for a thinner pump. Color touch screen Rechargeable lithium polymer battery 300-unit cartridge Compatible with Tandem infusion sets only	T:slim X2 with Basal-IQ feature reduces the frequency and duration of low-glucose events by predicting sensor glucose levels 30 minutes ahead and suspending basal insulin delivery if the sensor glucose levels are expected to drop below 80 mg/dL or if an actual glucose level of 70 mg/dL or less occurs. Basal insulin delivery restarts automatically once glucose levels begin an upward trend	Minimum insulin delivery: 0.1 units/h Maximum insulin delivery: 15 units/h Insulin delivery in increments of 0.001 units.	Minimum insulin delivery: 0.05 units Maximum insulin delivery: 25 units Insulin delivery in increments of 0.01-unit with an option for up to an additional 25 units.	The pump is watertight to 3 feet for up to 30 minutes The pump communicates with the Dexcom G6 CGM. The Tandem Device Updater is a Mac® and PC-compatible tool for the remote update of Tandem insulin pump software. T:slim insulin pump users (in-warranty) can upgrade their pumps' software to access new and enhanced insulin pump features on-line, real-time without the need to wait for the typical multi-year warranty cycle. The t:simulator™ App is a digital pump demo application to test the touchscreen interface of a Tandem insulin pump on a smartphone or a tablet.
Dana Insulin Pump	Pump 2.95 × 1.77 × 0.74 in. 2.15 oz. with battery and full reservoir the remote control is 75mm × 32mm × 20mm (43g). 3.6-volt DC lithium battery	300-unit cartridge Compatible with Sooil infusion sets only	Minimum insulin delivery: 0.04 units/h Maximum insulin delivery: 16 units/h Insulin delivery in increments of 0.01- or 0.1-units	Minimum insulin delivery: 0.1 unit Maximum insulin delivery: 80 units Insulin delivery in 0.1-, 0.5-, or 1-unit increments. Insulin-to-carbohydrate ratio in whole units only.	Pump is waterproof at 3.3 feet deep for 1 h. Wireless Bluetooth connection allows the pump to be operated by an Android smartphone via the Dana app

(continued)

Table 3.1. Insulin Pump Models and Their Technical Features (*continued*)

Insulin pump brand name, model	Pump size and technical specifications	Pump features, reservoir and infusion set	Basal insulin delivery	Bolus insulin delivery	Other features
Omnipod	Pod: 1.53 × 2.05 × 0.57 in. 0.88 oz. with empty reservoir Personal Diabetes Manager (PDM): 2.4 × 4.4 × 0.98 in. 4.4 oz. with batteries Pod: battery integrated PDM: 2 AAA battery	It is a patch pump without tubing. The pod is a single- use, disposable device that attaches to the body with an adhesive. There is a built-in, in-dwelling cannula extending directly beneath the pod that sits in the subcutaneous tissue. Each pod is worn up to for 72 h Personal Diabetes Manager (PDM) device controls the pod's functions remotely Pod is required to be within 5 feet of the PDM to deliver bolus doses. Once programmed, the pod continues to deliver basal insulin regardless of the PDM proximity. The PDM contains more than 1,000 common foods (with nutrition information) and stores up to 36 preset carbohydrate values. Insulin delivery must be suspended to change basal insulin dose settings. PDM has a built-in blood glucose meter. 200-unit reservoir built into pod.	Minimum insulin delivery:0.05 units/h Maximum insulin delivery: 30 units/h Insulin delivery in 0.05-unit increments	Minimum insulin delivery: 0.05 units Maximum insulin delivery: 30 units Insulin delivery in in increments of 0.05 units. Insulin- to-carbohydrate ratio in whole units only.	Approved for use by adults and children. Energy source: Pod: battery integrated The pod is waterproof for up to 25 feet deep for 60 minutes CGM: The Omnipod does not have direct integration with a continuous glucose monitor. The Omnipod DASH™ Insulin Management System consists of the pod and the PDM (locked-down, handheld, Android device) with touch-screen PDM interface, Bluetooth® wireless technology, and wireless internet connectivity. The PDM uploads data to the secure Insulet Cloud via WiFi, which can then be viewed on a personal cell phone using the Omnipod VIEW™ app and the Glooko® data management system. The PDM can communicate through Bluetooth® wireless technology to the Omnipod DISPLAY™ app installed on a personal cell phone.

(*continued*)

Device	Dimensions/Power	Description	Basal	Bolus	Notes
V-Go Patch Pump	2.4 × 1.3 × 0.5 in.; 0.7 to 1.8 oz. filled, depending on units of insulin used Pump has no battery; uses mechanical power source	It is a patch pump with no tubing. V-Go 20 insulin capacity: 56 units total V-Go 30 insulin capacity: 66 units total V-Go 40 insulin capacity: 76 units total Comes with a built-in 30-gauge, 4.6-millimeter stainless-steel needle with a 90-degree insertion angle. Needle retracts into the device after use to prevent sharps injury.	V-Go 20: 20 units basal insulin infusion over 24 h V-Go 30: 30 units basal insulin infusion over 24 h V-Go 40: 40 units basal insulin infusion over 24 h	V-Go 20,30,40: up to 36 units insulin bolus in 2-unit increments	The Omnipod could be uploaded using Glooko, Tidepool, and Diasend data-management systems. Pump is designed for use by adults with type 2 diabetes. It delivers bolus insulin with a manual button press (not an electronic system). Each disposable device is used for 24 h. V-go pump is waterproof up to a depth of 3 feet, 3 inches, for 24 h. Does not work with data-management software and doesn't connect with any glucometers or CGM.

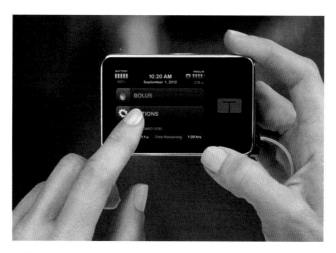

Figure 3.4. Tandem t:slim touch screen display.

PRINCIPLES OF CSII INSULIN DOSING: BASAL-BOLUS INSULIN DOSING

The pump delivers rapid-acting insulin similar to the way in which the human pancreas delivers insulin: through continuous basal insulin and bursts of insulin bolus delivery. The same rapid-acting insulin contained in a pump's reservoir is used for basal and bolus insulin infusion in precise amounts based on preprogrammed settings.

Basal Insulin Delivery

The insulin pump delivers a constant flow of insulin to counteract the steady of flow of glucose into the blood provided by the liver throughout the day. Basal insulin is essential to keep blood glucose levels consistent during periods of fasting. Basal insulin rates can be programmed in units per hour and are infused in minipulses every few minutes to deliver the programmed hourly totals. Insulin pumps can deliver multiple basal insulin delivery rates every hour throughout the day to account for the circadian variation in insulin needs that make them an appealing treatment method for patients with widely varying daily schedules, such as shift workers, athletes, or adolescents who go to bed late and sleep in on the weekends. Temporary basal rate adjustments accommodate transient changes in basal insulin needs and offer flexibility in managing insulin treatment when dealing with unexpected events, such as times during or after exercise (decrease in current rate), illness (increase in rate), stress (increase in rate), or prolonged hypoglycemia (decrease in rate) or hyperglycemia (increase in rate). Temporary basal rates can be programmed for 0.5–72 h depending on pump model. Pumps automatically resume normal basal rates at the end of a set time. The rate change could be entered in units or hour but more commonly are entered as a percentage of the current rates. Temporary dose adjustments should be clearly explained to the patients when making recommendations, particularly given that the terminology could be different based on the insulin pump model. A 100% increase in basal rate, namely, doubling the basal infusion rate, could be programmed either as +200% or +100% temporary basal rate depending on the pump mode. Conversely, decreasing the rate to 80% basal rate might require a pump command entry of either 80% basal rate or a 20% temporary basal rate reduction depending on the insulin pump model.[17–22] These minor differences in insulin pump command settings could potentially result in undesirable insulin dosing as well as unexpected glycemic response if patients are not well trained in the specifics of their own pump adjustments.

Bolus Insulin Delivery

The bolus insulin infusion is administered as a burst of insulin delivery to cover the carbohydrate amount in meals and snacks and to correct hyperglycemia. The bolus delivery requires manual user input and can be calculated either by a meal bolus calculator embedded in the pump memory or by user entry of bolus insulin unit amount. The pump meal bolus calculator is preprogrammed with an insulin-to-carbohydrate ratio (ICR), the grams of carbohydrate that 1 unit of insulin will cover, the insulin sensitivity factor (ISF) or correction factor, and the number of blood glucose points that is expected to drop per unit of insulin given to achieve a target blood glucose range. The target glucose level or range is set by the physician and the patient and is one of the factors the pump uses to calculate a bolus dose. Insulin pumps allow for multiple target glucose levels, and anecdotally, a higher blood glucose target is set for bedtime and overnight than for daytime to reduce the risk of overnight hypoglycemia.

When a patient enters total number of meal carbohydrates into the bolus calculator, the bolus calculator will determine a recommended dose of insulin based on the ICR and the additional dose to correct the blood glucose based on the ISF. The bolus dose is delivered only if the patient confirms delivery. The correction dose is calculated only if the blood glucose or CGM is entered in to the pump. Some insulin pumps facilitate direct communication between the patient's glucose meter and insulin pump and eliminate the need for manual blood glucose entry. The insulin bolus dose may be reduced by a meal bolus calculator, depending on the blood glucose level (negative correction to deliver less insulin if the blood glucose is below target range) and insulin on board (less insulin dose if the system detects that active insulin already is on-board). The pump also has multiple bolus profiles, including standard, split-dose, extended, and combined boluses.

Custom Bolus Functions

Typically, an insulin bolus is delivered by the insulin pump at a constant rate over a set period of time. The terminology of the advanced bolus options varies depending on the pump brand; "the extended bolus" (a.k.a. square-wave) is among the most commonly used, along with "the split bolus" (a.k.a multiple bolus) and "the combination bolus" (a.k.a dual-wave). These advanced bolus features offer alternative bolus delivery options by altering the timing and type of bolus.[23]

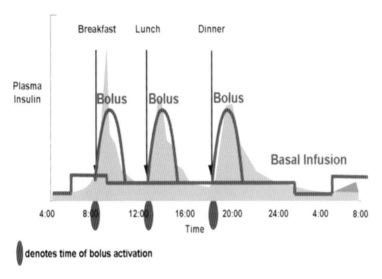

Figure 3.5. Basal and bolus insulin delivery.

Standard Bolus

The complete amount of insulin bolus is delivered without any delays at the insulin pump model specific rate (Figure 3.5). The speed of insulin bolus delivery varies depending on the insulin pump model. Contemporary insulin delivery devices are equipped with multiple insulin delivery rate features and offer two bolus speed options. The standard default setting is 1.5 units/min insulin; this is the same bolus speed as other commercially available pumps (Omnipod and Tandem t:slim; see Figures 3.3 and 3.4). The other standard default setting is a rapid bolus speed option of 15 units/min insulin. Although the rate of insulin bolus delivery is increased 10-fold, when insulin is infused using the new rapid bolus setting, limited data are available concerning the impact of insulin rapid bolus delivery rate on insulin pharmacokinetics and pharmacodynamics (ClinicalTrials.gov Identifier: NCT03542682).

Split-Wave Bolus

Insulin bolus delivery is split into two as a percentage of the whole, typically by 50% for one immediate delivery and a second delivery after a predetermined period of time from the first bolus (Figure 3.6). The split-wave bolus is used to better match the insulin delivered by the pump to the digestion of the meal, resulting in better blood glucose control.[23]

Extended (Square-Wave) Bolus

The extended bolus is consistently and evenly delivered over an extended set length of time (15–30 min up to 6–8 h). The user dials in the entire bolus insulin amount and then the period over which the bolus is to be delivered for the bolus to be infused in equal amounts and at regular intervals over the chosen period (Figure 3.6). The extended bolus profile is suggested for low-glycemic index or high-fiber meals or for situations in which eating is done over a prolonged period of time, such as with a buffet-type meal.

Combination (Dual-Wave) Bolus

The pump delivers a combination of an immediate standard bolus followed by an extended bolus (Figure 3.6). The combination bolus is often programmed as a percentage split (e.g., 50% immediate delivery and 50% over X h). It is commonly used with high-fat foods or meals in which the fat content of the food can significantly slow the absorption of the carbohydrate content and typically cause an additional rise in blood glucose levels several hours after eating. The Medtronic MiniMed 670G hybrid closed-loop system does not offer the use of extended boluses when in auto mode.[17]

Easy Bolus

The easy bolus function allows the user to more efficiently dial up the number of units and deliver the dose with fewer button presses. The insulin delivery is otherwise identical to the standard bolus.

CLINICAL OUTCOMES WITH CSII TREATMENT

Numerous randomized and nonrandomized studies have supported the efficacy and safety of CSII. A meta-analysis assessing CSII versus intensive insulin injection therapy via 12 RCTs showed a reduction of 0.44 in the HbA_{1c} (CI 0.20–0.69) in patients using CSII and with a concomitant total daily insulin dose reduction of 10% to 20%.[24,25] Multiple studies have shown that insulin pumps reduce the frequency of severe hypoglycemic events relative to MDI injections.[26]

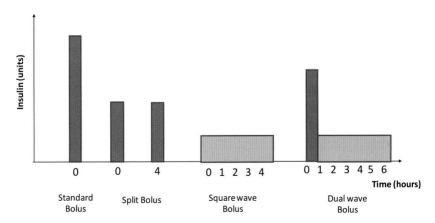

Figure 3.6. Standard, split, extended (square-wave), combination (dual-wave) bolus profiles.

The risk of diabetic ketosis during CSII treatment has long been in debate. Hyperglycemia and ketosis can occur during CSII treatment because of disruption of insulin delivery whether through a device, an infusion site problem, or patient errors in usage. Recent data from a population-based cohort study of 30,579 patients demonstrated significantly lower rates of diabetic ketoacidosis and severe ketoacidosis with pump therapy versus injection therapy in adolescents and young adults ages 16 to 19 years old but not in other age-groups.[27] It is fair to say that sustained improvements in insulin delivery fault detection algorithms and alerts would reduce the risk of ketosis and add another layer of safety for patients on CSII treatment.

Higher treatment satisfaction and improved quality of life with CSII use have been reported in people with T1D and greater lifestyle flexibility and decreased fear of hypoglycemia have been noted as the most significant factors with a favorable impact on patient reported outcomes.[28,29] CSII therapy should be discontinued if psychiatric or other contraindications emerge after the initiation of pump treatment, or if the patient has recurrent infusion site infections or allergic reactions. The CSII discontinuation rates have been 5% or less at most centers.[30] Evidence is growing that CSII is cost-effective, both in general and compared with MDI for children and adults with T1D.[31]

The CSII use in the type 2 diabetes (T2D) population has been gradually increasing and an insulin pump therapy may be used if patients with T2D have not achieved their HbA_{1c} goal despite intensive insulin therapy, use of oral agents and other injectable drugs, and lifestyle changes.[32] Findings from multiple multicenter clinical RCTs support the health benefits of insulin pump treatment as compared with MDI in the population with T2D.[33,34]

THE FUTURE OF INSULIN PUMP TREATMENT

Almost four decades ago, insulin pump therapy transformed the management of diabetes by introducing an innovative method of flexible insulin dosing, customized for user's lifestyle and needs.[1] The adoption of insulin pump treatment has not been swift; however, over the course of several years, the number of patients using CSII has been increasing.[35] Diabetes technology tools, along with the insulin pump technology, have been evolving at an extraordinary rate, with new technologies being created and existing technologies improving every year.[36] As technology has evolved, it has become apparent that insulin pumps have more to offer to improve diabetes treatment. Rather than functioning as a stand-alone device, insulin pumps are interconnected with multiple devices and can accomplish more with the integrated systems that adapt not only to the patient's characteristics but also to external disruptors, such as exercise and stress factors, for an ultimate personalized treatment approach. Next-generation insulin pumps complemented with new-generation faster-acting insulin analogs to keep up with the pace of real-time sensor glucose–driven insulin treatment will bring us a step closer to being able to mimic physiologic glycemic regulation.[7,37,38] Insulin pumps will continue to play a key role in the treatment of diabetes and will reach their full potential in improving clinical outcomes through their use in integrated, automated diabetes management systems along with the new-generation, insulin pump–compatible faster-acting insulin analogs.

REFERENCES

1. Tamborlane WV, Sherwin RS, Genel M, Felig P. Reduction to normal of plasma glucose in juvenile diabetes by subcutaneous administration of insulin with a portable infusion pump. *N Engl J Med* 1979;300(11):573–578

2. Pickup JC, Keen H, Parsons JA, Alberti KG. Continuous subcutaneous insulin infusion: an approach to achieving normoglycaemia. *Br Med J* 1978;1(6107):204–207

3. Home PD, Pickup JC, Keen H, et al. Continuous subcutaneous insulin infusion: comparison of plasma insulin profiles after infusion or bolus injection of the mealtime dose. *Metabolism* 1981;30(5):439–442

4. Zinman B, Tildesley H, Chiasson JL, et al. Insulin lispro in CSII: results of a double-blind crossover study. *Diabetes* 1997;46(3):440–443

5. Miller KM, Foster NC, Beck RW, et al. Current state of type 1 diabetes treatment in the U.S.: updated data from the T1D Exchange Clinic Registry. *Diabetes Care* 2015;38(6):971–978

6. DiMeglio LA, Pottorff TM, Boyd SR, et al. A randomized, controlled study of insulin pump therapy in diabetic preschoolers. *J Pediatr* 2004;145(3):380–384

7. Cengiz E, Bode B, Van Name M, Tamborlane WV. Moving toward the ideal insulin for insulin pumps. *Expert Rev Med Devices* 2016;13(1):57–69

8. Zijlstra E, Demissie M, Graungaard T, et al. Investigation of pump compatibility of fast-acting insulin aspart in subjects with type 1 diabetes. *J Diabetes Sci Technol* 2018;12(1):145–151

9. Colquitt J, Royle P, Waugh N. Are analogue insulins better than soluble in continuous subcutaneous insulin infusion? Results of a meta-analysis. *Diabetes Med* 2003;20(10):863–836

10. Swan KL, Dziura JD, Steil GM, et al. Effect of age of infusion site and type of rapid-acting analog on pharmacodynamic parameters of insulin boluses in youth with type 1 diabetes receiving insulin pump therapy. *Diabetes Care* 2009;32(2):240–244

11. Muchmore DB, Vaughn DE. Accelerating and improving the consistency of rapid-acting analog insulin absorption and action for both subcutaneous injection and continuous subcutaneous infusion using recombinant human hyaluronidase. *J Diabetes Sci Technol* 2012;6(4):764–772

12. Stickelmeyer MP, Graf CJ, Frank BH, et al. Stability of U-10 and U-50 dilutions of insulin lispro. *Diabetes Technol Ther* 2000;2(1):61–66

13. Lane WS, Weinrib SL, Rappaport JM, Przestrzelski T. A prospective trial of U500 insulin delivered by Omnipod in patients with type 2 diabetes mellitus and severe insulin resistance. *Endocr Pract* 2010;16(5):778–784

14. Bergenstal RM, Klonoff DC, Garg SK, et al. Threshold-based insulin-pump interruption for reduction of hypoglycemia. *N Engl J Med* 2013;369(3):224–232

15. Buckingham BA, Raghinaru D, Cameron F, et al. Predictive low-glucose insulin suspension reduces duration of nocturnal hypoglycemia in children without increasing ketosis. *Diabetes Care* 2015;38(7):1197–1204

16. Forlenza G, Li Z, Buckingham B, et al. Predictive low glucose suspend reduces hypoglycemia in adults, adolescents, and children with type 1 diabetes in an at-home randomized crossover study: Results of the PROLOG trial. *Diabetes Care* 2018;41(20):2155–2161

17. Medtronic 670G. Available from www.medtronicdiabetes.com/products/minimed-670g-insulin-pump-system. Accessed on 10 February 2019

18. Medtronic 630G. Available from www.medtronicdiabetes.com/products/minimed-630g-insulin-pump-system. Accessed on 10 February 2019

19. Medtronic 530G. Available from http://www.medtronicdiabetes.com/search?cq=Medtronic+530G. Accessed on 10 February 2019

20. t:slim. Available from www.tandemdiabetes.com/products/t-slim-x2-insulin-pump. Accessed on 10 February 2019

21. Cellnovo. Available from www.myomnipod.com/healthcareproviders/clinical-resources/provider. Accessed on 10 February 2019

22. Sooil. Available from www.sooil.com/eng/product. Accessed on 10 February 2019

23. Heinemann L. Insulin pump therapy: what is the evidence for using different types of boluses for coverage of prandial insulin requirements? *J Diabetes Sci Technol* 2009;3(6):1490–1500

24. Pickup J, Mattock M, Kerry S. Glycaemic control with continuous subcutaneous insulin infusion compared with intensive insulin injections in patients with type 1 diabetes: meta-analysis of randomised controlled trials. *BMJ* 2002;324(7339):705

25. Weissberg-Benchell J, Antisdel-Lomaglio J, Seshadri R. Insulin pump therapy: a meta-analysis. *Diabetes Care* 2003;26(4):1079–1087

26. Pickup JC, Sutton AJ. Severe hypoglycaemia and glycaemic control in type 1 diabetes: meta-analysis of multiple daily insulin injections compared with continuous subcutaneous insulin infusion. *Diabetes Med* 2008;25(7):765–774

27. Karges B, Schwandt A, Heidtmann B, et al. Association of insulin pump therapy vs insulin injection therapy with severe hypoglycemia, ketoacidosis, and glycemic control among children, adolescents, and young adults with type 1 diabetes. *JAMA* 2017;318(14):1358–1366

28. Nicolucci A, Maione A, Franciosi M, et al. Quality of life and treatment satisfaction in adults with type 1 diabetes: a comparison between continuous subcutaneous insulin infusion and multiple daily injections. *Diabetes Med* 2008;25(2):213–220

29. Hoogma RP, Hammond PJ, Gomis R, et al. Comparison of the effects of continuous subcutaneous insulin infusion (CSII) and NPH-based multiple

daily insulin injections (MDI) on glycaemic control and quality of life: results of the 5-nations trial. *Diabetes Med* 2006;23(2):141–147

30. Pickup JC. Insulin-pump therapy for type 1 diabetes mellitus. *N Engl J Med* 2012;366(17):1616–1624

31. Roze S, Smith-Palmer J, Valentine W, et al. Cost-effectiveness of continuous subcutaneous insulin infusion versus multiple daily injections of insulin in type 1 diabetes: a systematic review. *Diabetes Med* 2015;32(11):1415–1424

32. Pickup JC, Reznik Y, Sutton AJ. Glycemic control during continuous subcutaneous insulin infusion versus multiple daily insulin injections in type 2 diabetes: individual patient data meta-analysis and meta-regression of randomized controlled trials. *Diabetes Care* 2017;40(5):715–722

33. Reznik Y, Morello R, Zenia A, et al. Autonomy of patients with type 2 diabetes with an insulin pump device: is it predictable? *J Diabetes Sci Technol* 2014; 8(4):760–765

34. Reznik Y, Cohen O, Aronson R, et al. Insulin pump treatment compared with multiple daily injections for treatment of type 2 diabetes (OpT2mise): a randomised open-label controlled trial. *Lancet* 2014;384(9950):1265–1272

35. Renard E. Insulin pump use in Europe. *Diabetes Technol Ther* 2010;12(Suppl. 1): S29–S32

36. Cengiz E, Sherr JL, Weinzimer SA, Tamborlane WV. New-generation diabetes management: glucose sensor-augmented insulin pump therapy. *Expert Rev Med Devices* 2011;8(4):449–458

37. Heinemann L, Muchmore DB. Ultrafast-acting insulins: state of the art. *J Diabetes Sci Technol* 2012;6(4):728–742

38. Cengiz E. Undeniable need for ultrafast-acting insulin: the pediatric perspective. *J Diabetes Sci Technol* 2012;6(4):797–801

Chapter 4
Status of Continuous Glucose Monitoring Technology in Clinical Practice

CLARE O'CONNOR, MD, MPH,[1] AND GRAZIA ALEPPO, MD, FACE, FACP[1]

INTRODUCTION

In less than two decades, continuous glucose monitoring (CGM) systems have emerged from being used predominantly for office-based procedures to providing personal tools for daily glucose management. Professional societies, including the American Diabetes Association, the Endocrine Society, and the American Association of Clinical Endocrinologists, have published guidelines in the past few years endorsing CGM for use in people with type 1 diabetes (T1D) as well as acknowledging the potential benefits for people with type 2 diabetes (T2D) who are following an intensive insulin management plan.[1-3]

Self-monitoring of blood glucose (SMBG) via finger-stick offers limited information by providing glucose levels at only single points in time, whereas CGM can track the patterns and trends of glucose levels throughout the day. The most current systems available are even able to offer predictive alerts for impending hypoglycemia.

CGM systems available today are divided in two main categories: professional and personal. Diagnostic (professional) CGM procedures, performed with practice-owned systems, include the placement of a sensor on patients during office visits, providing them with instructions that are specific for the systems used. Depending on the system brand, patients wear them for 6, 7, or up to 14 days. Data collected from the sensors are uploaded and reviewed with the patient. Professional CGM systems also can be worn in a "blinded" fashion, which means that patients wear the sensors but are not able to see their glucose levels until the system is removed and uploaded; or in an "unblinded" fashion, in which the patient essentially is wearing a real-time CGM system and receiving alerts and alarms to view glucose levels for the duration of the procedure.

These procedures offer healthcare providers with the opportunity to gain a greater understanding of their patients' glycemic trends and patterns, while also formulating personalized therapy adjustments based on analysis and review of the CGM data.

Several CGM systems are also available commercially for personal use, whether as stand-alone or integrated systems with insulin pumps. Most CGM systems measure glucose levels in the interstitial fluid by using an enzymatic

[1]Division of Endocrinology, Metabolism and Molecular Medicine, Feinberg School of Medicine, Northwestern University, Chicago, IL.

reaction with glucose oxidase as the substrate; other systems, such as the implantable Eversense system from Senseonic, uses fluorescence sensing technology.[4] The information recorded by the sensor is sent by a transmitter to various display devices. Stand-alone CGM systems display the information on either a receiver (Dexcom G4 PLATINUM/Dexcom G5/G6) or through mobile applications on smartphones and smartwatches (Apple/Android for Dexcom G5/G6 Mobile; Apple for Medtronic Guardian Connect Mobile).[5]

CGM systems integrated with insulin pumps display the CGM data directly on the insulin pump screen, such is the case for Medtronic MiniMed pump systems (530G, 630G, and 670G) or Tandem pump systems (t:slim, t:slim X2, and t:slim with basal-IQ);[6] the latter is also able to display CGM data on smartphones or smartwatches at the same time.

The way Abbott FreeStyle Libre's sensor glucose (SG) levels retrieve data is different. Data can be viewed only when the user "scans" the reader over the sensor or transmitter unit. For this reason, FreeStyle Libre is also referred to as a flash CGM (FCGM) or intermittently scanned CGM (is-CGM) versus a real-time CGM (rt-CGM), as all other systems are known. Other than the Abbott FreeStyle Libre, which records values every 15 min and has no audible alarms (an audible tone is provided with alerts to perform finger-stick testing), all other CGM systems provide glucose readings every 5 min and have audible alerts and alarms that can be set with the healthcare providers and customized according to the user's needs.

CGM technology has substantially evolved over time; newer systems have increased accuracy and longer sensor duration. Although some of the commercially available systems continue to require finger-sticks before using the CGM information to dose insulin (such as is the case for systems using Medtronic Guardian Sensor 3 and Senseonic Eversense systems), others have received approval from the U.S. Food and Drug Administration (FDA) for nonadjunctive use, which means they can be used independently to dose insulin from the information provided by the display device (Dexcom G5/G6 and Abbott FreeStyle Libre).[6] Newest versions, such as the Dexcom G6 and FreeStyle Libre, are factory calibrated and can be used for up to 10 and 14 days, respectively, whereas the implantable sensor Senseonic's Eversense, is approved for use up to 90 days. Traditionally, the mean absolute relative difference (MARD) has been used to assess sensor accuracy, with lower MARD values suggesting greater accuracy.[7] MARD and features of available personal CGM systems are given in Table 4.1.

For Dexcom CGM systems and Medtronic Guardian Connect Mobile, a "share" feature allows users to choose designated individuals (whether a parent, spouse, or friend) to "follow" their CGM data on smartphones and receive alerts and alarms for hypo- or hyperglycemia set up by the user. Other CGM systems have available "share" features, but these are not yet available in the U.S.

Each CGM system shows glucose rate-of-change trend arrows on the various display devices, apps, and insulin pumps. Therapy adjustments can be made based on these trend arrows, in particular, for CGM systems approved for nonadjunctive use. Many approaches to rate-of-change trend arrows have been published that suggest modifications of insulin doses based on a variety of algorithms, but these methods have not been validated in randomized controlled clinical trials (RCTs)

Table 4.1. Features of Selected FDA-Approved and Commercially Available Personal CGM Systems

	Dexcom G4 PLATINUM	Dexcom G5	Medtronic Enlite 2	Medtronic Guardian Sensor 3	FreeStyle Libre	Dexcom G6	Eversense Senseonic
MARD	13%	9%	13.6%	9.1%[a]–10.6%[b] 8.7%[a]–9.6%[b]	9.7%	9%	8.5%
Warm-up time	2 h	2 h	2 h	2 h	1 h	2 h	24 h
Sensor Wear Duration	Up to 7 days	Up to 7 days	Up to 6 days	Up to 7 days	Up to 14 days	Up to 10 days	Up to 90 days
Calibrations	Every 12 h	Every 12 h	Every 12 h	Every 12 h 2 calibrations/day 4 calibrations/day	None[c]	None	Every 12 h
Audible Alarms, Alerts	Yes	Yes	Yes Predictive alerts	Yes Predictive alerts	No	Yes Hypoglycemia predictive alerts	Yes Hypoglycemia predictive alerts
Labeling	Requires finger-stick confirmation	Nonadjunctive	Requires finger-stick confirmation	Requires finger-stick confirmation	Nonadjunctive	Nonadjunctive	Requires finger-stick confirmation
Pump Integration	Animas Vibe Tandem t:slim G4	Tandem t:slim X2	MiniMed 530G, 630G	MiniMed 670G hybrid closed-loop system	None	Tandem t:slim Basal-IQ (PLGS)	None
Software and Compatible Devices	Dexcom G4 platinum receiver and Share 2 app (Apple) with Follower app (Apple/ Android) Animas Vibe Tandem t:slim	Dexcom G5 receiver and Dexcom Mobile app (Apple, Android) Tandem t:slim X2	Medtronic MiniMed 530G, 630G	Medtronic MiniMed 670G hybrid closed-loop system Guardian Connect Mobile (Apple)	FreeStyle Libre Reader	Dexcom G6 receiver and Dexcom Mobile app (Apple, Android) Tandem t:slim Basal-IQ (PLGS)	Eversense app (Apple/Android)
Population	>2 years old	>2 years old, including CMS patients	>18 years old	>7 years old	>18 years old, including CMS patients	>2 years old	>18 years old
Acetaminophen interference	Yes	Yes	Yes	Yes	No	No	No

CMS, U.S. Centers for Medicare and Medicaid Services.

[a]Arm; [b]abdomen; [c]Patients are encouraged to check glucose by finger-stick if their symptoms do not match the sensor glucose value on the Libre Reader or if prompted to do so by the Libre Reader (see the FreeStyle manual).

and should be considered primarily as starting points for personalized insulin dose adjustments.[8–10] Of note, rates of glucose change depicted by trend arrows are different between devices, and to make safe changes in therapy, it is necessary for patients and healthcare providers to learn the differences between these systems and apply algorithms designed for specific systems. Comparisons of glucose rate of change trend arrows are outlined in Table 4.2.

The clinical benefits of CGM therapy on glycemic control have been demonstrated in multiple clinical trials over the last decade both in patients on insulin pump and multiple daily injections. At least 27 published RCTs have assessed the outcomes of CGM in T1D and T2D, most consistently showing reductions in HbA_{1c} as well as reductions in hypoglycemia.[11]

Patient Selection

Any person with diabetes could be a potential candidate for CGM therapy, and in particular, all people with T1D should consider using CGM as part of their therapy in addition to insulin therapy. To achieve the full benefits from CGM therapy and to successfully improve glucose metrics, however, it is imperative to identify appropriate candidates.

Although increasing, the overall use and uptake of CGM technology in people with diabetes is still not widespread. The T1D Exchange Registry Clinic Network has more than 30,000 individuals with T1D from more than 80 clinics across the U.S. In the Exchange's most recent report (2016–2018), CGM users accounted for 30% of the enrolled participants, substantially increasing from 7% in 2010–2012 and correlating with FDA approval for younger ages. Among the CGM users, 83% were also using insulin pump systems, whereas 17% were on multiple daily injections (MDIs).[12] This estimate of CGM users is increasing, especially when compared to data obtained from the T1D Exchange just a few years ago, which found that only 13% of patients on an insulin pump and 2% of patients using MDIs of insulin also used CGM.

Traditionally, barriers to CGM use have included perceived poor accuracy, cost, discomfort, alarm fatigue, and short sensor duration. Thankfully, most of these barriers have been overcome: accuracy has greatly improved; sensor duration has been extended to 7, 10, 14, or even 90 days; and newer sensors are easier to insert and more comfortable to wear. Users who are concerned about alarm fatigue have the option of using the FreeStyle Libre Flash, which provides audible alerts only if the reader is scanned during a hypo- or hyperglycemic episode for glucose levels that are <70 mg/dL or >240 mg/dL.[9] For other patients, the root cause of alarm fatigue should be evaluated, and alerts and alarms should be adjusted accordingly to enhance the patient experience and receive all of the benefits of CGM therapy.

In January 2017, CGM coverage was extended for the first time to Center for Medicare and Medicaid Services (CMS) beneficiaries with diabetes, treated with at least three insulin injections per day, measuring glucose levels by finger-stick four times per day, and requiring frequent insulin adjustments. Today, Medicare has approved two systems: Dexcom G5 and Abbott FreeStyle Libre. Cost, however, remains a persistent barrier even though most insurance plans cover these tools; hopefully, in the future, the cost will decrease as well and make these systems affordable to all who wish to use them.

Table 4.2. CGM System Differences in Glucose Rate-of-Change Trend Arrows

	Free Style Libre	Dexcom G4 PLATINUM/G5 Mobile/G6 Mobile	Medtronic MiniMed Enlite 2 (530G)	Medtronic MiniMed Guardian Sensor 3 (670G)/Enlite 2 (630G)/Guardian Connect	Senseonic Eversense
↑↑↑	N/A	N/A	N/A	Glucose is rising at a rate of ≥3 mg/dL per min	N/A
↑↑	N/A	Glucose is rapidly rising >3 mg/dL per min	Glucose is rising at a rate of ≥2 mg/dL per min	Glucose is rising at a rate of ≥2 but <3 mg/dL per min	N/A
↑	Glucose is rising quickly (>2 mg/dL per min)	Glucose is rising 2–3 mg/dL per min	Glucose is rising at a rate of 1–2 mg/ dL per min	Glucose is rising at a rate of ≥1 but <2 mg/dL per min	Very rapidly rising glucose levels, rising at a rate of >2 mg/dL per min
↗	Glucose is rising (1–2 mg/dL per min)	Glucose is slowly rising 1–2 mg/dL per min	N/A	N/A	Moderately rising glucose level, rising at a rate between 1 and 2 mg/dL per min
→	Glucose is changing slowly (<1 mg/dL per min)	Steady glucose is not increasing/decreasing >1 mg/dL per min	N/A	N/A	Gradually rising or falling glucose levels, falling or rising at a rate between 0 and 1 mg/dL per min
↘	Glucose is falling (1–2 mg/dL per min)	Glucose is slowly falling 1–2 mg/dL per min	N/A	N/A	Moderately falling glucose levels, falling at a rate between 1 mg/dL and 2 mg/dL per min
↓	Glucose is falling quickly (>2 mg/dL per min)	Glucose is falling 2–3 mg/dL per min	Glucose is falling at a rate of 1–2 mg/dL per min	Glucose is falling at a rate of ≥1 but <2 mg/dL per min	Very rapidly falling glucose levels, falling at a rate >2 mg/dL per min
↓↓	N/A	Glucose is rapidly falling >3 mg/dL per min	Glucose is falling at a rate of ≥2 mg/dL per min	Glucose is falling at a rate of ≥2 but <3 mg/dL per min	N/A
↓↓↓	N/A	N/A	N/A	Glucose is falling at a rate of ≥3 mg/dL per min	N/A

For patients to achieve the full benefits of CGM therapy, it is important that patients receive adequate training, understand calibration techniques for the systems that require it, use the CGM on a nearly daily basis, and be active participants in their diabetes management.

CGM System Selection

CGM system selection is a newer concept, driven by the fact that in the last year multiple devices have become available. Although most of the systems have great similarities, important differences exist among them and these dictate careful consideration when recommending CGM therapy.

First, the argument of "CGM after insulin pump" is no longer valid. Many studies have clearly shown that CGM use in patients with T1D and T2D on intensive insulin therapy using MDI is at least as effective as insulin pump therapy in conjunction with or followed by CGM therapy.[13] Therefore, patients with T1D should be counseled to consider CGM therapy as soon as possible; ideally, right after diagnosis whether the patients are adults or of pediatric age and regardless of the insulin delivery method. The same approach should be considered for patients with T2D on MDIs who are at increased risk for and fearful of hypoglycemia.

Second, although patients generally should be allowed to choose their devices, it is important to determine what is the most appropriate device based on the patient's medication regimen, comorbidities, risk of hypoglycemia, presence of hypoglycemia unawareness, or history of severe hypoglycemic episodes requiring the assistance of others. For the latter group of patients, it is appropriate to consider a system that can provide audible alerts and alarms for impending hypoglycemia or with predictive hypoglycemia alerts to reduce the frequency and severity of hypoglycemia. For this type of patient, likely a patient with T1D or long-standing T2D on MDI, such CGM devices as the Dexcom family of G5-G6 generations; Medtronic Guardian Connect Mobile; Senseonic Eversense; or an insulin pump with threshold, low-predicted glucose suspend features or a hybrid closed-loop system would be appropriate. For patients who have preserved hypoglycemia awareness or for patients on a regimen that would unlikely cause hypoglycemia, such as a patient with T2D taking oral medications with or without long-acting insulin or glucagon-like peptide 1 (GLP-1) receptor agonist, Abbott FreeStyle Libre would offer great advantages.[14] With this system, patients are able to view their glucose levels by painlessly scanning the reader over the sensor multiple times per day for up to 14 days without the need to calibrate the system. Similarly, Dexcom G5 or G6 CGM systems, both approved for nonadjunctive use, with a sensor duration of up to 7 and 10 days, respectively, would reduce in these patients the burden of blood glucose measurements to either two per day or none, as is the case of the Dexcom G6 system, which requires no calibrations.

CGM Use in Clinical Practice

CGM systems are used in clinical practice as professional procedures and for personal use. To date, no standardized approach is available to the interpretation of professional or personal CGM reports. The primary obstacles include brand-specific reports, a lack of cohesiveness on which data are reported, a perceived lack of time during office visits, lack of dedicated personnel uploading the data and preparing it for the healthcare provider to review, and the lack of a systematic approach to the data available. Also, many providers have not received training in interpreting CGM reports and may feel overwhelmed by the amount of information available without a systematic approach to the data. Efforts have been made in the past several years to simplify the reports to better understand patient progress and to make therapeutic plans during an office visit or when reviewing patient CGM data remotely. In the following paragraphs, we discuss several aspects that are important for the clinician to be familiar with when reviewing CGM data.

The ambulatory glucose profile (AGP) is one of the most helpful reports for the provider and is an excellent place to start the CGM review.[15] This type of report is used by several systems, including Dexcom CLARITY, Diasend-Glooko, Tidepool, Abbott Libreview, Tandem T:Connect, and Medtronic CareLink software. Ideally, at least 14 days of data should be reviewed, as this has been shown to provide a good estimate of glycemic values for a 3-month period.[16] The most important measures to review include the SG average and standard deviation (SD); the percentage of time spent in euglycemia (70–180 mg/dL), hypoglycemia (<70 mg/dL and <54 mg/dL), or hyperglycemia (>180 mg/dL and >250 mg/dL); and the coefficient of variation (CV).

The CV is a measure of glycemic variability (GV). It is an important element to review because increased variability is associated with an increased risk of hypoglycemic events. It is calculated by dividing the mean SG average by the SD. A CV of <36% is desirable and correlates with the frequency of hypoglycemia—that is, the lower the CV, the lower the hypoglycemia frequency.[17]

Time spent in hypoglycemia, hypoglycemic trends, and repeating patterns should be reviewed next, paying particular attention to nocturnal hypoglycemia and the duration of each hypoglycemic episode. Time spent in hyperglycemia and postprandial excursions should be reviewed as well. Interventions should be made to adjust therapy as needed, whether related to basal insulin (or basal rates if using insulin pump therapy) or mealtime insulin doses as well as insulin sensitivity factors.

Finally, it is important to review the effects of activities and lifestyle (e.g., exercise, diet, alcohol use) that will be unique to each patient.[18] Attention should be paid to alert settings, so that alarm fatigue is minimized, and alerts should be set appropriately according to the patient's specific needs.

The key to the successful use of CGM data for both patients and providers is in its analysis on a regular basis, especially for the CGM user between visits.

Studies evaluating the most effective interventions incorporate all components of the feedback loop. This includes connecting patients to their healthcare team with two-way communication, analyzing patient generated data, and tailoring feedback and intervention based on patient feedback and data trends.[19] Various systems available today can send users weekly messages with trends or even suggestions for repeating trends.

PRACTICAL APPROACH TO CGM DATA INTERPRETATION USING CLINICAL VIGNETTES

A picture is worth ten thousand words.

Fred R. Barnard (1927)

This section provides clinical examples of specific trends and patterns noted on patients reports and provides readers with practical applications to enhance their understanding of CGM and improve patient outcomes.

Usefulness of AGP Report, Time in Ranges, and CV versus HbA$_{1c}$

A 30-year-old woman with T1D since she was 7 years old, on MiniMed 530G insulin pump and Dexcom G5 rt-CGM, presents to the office for a routine appointment. She reports both significant hyperglycemia and hypoglycemia over the past few weeks. She notes several new variables to her schedule, including recent travel, changes in her work shift from night to daytime, and a more sedentary work schedule. While on vacation, she noted a significant increase in overnight hypoglycemia and attributed it to increased alcohol intake. Her most recent HbA$_{1c}$ is 6.8%. A detailed review of her insulin pump and CGM data was performed.

Her rt-CGM AGP summary (Figure 4.1) shows an average glucose of 162 mg/dL and time in target range (70–180 mg/dL) of 56.5%. Her time spent in hypoglycemia is 9.2% (ideal goal <4%) and she spends 47.2% in hyperglycemia, with a CV of 42.9% (goal <36%), showing significant glycemic variability despite an HbA$_{1c}$ of 6.8%.

Further review of her Daily Glucose Profile and Daily View Reports in the Dexcom CLARITY software shows global hyperglycemia during the day as well as postprandial hyperglycemia, both likely induced by her new sedentary work schedule with increased insulin requirements, and insufficient insulin doses at mealtimes. Her insulin-to-carbohydrate ratio (ICR) was adjusted from 1:9 (1 unit per 9 g carbohydrate) to 1:8, and her insulin pump basal rates were increased accordingly.

She returned 2 months later, and her AGP profile showed significant improvement with a lower average glucose from 162 mg/dL to 135 mg/dL, increased time in target range from 56.4% to 75.4%, and a decrease of time in hyperglycemia >180 mg/dL and >250 mg/dL from 47.2% to 19.2%. Her CV also improved from 42.9% to 36.8%. Despite the improvement of time in target range and a reduction of time in hyperglycemia, however, this patient has persistent excessive time spent in hypoglycemia (~147 min/day), which is mainly present overnight, as shown in Figure 4.2.

Usefulness of CGM Daily View Reports in Identifying Alcohol-Induced Hypoglycemia Patterns

The patient discussed previously (Figures 4.1 and 4.2) reports an increased frequency of nocturnal hypoglycemia despite an improvement in her time in target range and a decrease in her glycemic variability represented by the CV of 36.8%. A detailed review of Daily View Reports on Dexcom CLARITY revealed an increased frequency and severity of hypoglycemia on weekend nights after moderate consumption of alcoholic beverages (Figure 4.3).

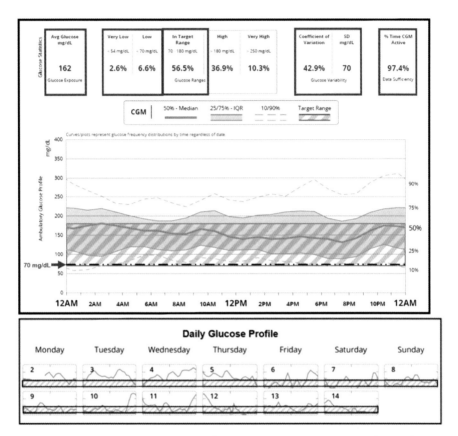

Figure 4.1. Usefulness of the CGM reports in identifying glycemic trends for intervention during clinic visit. A 30-year-old woman with T1D on MiniMed 530G insulin pump and Dexcom G5 rt-CGM reports more frequent hyperglycemia and hypoglycemia in the setting of many new variables (travel, working day shift instead of night shift, and change from active to sedentary job). **Top panel:** AGP preintervention shows time in target range of 56.5% followed by 9.2% time spent in hypoglycemia and elevated CV at 42.9% (target <36%). **Lower panel:** Daily glucose profile with global hyperglycemia and postprandial hyperglycemia. Based on these reports daytime pump basal rates were increased and the ICR was changed from 1:9 to 1:8.

As seen in Figure 4.3, on a Friday night, she ate a meal at a restaurant, followed by consumption of three servings of alcohol. At bedtime, her CGM system alerted her to a high SG. She took a correction bolus per her insulin pump bolus calculator for an SG of 240 mg/dL, and then went to bed without further insulin

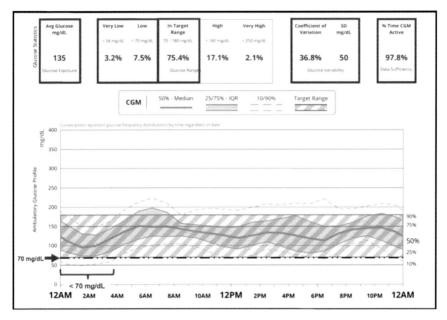

Figure 4.2. Postintervention rt-CGM review. Patient returns after the changes were made. AGP shows increase of time in target range (70–180 mg/dL) to 75.4% and improved CV from 42.9% to 36.8%. An increase in time spent in hypoglycemia is now seen at 10.7%, however, especially overnight. This prompted further assessment during the clinic visit to identify etiology of nocturnal hypoglycemia (see Figure 4.3).

adjustments. She experienced hypoglycemia at <54 mg/dL in the early morning hours, required correction of hypoglycemia with rapid-acting carbohydrates, and experienced hyperglycemia thereafter, with glucose levels >150 mg/dL the following morning. She reports that these patterns have happened regularly when she consumes alcohol in the evenings.

Alcohol-induced hypoglycemia is thought to be due to the inhibition of gluconeogenesis and has been associated with impaired counter-regulatory response, impaired cognition, and impaired hypoglycemia awareness.[20] For people with diabetes, this combination of effects can be dangerous. RT-CGM is a helpful tool to alert patients to alcohol-related nocturnal hypoglycemia events, as demonstrated in Figure 4.3. Evidence on how to prevent alcohol-induced hypoglycemia is fairly limited.[20] Recommendations include advising patients to always eat food when consuming alcohol, have a bedtime snack (without insulin coverage), and limit alcohol intake to no more than the recommended amounts (one serving for women per day and two servings for men per day).[20] For our patient, in addition to recommending a 20-g carbohydrate bedtime snack (without insulin coverage) and using a conservative correction bolus for hyperglycemia, we also recommended a reduction of basal rates overnight by 25–40% for 4–6 h on nights when

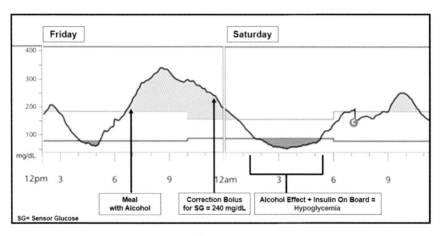

Figure 4.3. Usefulness of the CGM Daily View Report to identify alcohol-induced nocturnal hypoglycemia. After identifying nocturnal hypoglycemia on the AGP report (Figure 4.2), review of the Daily Trends in the rt-CGM report reveals that nocturnal occurs primarily on weekend nights. The patient states that she had a meal with three alcoholic beverages on Friday evening, followed by postprandial hyperglycemia. She took a correction insulin bolus for an SG of 240 mg/dL without any further modifications of insulin pump settings. Subsequently, she developed nocturnal hypoglycemia as low as <54 mg/dL early Saturday morning. To reduce the risk of hypoglycemia, the following strategy was recommended on evenings when alcohol is consumed: eat a carbohydrate snack (20 g) at bedtime without insulin coverage, use a conservative correction bolus, and set a temporary basal rate reduction overnight by 25–40% for 4–6 h at bedtime.

consuming alcohol. For patients using MDI, similar recommendations can be made, and patients can either lower the long-acting insulin dose overnight by 25%, or decrease the evening meal insulin dose and eat a 20-g carbohydrate bedtime snack without coverage with insulin to avoid nocturnal hypoglycemia induced by alcohol consumption.

Using rt-CGM Data to Guide Mealtime Insulin

Case Study 1: Identify the Need for Prandial Insulin Dose Adjustment. A 28-year-old woman with T1D diagnosed at age 12 presents for a routine visit. She manages her diabetes with a MiniMed Medtronic 723 Paradigm Revel insulin pump and Dexcom G5 rt-CGM. Her most recent HbA$_{1c}$ is 6.6%. She is frustrated by daily postmeal hyperglycemia, especially at lunchtime. Review of her rt-CGM data on the Dexcom CLARITY confirms postprandial hyperglycemia primarily after lunch (Figure 4.4*A*). On the basis of this information, her ICR is changed from 1:15 to 1:10 and she is encouraged to try more accurate carbohydrate counting.

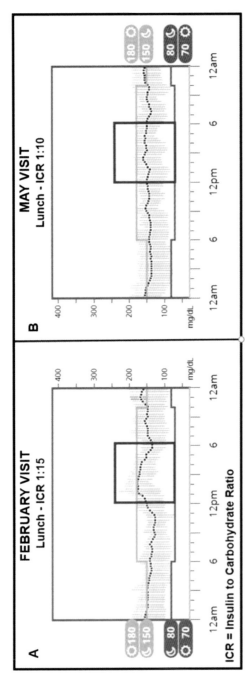

Figure 4.4. Usefulness of CGM data to identify the need for prandial insulin dose adjustment. A 28-year-old woman with T1D managed with MiniMed Medtronic 723 Paradigm Revel insulin pump and Dexcom G5 rt-CGM reports postprandial hyperglycemia. *A*: Summary view in Dexcom CLARITY identifies postprandial hyperglycemia after lunch (red box) during February visit. Based on this information, her ICR is changed from 1:15 to 1:10 and patient is further educated on accurate carbohydrate counting. *B*: Summary view of rt-CGM at return visit (May) shows improvement in postprandial glucose (red box) after the modification in ICR was implemented.

On her return visit, she reports having successfully improved her post-lunch glucose levels, confirmed by CGM review (Figure 4.4*B*), suggesting that the intervention was effective.

Case Study 2: Identify Challenges with Insulin Timing and Appropriate Dosing for Meal Bolus. A 67-year-old man with a 28-year history of T1D complicated by neuropathy, microalbuminuria, nonproliferative diabetic retinopathy, myocardial infarction, and hypoglycemia unawareness presents for a follow-up. His HbA$_{1c}$ is 7.3%. He recently started CGM therapy, after CMS began covering CGM systems. Before initiating Dexcom G5, he was managing his diabetes with MDI and SMBG; he had experienced multiple episodes of severe hypoglycemia requiring assistance of others in the past 3 years. His current regimen is a glargine SoloStar pen 26 units daily, insulin aspart FlexPen 9 units with meals plus a correction factor (CF) of 50 with a glucose target of 150 mg/dL. Shortly after starting CGM therapy, he contacted our office to report significant postprandial hyperglycemia. On review of his AGP report (Diasend-Glooko, Figure 4.5*A*), it was noted that his SG average was blood glucose of 200 mg/dL, with an SD of 68 (CV = 34%); time in target range (70–180 mg/dL) was at 41%, time in hyperglycemia was at 58%, and he had minimal time spent in hypoglycemia at 1%. Of note, overnight and post-breakfast hyperglycemia was evident as well as hyperglycemic trends post-dinner into bedtime (Figure 4.5*A*). On further questioning, he reports he frequently eats cereal for breakfast and takes the breakfast insulin dose after eating. He reports eating a smaller lunch and being more active during the day; however, he eats a larger dinner and doses insulin postmeal.

On the basis of the information gathered and the CGM trends, he was advised to increase the breakfast insulin dose and to take the meal bolus at least 15–20 min before eating. He also was advised to add some type of protein to his breakfast and to eat the protein before the carbohydrates. Similarly, his dinnertime insulin dose was increased, and he was advised to take the insulin before eating as well.

Upon returning 1 month later (Figure 4.5*B*), significant improvements in his CGM tracing were noted. His SG average had decreased to 169 mg/dL, with an SD of 54 (CV = 31.9%); time in target range had increased to 57%. Comparing the two graphs, it was evident that postprandial hyperglycemia for all meals had significantly improved without increasing time spent in hypoglycemia (1%).

Case Study 3: Usefulness of CGM in Identifying Effects of a Complex Meal on Glucose Levels. A 26-year-old woman with a 6-month history of T1D, managed with Insulet Omnipod insulin pump and Dexcom G5, presents for a routine visit. Her most recent HbA$_{1c}$ is 6.7%, which significantly improved since diagnosis (13.1%). Her AGP shows time in target range at 64%; however, she reports hypoglycemia 1–2 h post-dinner, requiring hypoglycemia correction with rapid-acting carbohydrates, followed by overnight and morning hyperglycemia. She notices these trends when she eats pizza or meals rich in fat or protein.

This case illustrates the effect that a complex meal with fat, protein, and carbohydrates has on postprandial glucose trends. The addition of fat to carbohydrates leads to slowing of gastric emptying as well as decreased insulin sensitivity. The resulting effect is early postprandial hypoglycemia followed by late postprandial hyperglycemia because of a mismatch of insulin action and food absorption, as shown in Figure 4.6*A*. With these meals, in general, a higher insulin dose is necessary to account for fat, sometimes requiring up to a twofold increase

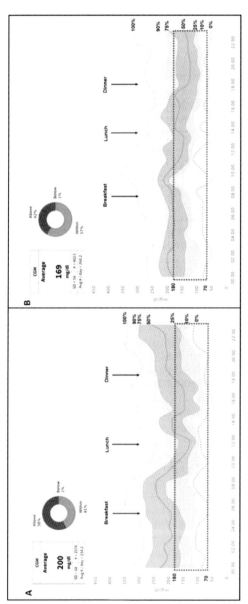

Figure 4.5. Role of AGP summary of Dexcom G5 rt-CGM data (Diasend-Glooko) in identifying the need for postprandial insulin adjustment. A 67-year-old man with long-standing T1D on MDI has recently started using rt-CGM (Dexcom G5). *A:* Preintervention AGP report shows high average SG of 200 mg/dL, TIR 41% of the time, and prominent nocturnal and post-breakfast/post-dinner hyperglycemia (thick blue band that extends well above goal range, which is indicated by dotted red box). He admitted to eating a high-carbohydrate breakfast (cereal) and often delaying insulin boluses until after the meal. Interventions included increasing mealtime insulin with breakfast and dinner, instructing patient to bolus 15–20 min before meal and adding protein to breakfast at beginning of the meal. *B:* Postintervention AGP report at return visit demonstrates improved average SG of 169 mg/dL, improved time in range to 57% without increase in hypoglycemia (1% vs.1%), and noticeably lower postmeal hyperglycemia peaks (lower peak blood glucose values and smaller width blue band suggesting decreased glycemic variability).

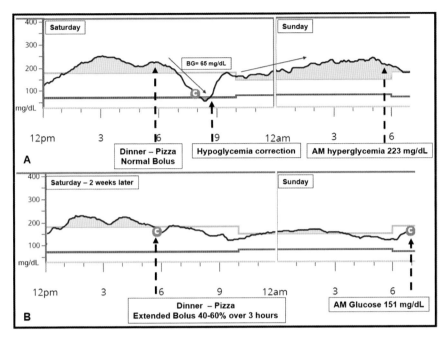

Figure 4.6. Effect of complex meals (deep-dish pizza) on absorption of food and timing of insulin. A 26-year-old woman with recently diagnosed T1D (managed by Omnipod insulin pump and Dexcom G5). *A*: Review of daily trend report shows the patient took a normal bolus for pizza that caused early postprandial hypoglycemia (blood glucose at calibration 65 mg/dL), necessitating the intake of extra carbohydrates to correct hypoglycemia. Hypoglycemia was followed by prolonged hyperglycemia overnight with morning hyperglycemia and blood glucose of 223 mg/dL. Complex meals (the addition of fat to carbohydrate) can cause slower gastric emptying and decreased insulin sensitivity. Giving a normal insulin bolus can cause early postprandial hypoglycemia followed by late postprandial hyperglycemia because of a mismatch of insulin action and food absorption, as this example shows. The patient was instructed to use an extended bolus over 3 h for complex meals. *B*: On her return visit, review of a daily trend report shows improved glycemic control after a similar complex meal of pizza. There is no further evidence of early postmeal hypoglycemia and improvement of the delayed postprandial hyperglycemia overnight after using an extended bolus set at 40–60% over 3 h. For patients using MDI, another option could be to manually split the insulin bolus into two separate doses (one at the start of meal and another 1–2 h later).

in insulin compared to the dose calculated for carbohydrate intake alone. The addition of protein to a high-fat meal appears to be additive and also can lead to delayed postprandial hyperglycemia.[21,22]

Strategies to overcome this challenge require the use of advanced bolus features in insulin pumps, such as dual-wave or extended boluses (depending on insulin pump brand), or to split the insulin bolus in two separate doses for patients using MDI (one at the start of a meal and another dose 1–2 h later, or as needed based on CGM trends). We asked our patient to use an extended bolus over 3 h and to let us know if she found a difference. A subsequent CGM review showed us that using the advanced bolus features resulted in better postprandial and overnight glucose profiles (Figure 4.6*B*).

Advanced boluses need to be individualized based on patient needs. These boluses are particularly useful in patients with known delayed gastric emptying or a history of gastroparesis, in which case a longer duration or different advanced bolus set-up (i.e., 30–70% for 3–4 h or longer) may need to be employed.

Using CGM Data to Help Manage Exercise-Induced Hypoglycemia

A 32-year-old woman with a 15-year history of T1D and postablative hypothyroidism presents to the endocrinology office. She manages her diabetes with Dexcom G4 rt-CGM integrated in an Animas Vibe insulin pump. She is physically active and usually runs in the morning, and occasionally in the evenings. She reports frequent hypoglycemic episodes with exercise and would like to learn how to avoid them. Review of insulin pump and rt-CGM data was performed using Diasend-Glooko software. The Comparison Report (Day-by-Day Overview) was used to identify hypo- and hyperglycemia patterns and their relation to insulin boluses and pump settings in one useful screen. Review of her data showed hyperglycemia before exercise close to 300 mg/dL (Figure 4.7), for which the patient took a full correction dose via insulin pump. Upon exercise started shortly thereafter, she experienced a rapid decrease of glucose levels with hypoglycemia close to 40 mg/dL. The lower panel in Figure 4.7 shows that no modifications to basal rates were made before exercise, nor during or after exercise, to prevent exercise-induced hypoglycemia. Combined with the correction dose given before physical activity and the presence of active insulin on-board, the overall insulin amount became excessive for this patient in the setting of increased glucose utilization and increased insulin sensitivity driven by aerobic exercise. The patient ingested rapid-acting carbohydrates while exercising, followed by another snack following exercise for which she took 2.8 units. At lunchtime, she again took 4.3 units with her meal. Shortly thereafter, she noticed significant hyperglycemia with rapid up-trending arrows and hyperglycemia alarms and decided to give an additional dose of insulin of 3.8 units overriding the bolus calculator. As expected, unfortunately, aggressive postprandial correction of hyperglycemia in the presence of active insulin on board from a recent meal bolus caused a rapid and significant drop of glucose because of insulin stacking, requiring small and frequent snacks throughout the afternoon into the evening. This patient was retrained on how to appropriately reduce insulin before aerobic activity, such as by employing the use of temporary basal with variable duration, and to avoid having active insulin on board before exercise. Additionally, she was encouraged to avoid aggressive correction of postmeal

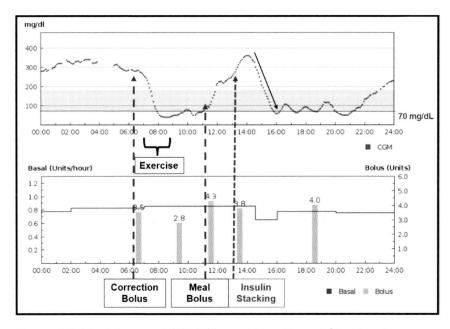

Figure 4.7. Usefulness of CGM Comparison Report (day-by-day over-view) to identify hypo- and hyperglycemia patterns and their relation-ship to insulin boluses and pump settings. Review of the report in a 32-year-old woman with T1D managed with Dexcom G4 rt-CGM integrated in an Animas Vibe insulin pump, who is an avid runner, shows pre-exercise hyperglycemia of 300 mg/dL for which patient took full correction bolus (solid vertical blue line in lower panel), followed by exercise with rapid descent into hypoglycemia as a result of exercising with active insulin on board and lack of temporary basal (basal insulin seen as horizontal blue line in the lower panel). After exercise routine, she ingested a snack blousing with 2.8 units of insulin; she then ate lunch and bolused with 4.3 units of insulin. She noted hyperglycemia with up-trending arrows shortly after and took an additional 3.8 units of insulin overriding the bolus calculator and leading to insulin stacking. The added insulin dose, along with recent exercise and increased insulin sensitivity from aerobic exercise, led to a rapid drop in glucose and prolonged hypoglycemia into the evening, which required multiple snacks to avoid further hypoglycemia. She was retrained to reduce insulin before aerobic activity, including use of a lower temporary basal rate and avoiding having insulin on board preceding aerobic activity. She was instructed to avoid insulin stacking and overriding the bolus calculator. Reviewing the CGM data in this setting allows the provider to understand exactly how patients are dosing insulin in relation to their glucose levels, which can be revealing to help identify the most appropriate interventions and behavioral changes, as seen in this case.

hyperglycemia and to follow the suggestions of the bolus calculator to avoid insulin stacking.

Exercise has complex effects on glucose levels and metabolism; its effects vary with the type of exercise, duration, and intensity. Aerobic exercise (walking, swimming, running, cycling) often leads to cellular glucose uptake in an insulin-independent mechanism and increased insulin sensitivity, which can lead to acute or delayed hypoglycemia with variable duration (up to 24 h).[23] Anaerobic exercise (strength training, weight lifting, high-intensity interval training) can lead to acute hyperglycemia and increased risk for delayed nocturnal hypoglycemia. These complexities understandably lead to many barriers to exercise for patients with diabetes, including fear of hypoglycemia and lack of confidence in modifications needed for exercise. Strategies for modifications of insulin dosing in preparation for exercise have been reported,[23] and suggestions on how to prepare for exercise with changes in insulin doses are available at ExCarbs.[24]

Usefulness of FreeStyle LibreView Reports in the Management of Diabetes

Case Study 1: Benefit of Using Diagnostic CGM in a Patient with T2D. A 71-year-old man with a history of T2D diagnosed 20 years ago, complicated by peripheral neuropathy, presents for a routine follow-up visit. His current diabetes regimen includes glargine SoloStar pen 15 units daily at bedtime, repaglinide 3 mg with meals, and metformin XR 1,000 mg twice daily. He has declined past recommendations to use MDIs of insulin because of cost. He usually performs SMBG once daily in the morning and his glucose levels are between 100 mg/dL and 120 mg/dL. His latest HbA_{1c} is 9.3%, however, and it has increased from 8.9% since his last visit. A diagnostic CGM procedure was performed with a FreeStyle Libre PRO to better understand this patient's glucose trends as well as the pattern of and discrepancy between blood glucose levels and HbA_{1c}. The patient was instructed to monitor glucose at least twice daily during the procedure. An upload of the glucose meter data via Diasend-Glooko showed a blood glucose average of 125 mg/dL. However, hyperglycemia was noted in the evening (Figure 4.8). Review of the FreeStyle LibreView CGM tracing showed an AGP summary with time in target range of 39% and time in hyperglycemia at 55% with 6% time in hypoglycemia. The AGP SG average was 193 mg/dL, which was much higher than the average blood glucose reported by SMBG of 125 mg/dL.

The AGP graph showed a downward trend overnight with normal glucose levels in the morning, followed by sustained hyperglycemia throughout the day (Figure 4.9, upper panel). Upon review of the food diary he kept during the procedure, it appeared that the patient consumed large amounts of carbohydrates with meals and was consuming sweetened beverages on a regular basis, multiple times per day, which contributed to hyperglycemia.

Figure 4.9 (lower panel) shows 2 days of data highlighting the significant postprandial hyperglycemia seen after meals and snacks followed by a hypoglycemia trend overnight because of the extra intake of repaglinide at bedtime for hyperglycemia. The plan of care for this patient included modification of his meal plan to substantially reduce carbohydrates and sweetened beverages as well as to increase the repaglinide with meals only (avoiding taking repaglinide at bedtime

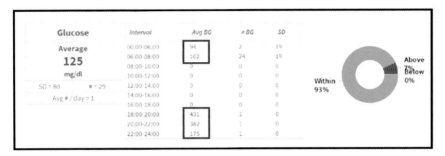

Figure 4.8. Benefits of Diagnostic CGM use in a patient with T2D.
Data from a glucometer upload (Diasend-Glooko) during diagnostic CGM
review. Target glucose levels are noted in the morning; however, hyperglycemia is noted between 6 and 10 P.M.

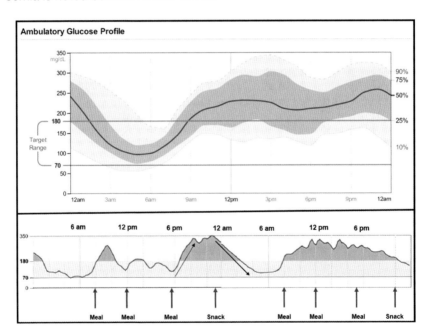

Figure 4.9. Diagnostic CGM review. *Upper panel*: AGP shows overnight
down-trending pattern of sensor glucose levels, with normal fasting glucose levels in the morning. These are followed by sustained hyperglycemia for the rest of the day with down-trending SG levels overnight, as a
result of the patient taking additional repaglinide at bedtime. *Lower panel*:
usefulness of food intake record with daily review of glycemic trends to
identify the etiology of hyperglycemia. The patient reported eating large
amounts of carbohydrates with meals and ingestion of sweetened beverages contributing to his hyperglycemia.

if not eating a full meal). Using professional CGM in this patient with T2D revealed unexpected glucose patterns that explained the discrepancy between his baseline glucose levels and his HbA_{1c}. This tool can be extremely helpful to help patients make behavior modifications and implement targeted interventions to improve glycemia.

Case Study 2: Usefulness of FreeStyle FCGM to Reveal the Correlation between Glucose Control and Number of Daily Scans. A 36-year-old woman with T1D diagnosed at age 10 recently initiated therapy with a MiniMed 670G hybrid closed-loop system. On a routine follow-up appointment, she is tearful and states that she is overwhelmed by the number of alarms and the perceived excessive interaction with her new pump/CGM. She spends most of the time in Manual Mode because of alarm fatigue. Even though her most recent HbA_{1c} is 7.1%, she has significant glycemic variability and would greatly benefit from CGM therapy. She opts for FreeStyle Libre because there is no need for calibration and there are no audible alarms and she understands the need to scan the reader at least 8–10 times per day to reduce glycemic variability. Upon her return visit, the reader is uploaded to LibreView software. As seen in Figure 4.10, the AGP report shows significant glycemic variability and frequent hypoglycemic episodes. Upon further review, she reveals that she scans the reader on average only 4–5 times per day and on some days only once. The patient was retrained on the importance of multiple scans per day to obtain the CGM benefits of reducing glycemic fluctuations and to avoid extreme hypo- and hyperglycemia. The benefits of the FreeStyle Libre Flash have been described, and successful use of this system correlates with the frequency of reader scans.[25] More specifically, recent studies using FCGM found an average number of scans per day of 15 for T1D and 8 for T2D.[26,27] As part of CGM review, it is important to address frequency of reader scans per day, as the number of scans per day appears to positively correlate with more time spent in the target range and less time spent in hypo- or hyperglycemia.[27] The ideal number of scans per day should be decided on an individual basis and modified based on trends noted during data review.

Usefulness of CGM in Identifying Causes and Effects of Insulin Stacking

A 34-year-old woman with T1D, Addison's disease, and Hashimoto-induced hypothyroidism presents for a routine follow-up appointment. She uses Animas OneTouch Ping insulin pump and Dexcom G5 CGM to manage her diabetes. Her most recent HbA_{1c} is 6.8%; however, on review of her CGM data, significant glycemic variability is noted (43.75%, goal <36%) (Figure 4.11, upper panel, AGP). Her time in target range is 60%, but her time in hypoglycemia is excessive at 7% (>100 min/day). On closer review of her pump/CGM data via the Diasend-Glooko software depicted in Figure 4.12, it is noted that the mealtime boluses are given after eating, with subsequent postprandial hyperglycemia; postprandial glucose elevations are followed by multiple correction boluses, leading to insulin stacking and hypoglycemia, often with values <54 mg/dL. This patient's hypoglycemia is particularly problematic in view of her Addison's disease, with blunted or absent response to steroid-induced glycogenolysis in the setting of level-two hypoglycemia. Careful review of specific reports, such as the Day-to-Day Comparison Report, can help the clinician and the patient reveal the causes

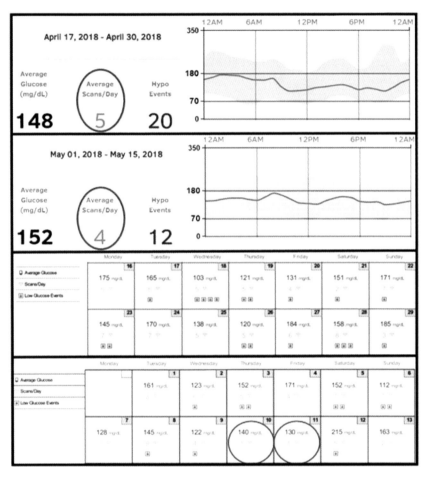

Figure 4.10. Usefulness of LibreView software in revealing number of scans/day performed by users. A 36-year-old woman with T1D managed with a MiniMed 670G hybrid closed-loop system is overwhelmed with frequent alarms and opts to switch to FreeStyle Libre (no audible alarms and no calibration required). She is instructed to scan the reader at least 8–10 times per day. Review of daily scans shows an average of 4–5 scans per day (top red circles) and only 1 scan on some days (bottom red circles). The report shows significant hypoglycemia and hyperglycemia despite an average blood glucose of 148–152 mg/dL, suggesting significant glycemic variation and inadequate glycemic control. She was instructed to increase the number of glucose scans per day, as the successful use of this system correlates with the frequency of reader scans. It is important for the provider to review how often patients are scanning the FreeStyle Libre Reader.

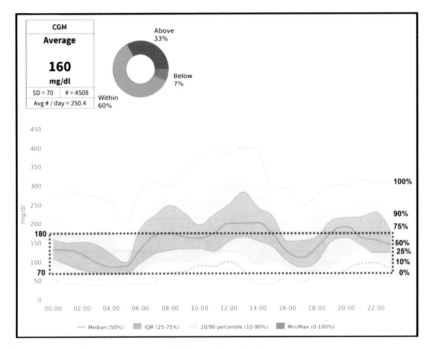

Figure 4.11. Usefulness of CGM in identifying causes of glycemic variability. A 34-year-old woman with T1D, Addison's disease, and Hashimoto-induced hypothyroidism manages her diabetes with Animas One-Touch Ping insulin pump and Dexcom G5. Her most recent HbA$_{1c}$ is 6.8%. Review of AGP summary report shows an average blood glucose of 160 mg/dL, but significant glycemic variability as evidenced by a CV of 43.75% (goal <36%). Her time in target range is 60%, but her time in hypoglycemia is excessive at 7%.

of wide glycemic fluctuations, as well as hypoglycemia. These reports can give the clinician the opportunity to provide feedback on optimizing premeal insulin dosing (ideally 15 min before eating), adjusting the ICR or even recommending the use of the rate-of-change arrow method to improve overall glycemia without "chasing" glucose levels.[8] With the approval of Dexcom G5/G6 systems for nonadjunctive insulin dosing, by paying attention to trend arrows and adjusting insulin doses based on their direction, patients can proactively modify their insulin dose to improve overall glycemia (Figure 4.13).[8]

Adjusting Correction Insulin Dose Using the Endocrine Society Approach to CGM Trend Arrows

A 42-year-old man with T1D diagnosed at age 24 presents for a routine appointment. His diabetes is managed with MDI. His regimen includes glargine

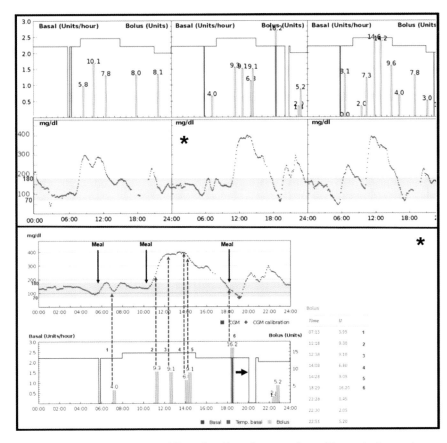

Figure 4.12. Importance of Day-by-Day Comparison Reports to understand cause of glycemic variability. On further review of data (Figure 4.11), it is noted that patient is often giving a mealtime bolus after eating (lower panel with timing of mealtime boluses relative to meals indicated with red arrows). This is followed by additional insulin boluses (solid blue vertical bars in lower panel) leading to insulin stacking and subsequent hypoglycemia despite attempts to mitigate it with the use of temporary basal at 0% for almost 1 h. *Time period in upper panel is magnified in the lower panel.

SoloStar pen, 20 units at bedtime, and lispro KwikPen with an ICR of 1:15 for meals and a CF of 50 and a blood glucose target of 150 mg/dL.

He is also using Dexcom G5 CGM system nonadjunctively, calibrating twice daily and using the SG levels to dose insulin. His latest HbA$_{1c}$ is 7%. On review of the AGP report (Figure 4.14, left panel), he has an average glucose of 174 mg/dL, time in target range 55.6%, time in hyperglycemia (>180 mg/dL and >250 mg/dL

New Approach to Adjusting Insulin Doses Using Trend Arrows in Adults: Pre-meal and Corrections ≥4 Hours Post-meal

Trend Arrows		Correction Factor* (CF)	Insulin Dose Adjustment (U)
Receiver	App		
↑↑	◯	<25	+4.5
		25–<50	+3.5
		50–<75	+2.5
		≥75	+1.5
↑	◯	<25	+3.5
		25–<50	+2.5
		50–<75	+1.5
		≥75	+1.0
↗	◯	<25	+2.5
		25–<50	+1.5
		50–<75	+1.0
		≥75	+0.5
➡	◯	<25	No adjustment
		25–<50	No adjustment
		50–<75	No adjustment
		≥75	No adjustment
↘	◯	<25	-2.5
		25–<50	-1.5
		50–<75	-1.0
		≥75	-0.5
↓	◯	<25	-3.5
		25–<50	-2.5
		50–<75	-1.5
		≥75	-1.0
↓↓	◯	<25	-4.5
		25–<50	-3.5
		50–<75	-2.5
		≥75	-1.5

Insulin adjustments using trend arrows do not replace standard calculations using ICR and CF. Adjustments are increases or decreases of rapid-acting insulin in addition to calculations using ICR and CF. Adjustments using trend arrows are an additional step to standard care.

Considerations:
For the 4 hours following a meal, avoid adjusting insulin dose using trend arrows. Refer to REPLACE-BG recommendations, summarized in Figure 4, for an approach to minimize hypo- and hyperglycemia during this timeframe.

For frail or older adults, start conservatively to reduce hypoglycemia risk:
  ▸ Upward arrows: reduce dose increase by at least 50% (e.g., +1.0 U may become +0.5 U or no insulin increase)
  ▸ Downward arrows: increase dose reduction by least 50% (e.g., -1.0 U may become -1.5 or -2.0 U)

For rapidly rising sensor glucose (2 UP arrows; ↑↑) at pre-meal, consider administering insulin 15–30 minutes before eating.

For rapidly falling sensor glucose (2 DOWN arrows; ↓↓):
  ▸ Pre-meal: consider administering insulin closer to the meal
  ▸ Near or lower than 150 mg/dL: consider holding pre-meal insulin dose until glucose trends have stabilized

*Correction factor (CF) is in mg/dL and indicates glucose lowering per unit of rapid-acting insulin.

Figure 4.13. Adjusting insulin doses using rt-CGM trend arrows.
In addition to adjusting premeal bolus timing and ICR (Figures 4.12 and 4.14), patients can be instructed to adjust insulin doses based on CGM trend arrows. By following the table and adding or subtracting to the total insulin dose (carbohydrates bolus plus correction bolus if needed), the suggested insulin doses in units are based on the patient's CF (or insulin sensitivity) units as indicated by the direction of the trend arrows. *Source*: Reproduced with permission from Aleppo et al.[8]

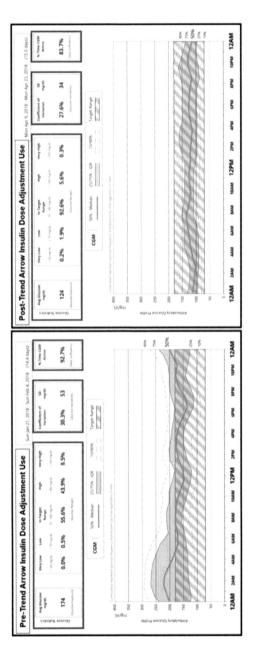

Figure 4.14. Use of Insulin dose adjustment based on CGM trend arrows. A 42-year-old man with a history of T1D managed with MDI (glargine SoloStar insulin pen 20 units at bedtime, mealtime lispro KwikPen ICR 1:15 and CF 50 for every 50 mg/dL > 150mg/dL) and Dexcom G5 presents for follow-up. *A:* AGP summary before incorporating Endocrine Society method using CGM trend arrows. The AGP shows time in target range of 55.6% of the time (goal >70%), and hyperglycemic 43.9% of the time. He was instructed to increase his glargine insulin and dinner ICR ratio was made more aggressive. He was also told to start following Endocrine Society guide for incorporating CGM trend arrows (Figure 4.13). HbA$_{1c}$ 7%. *B:* AGP summary after incorporating Endocrine Society method using CGM trend arrows to adjust premeal and >4 h postmeal insulin dosing. Return visit shows improved time in target range to 92.6% with a low coefficient of variation 27.6% (goal <36%) suggesting excellent glycemic control. HbA$_{1c}$ 6.3%.

combined) of 52.4%, and a CV of 30.3% (goal <36%). The graph shows overall global hyperglycemia even in the setting of HbA_{1c} of 7%.

After review of the CGM profiles, modifications to his regimen were made, increasing the glargine dose to a fasting glucose of 80–120 mg/dL and changing ICR to 1:10. Additionally, he was instructed to use the Endocrine Society approach to CGM trend arrows depicted on Figure 4.13.[8] By using this method, patients calculate their usual insulin dose by counting carbohydrates and adjusting glucose levels by their CF. In addition, they take into consideration the need for further insulin dose adjustment based on the direction of the trend arrows and using the corresponding dose adjustment (whether increase or decrease) based on their CF.

The patient returns to the clinic 3 months later. He shares that has been using the trend arrow method and has noted subjective improved glucose levels. Review of his latest CGM data (Figure 4.14, right panel) shows an improved SG average of 124 mg/dL (compared to 174 mg/dL), improved time in target range to 92%, minimal time spend in hypoglycemia <70 mg/dL of 0.5%, reduced time spent in hyperglycemia from 52.4% to 5.9%, and excellent CV of 27.6%. He also reports that using the trend arrows approach has empowered him to pay more attention to the types of meals eaten, modifying his insulin dose to reduce the frequency of a rapid SG increase or decrease (one or two arrows up-trending or down-trending). His most recent HbA_{1c} is 6.3%. This case emphasizes how incorporating CGM dynamic trend arrows for insulin dose fine-tuning can empower patients to implement successful strategies for their glucose management.

Usefulness of CGM Reports to Understand Challenges with MiniMed 670G Hybrid Closed-Loop System

Case Study 1. A 24-year-old woman with a 12-year history of T1D has initiated therapy with the MiniMed 670G hybrid closed-loop insulin pump system. Her HbA_{1c} before starting the 670G was 13.0% and has improved to 9.2% in 4 months. She is frustrated because she is finding it challenging to remain in auto mode, and the system exits auto mode at least 50% of the time during any given day. The system was uploaded to the Medtronic CareLink software and reviewed systematically (Figure 4.15).

Medtronic Smart Technology Best Practices suggest that users spend >80% of time in auto mode and wear their sensor at least 85% of the time. They also suggest spending at least 70% of the time in target range (70–180 mg/dL), with <4% of the time spent in hypoglycemia.[28] As seen in Figure 4.15, she spends 74% of the time in auto mode (A-blue pattern), which is gradually improving from 50% in the previous time frame (B-pink pattern), but both below the goal of 80%. Her time in range in the most recent weeks is only at 38%, with total time in hyperglycemia of 61%.

The Assessment and Progress Report from CareLink helps assess hypo- and hyperglycemic patterns (blue numbered circles) and also lists reasons for exiting auto mode. The Weekly Review report allows for a more in-depth analysis of the potential causes of auto-mode exits.

For this patient (Figure 4.16), it was noted that the majority of auto-mode exits were the result of high SG levels for >1 h due to postprandial hyperglycemia. She was advised to reduce simple carbohydrates, to add protein to her meals

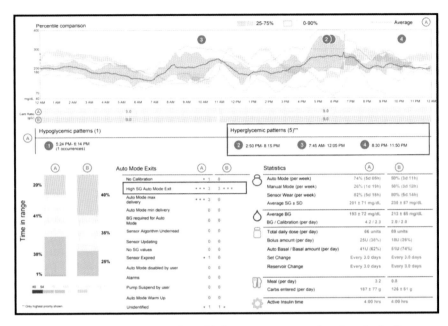

Figure 4.15. Usefulness of CareLink reports to understand challenges with using MiniMed 670G hybrid closed-loop system. A 24-year-old woman with T1D recently started 670G Medtronic insulin pump hybrid closed-loop system. Her HbA$_{1c}$ before initiation was 13% with an improvement to HbA$_{1c}$ 9.2% since transition. She reports concerns because of difficulty remaining in auto mode. Important elements to review include time in auto mode per week (goal >80%), sensor wear time per week (goal >85%), time in range (70–180 mg/dL; goal >70%), hypoglycemia (goal <3%), and patterns of hypo- and hyperglycemia that lead to exiting auto mode.

(eating carbohydrates last), and to use an ICR of 1:7 instead of 1:9 to reduce postprandial hyperglycemia. MiniMed 670G system users have found that taking insulin at least 15 min before eating and optimizing ICR are important components to increase time spent in auto mode.

Case Study 2. A 55-year-old man with 40 years history of T1D is seen in the endocrinology practice 1 month after initiating therapy with the MiniMed 670G hybrid closed-loop system. His most recent HbA$_{1c}$ is 8.3%. A detailed review of his CareLink data was performed at the return office visit.

He spends 97% of the time in auto mode and wears the sensor >90% of the time. Time in target range is below the Medtronic benchmark (70%) at 62% and he spends 36% of the time in hyperglycemia with 2% of time spent in hypoglycemia. Detailed analysis of the Weekly Review report shows postprandial hyperglycemia from premeal bolus, followed by multiple mini boluses over 1–2 h and

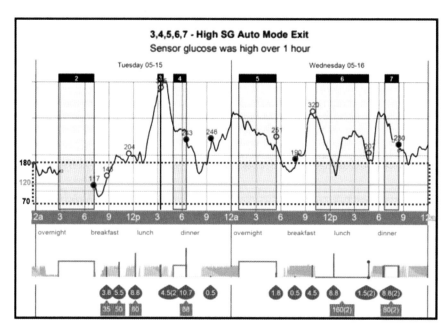

Figure 4.16. CareLink Weekly Review Report. The weekly report shows sensor glucose values (upper portion) with calibration glucose points, with shadowed areas indicating the patient's reason for exiting auto mode. For this patient, the majority of reasons for exiting auto mode were high SG glucose exits, resulting from SG levels in hyperglycemia for >1 h/episode. The lower portion shows the manual-mode basal rate settings as well as auto-mode microbolus (automated basal) delivery with meal boluses (orange and purple) and correction boluses (purple only). On the basis of this report, ICRs were modified from 1:9 to 1:7 and the patient was retrained to take insulin at least 15 min before meals.

subsequent rapid SG descent in hypoglycemia (70 mg/dL) despite an interruption of automated basal delivery (Figure 4.17). This phenomenon is quite common in 670G users, caused by the implementation of what has been called "phantom meal" boluses or "fake carbohydrate" boluses. Users often enter a carbohydrate amount but do not consume any carbohydrates to overcome persistent hyperglycemia.[28] Unfortunately, this behavior often causes wider glycemic fluctuations and increased rate of hypoglycemia. This patient was advised to optimize a premeal bolus, and his ICRs were changed to better match his insulin requirements.

CONCLUSION

CGM technology has advanced substantially in the past few years. The clinical benefits of CGM therapy are now established for patients with diabetes using

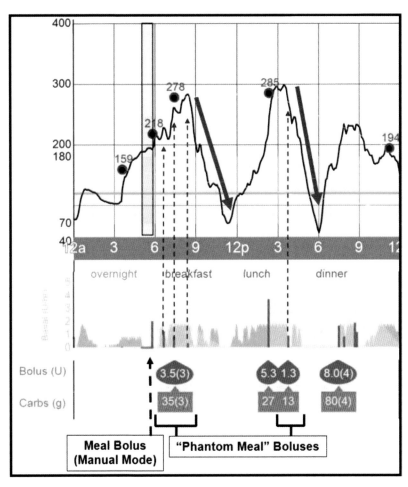

Figure 4.17. Usefulness of weekly review report in identifying "phantom meal" boluses and understanding causes of hyper/hypoglycemia. A 55-year-old man with a 40-year history of T1D is seen in the endocrinology practice 1 month after initiating therapy with MiniMed 670G system. His most recent HbA$_{1c}$ is 8.3%. Detailed analysis of the weekly review report shows postprandial hyperglycemia from insufficient premeal bolus (dotted black arrow), followed by multiple "mini" boluses (dotted blue arrows) over 1–2 h and subsequent rapid SG descent into hypoglycemia (<70 mg/dL) despite interruption of an automated basal delivery. Entering "fake carbohydrate" boluses often is employed by 670G users to override the bolus calculator. This patient's ICR was adjusted to provide more insulin for meals and he was retrained on the timing of insulin boluses and avoidance of using "phantom meal" boluses.

MDIs, sensor-augmented insulin pumps with or without low predicted-glucose suspend thresholds, and hybrid closed-loop systems already available or in development. Future automation of insulin delivery is becoming closer and closer thanks to the improved accuracy of CGM systems. Most important, combining a CGM data review with clinical evaluation during office visits is of paramount importance to enhance ongoing care for people with diabetes using CGM and to make personalized changes to medication regimens. Finally, training patients to understand their CGM reports and encouraging frequent review of these reports empowers patients to optimize their glucose levels in between visits and to reach their glycemic goals.

REFERENCES

1. Fonseca VA, Grunberger G, Anhalt H, et al. Continuous glucose monitoring: a consensus conference of the American Association of Clinical Endocrinologists and American College of Endocrinology. *Endocr Pract* 2016; 22(8):1008–1021

2. American Diabetes Association. Standards of medical care in diabetes, 2018. *Diabetes Care* 2018;41(Suppl.1):S126–S133

3. Peters AL, Ahmann AJ, Battelino T, et al. Diabetes technology-continuous subcutaneous insulin infusion therapy and continuous glucose monitoring in adults: an Endocrine Society clinical practice guideline. *J Clin Endocrinol Metab* 2016;101(11):3922–3937

4. FDA approves first continuous glucose monitoring system with a fully implantable glucose sensor and compatible mobile app for adults with diabetes [news release], 21 June 2018. U.S. Food and Drug Administration. Available from www.fda.gov/NewsEvents/Newsroom/PressAnnouncements/ucm611454.htm. Accessed 8 July 2018

5. Guardian Connect System—P160007. U.S. Food and Drug Administration. Available from www.fda.gov/MedicalDevices/ProductsandMedicalProcedures/DeviceApprovalsandClearances/Recently-ApprovedDevices/ucm604253.htm. Accessed 8 July 2018

6. Tandem Diabetes Care announces FDA approval of t:slim X2 insulin pump with basal-IQ technology, 21 June 2018. BusinessWire. Available from www.businesswire.com/news/home/20180621006260/en/Tandem-Diabetes-Care-Announces-FDA-Approval-tslim. Accessed 8 July 2018

7. Chamberlain JJ. Continuous glucose monitoring systems: categories and features. In *Role of Continuous Glucose Monitoring in Diabetes Treatment*. Arlington, VA: American Diabetes Association, 2018, p. 8–10

8. Aleppo G, Laffel LM, Ahmann AJ, et al. A practical approach to using trend arrows on the Dexcom G5 CGM System for the management of adults with diabetes. *J Endocr Soc* 2017;1(12):1445–1460

9. Aleppo G. Approaches for successful outcomes with continuous glucose monitoring. In *Role of Continuous Glucose Monitoring in Diabetes Treatment*. Arlington, VA: American Diabetes Association, 2018, p. 13–18

10. Kudva YC, Ahmann AJ, Bergenstal RM, et al. Approach to using trend arrows in the FreeStyle Libre flash glucose monitoring systems in adults. *J Endocr Soc* 2018;2(12):1320–1337

11. Peters A. The evidence base for continuous glucose monitoring. In *Role of Continuous Glucose Monitoring in Diabetes Treatment*. Arlington, VA: American Diabetes Association, 2018, p. 3–7

12. Foster NC, Beck RW, Miller KM, et al. State of type 1 diabetes management and outcomes from the T1D Exchange in 2016–2018. *Diabetes Technol Ther* 2019;21(2):66–72

13. McGill JB, Ahmann A. Continuous glucose monitoring with multiple daily insulin treatment: outcome studies. *Diabetes Technol Ther* 2017;19(S3):S3–S12

14. Edelman SV, Argento NB, Pettus J, et al. Clinical implications of real-time and intermittently scanned continuous glucose monitoring. *Diabetes Care* 2018;41(11):2265–2274

15. Bergenstal RM, Ahmann AJ, Bailey T, et al. Recommendations for standardizing glucose reporting and analysis to optimize clinical decision making in diabetes: the Ambulatory Glucose Profile (AGP). *Diabetes Technol Ther* 2013;15(3):198–211

16. Riddlesworth TD, Beck RW, Gal RL, et al. Optimal sampling duration for continuous glucose monitoring to determine long-term glycemic control. *Diabetes Technol Ther* 2018;20(4):314–316

17. Monnier L, Colette C, Wojtusciszyn A, et al. Defining the threshold between low and high glucose variability in diabetes. *Diabetes Care* 2017;40(7):832–883

18. Klonoff DC, Ahn D, Drincic A. Continuous glucose monitoring: a review of the technology and clinical use. *Diabetes Res Clin Pract* 2017;133:178–192

19. Greenwood DA, Gee PM, Fatkin KJ, Peeples M. A systematic review of reviews evaluating technology-enabled diabetes self-management education and support. *J Diabetes Sci Technol* 2017;11(5):1015–1027

20. Tetzschner R, Nørgaard K, Ranjan A. Effects of alcohol on plasma glucose and prevention of alcohol-induced hypoglycemia in type 1 diabetes: a systematic review with GRADE. *Diabetes Metab Res Rev* 2018;34(3):e2965–e2968

21. Smart CE, Evans M, O'Connell SM, et al. Both dietary protein and fat increase postprandial glucose excursions in children with type 1 diabetes, and the effect is additive. *Diabetes Care* 2013;36(12):3897–3902

22. Bell KJ, Toschi E, Steil GM, Wolpert HA. Optimized mealtime insulin dosing for fat and protein in type 1 diabetes: application of a model-based approach to derive insulin doses for open-loop diabetes management. *Diabetes Care* 2016;39(9):1631–1634

23. Riddell MC, Gallen IW, Smart CE, et al. Exercise management in type 1 diabetes: a consensus statement. *Lancet Diabetes Endocrinol* 2017;5(5):377–390

24. ExCarbs. Available from http://excarbs.com. Accessed 8 July 2018

25. Dunn TC, Xu Y, Hayter G, Ajjan RA. Real-world flash glucose monitoring patterns and associations between self-monitoring frequency and glycaemic measures: a European analysis of over 60 million glucose tests. *Diabetes Res Clin Pract* 2018;137:37–46

26. Haak T, Hanaire H, Ajjan R, et al. Flash glucose-sensing technology as a replacement for blood glucose monitoring for the management of insulin-treated type 2 diabetes: a multicenter, open-label randomized controlled trial. *Diabetes Ther* 2017;8(1):55–73

27. Bolinder J, Antuna R, Geelhoed-Duijvestijn P, et al. Novel glucose-sensing technology and hypoglycaemia in type 1 diabetes: a multicentre, non-masked, randomised controlled trial. *Lancet* 2016;388(10057):2254–2263

28. Aleppo G, Webb K. Integrated insulin pump and continuous glucose monitoring technology in diabetes care today: a perspective of real-life experience with the MiniMed 670G hybrid closed-loop system. *Endocr Pract* 2018;24(7):684–692

Chapter 5

Apps for Diabetes Management and Communication between Patients and Providers

David Ahn, MD[1]

Apple's introduction of the iPhone App Store in 2008 created an opportunity for software developers to create smartphone applications (apps) promising to assist in the management of diabetes. Despite numbering in the tens of thousands, only a small percentage of diabetes apps stand out as valuable clinical tools that might benefit a diabetes practitioner or person living with diabetes. Even then, evidence documenting clinical efficacy of diabetes apps is admittedly limited. A 2016 meta-analysis of 14 diabetes app studies showed a mean reduction in HbA_{1c} of 0.49%, with most studies being not blinded and limited in sample size.[1]

As trusted members of the care team and references for reliable and accurate information, physicians and providers owe it to their patients to support the clinically beneficial features and advantages of using diabetes apps, just as much as we need to caution them regarding their shortcomings and potential pitfalls.

Of note, the ever-changing nature of mobile apps presents challenges when recommending and highlighting specific apps within the static pages of a textbook. Without any advanced notice, an app can be completely removed from an App Store, introduce a crippling or deleterious bug via software update, or change pricing models on a whim. Furthermore, many of the apps discussed in this chapter are created by independent or smaller software developers rather than by pharmaceutical or medical device companies and therefore have more ephemeral commitments to the longevity of their products.

THE CASE FOR MOBILE APPS

Given these challenges presented by apps and software developers, why should clinicians and patients concern themselves with smartphone apps when managing diabetes?

The first advantage of using apps lies in the fact that most every patient (and clinician) has a smartphone nearby at all times. Smartphones are seemingly ever-present in contrast to glucose meters, which tend to be frequently left behind during outings to restaurants or the doctor's office. In fact, the cofounder of one glucose meter manufacturer (Sonny Vu) dubbed this phenomenon the "turn-around test": if you realized you left your device at home, would you turn around, go home, and get it? Smartphones pass the "turnaround test" with flying colors. Glucose meters do not even pass the "get it from the car" test.

---

[1]Program Director, Mary and Dick Allen Diabetes Center, Hoag Memorial Hospital Presbyterian, Newport Beach, CA.

Contributing to the ubiquity of smartphones is their appeal and usage across all ages and demographics. Although many people assume that older patients do not utilize smartphones and apps, a 2017 Pew Study found that 42% of adults age 65 years and older own a smartphone, 67% of senior citizens have or use the Internet, and 34% have or use social media. They concluded that smartphone usage in the elderly has quadrupled over the past 5 years. Those statistics are even higher when focusing in on the 65- to 75-year-old demographic.[2]

Not only are smartphones more prevalent than other analog diabetes tools, but they also are exponentially more powerful and have advanced capabilities. Diabetes logbook apps can generate beautiful charts, precise and live-updating statistics, and color-coded tables that previously were accessible only to the most computer-savvy users. Nutrition apps can instantly search databases consisting of millions of food entries, and social network apps can connect users to hundreds of thousands of others across the globe. Smartphones are literally supercomputers in our pockets. (For reference, a 2014 Apple iPhone 5 has 2.7 times the processing power of the 1985 Cray-2 supercomputer.[3])

Smartphones also offer benefits when it comes to transferring diabetes data, especially when compared with paper logbooks, which have been shown to be unreliable.[4] Electronic data exchange eliminates the biochemical hazards of handling paper logbooks stained by blood drops and preserves the integrity of the data by removing possible sources of error, such as illegible handwriting and fictitious or incomplete data entries. Last, while in-office glucose meter downloads also transfer data electronically, they require special software and proprietary cables that can dramatically slow down clinic workflows. Most smartphone apps can easily generate and share reports via e-mail and even by fax. Alternatively, providers can access their patient's data on their workstations via cloud-based web portals or, when all else fails, directly by viewing the smartphone screen.

Apps for Counting Carbohydrates and Creating Food Diaries

One of the most universally useful app categories for people with diabetes was not built specifically for diabetes but rather for healthy eating in general. Apps like MyFitnessPal, CalorieKing, and FatSecret offer exhaustive libraries of nutrition information, including carbohydrates, calories, and serving size. By serving both as references and logging tools, these apps play a vital role in managing weight and blood glucose.

Thanks to the fact that smartphones are usually kept within arm's reach, nutrition reference apps allow users to quickly look up carbohydrate and other information in real time while browsing a menu or walking down the supermarket aisle. The apps can display nutrition information from restaurants and cooking ingredients and can even provide rough estimates for home-cooked meals (e.g., a generic listing for "homemade tuna casserole" can be found on MyFitnessPal and FatSecret). Users can even search for entries using keywords or by scanning barcodes when available. These apps also remember and prioritize previously discovered food items, speeding up searches and logging with consistent usage over time.

Carbohydrate information can help users make healthy choices when selecting options at eating establishments and can increase the accuracy of counting carbohydrates for diet management or insulin dose calculations. In addition to serving purely as a reference, these apps can create a food diary or record of what users have eaten, which can better inform future analyses of glucose patterns with their care team.

Among the previously mentioned apps, each employs a different philosophy for establishing extensive libraries of nutrition information. MyFitnessPal's database first originated in 2005 and has been steadily expanding with a combination of verified and unverified (user-submitted) entries. In fact, the MyFitnessPal app has grown to become the most widely used health app of all time, with more than 150 million users as of February 2018.[5] Their thriving user community has built the most comprehensive food database available, including ethnic foods and highly specific menu permutations (e.g., Starbucks tall soy skinny vanilla latte). The accuracy of the data, however, is not 100% reliable and can be redundant with duplicate entries, and sometimes with differing nutrition information because of recipe changes over time or submission errors. FatSecret also combines verified and user-submitted information, with similar strengths and weaknesses.

In contrast to these apps, CalorieKing prioritizes accuracy over robustness by verifying every listing and committing to removing duplicate or outdated entries. Although CalorieKing's nutrition information is more reliable when available, their food database is noticeably smaller, with fewer results when searching for certain ethnic foods and smaller, regional restaurant chains.

The strengths and weaknesses of each app's approach to building their food databases potentially can be remedied by using both apps in tandem, although this can be tedious and creates multiple incomplete logbooks.

Using apps for counting carbohydrates should be done in conjunction with, not as a replacement for, proper dietary counseling. Because the core functionality of these apps is to display nutrition labels, users must know how to interpret nutrition labels and how to properly visually estimate portion sizes. Therefore, an ideal diabetes nutrition counseling session should train a user how to best incorporate these apps into the routine of choosing what to eat and recording a food diary.

Apps Centered around Self-Monitoring of Blood Glucose

By far, the most common type of diabetes app centers on self-monitoring of blood glucose (SMBG). Such diabetes life-logging apps allow patients to keep an ongoing record of their glucose measurements and other health parameters, such as medication administration, food diaries, workouts, and even mood. Regarding life-logging apps, two options stand out in terms of their reliability, features, and wide compatibility with both iPhone and Android smartphones and with various glucose meter manufacturers.

mySugr, founded in 2012, has grown to be one of the largest and most trustworthy diabetes life-logging apps and has been registered as a Class I medical device in Europe and the U.S. The mySugr app is available for both Apple and Android smartphones and allows users to record many types of diabetes data, including finger-stick glucose, CGM, nutrition, and activity data. The app's home screen displays a constantly updated average blood glucose, standard deviation, and a historical graph of blood glucose over time (see Figure 5.1A). Users also can see their estimated HbA$_{1c}$, which can help them translate their day-to-day glucose values into a long-term metric that they are familiar with.

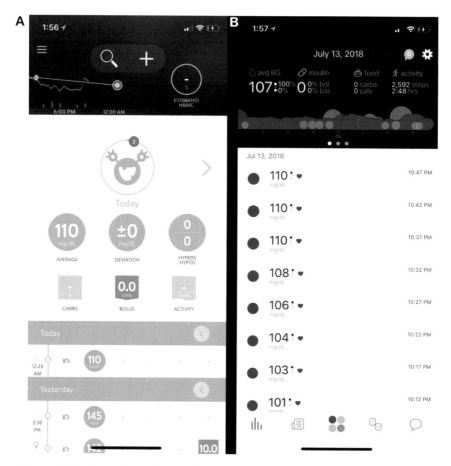

Figure 5.1. A: mySugr. **B:** One Drop.

mySugr is free to download and available on the iOS App Store and Google Play store for Android. Users can enable additional features, such as automated reminders and higher quality reports, for $2.99/month or $27.99/year.

Another popular free life-logging diabetes app for Android and iOS, One Drop, has rapidly grown in popularity since its launch in 2015. Like mySugr, One Drop allows for robust life-logging of many of the same parameters, such as glucose, medications, food, and activity. One Drop (Figure 5.1B) similarly displays real-time statistics on the home screen, including the estimated HbA$_{1c}$. A distinction with One Drop is that the app includes a food library for quickly looking up and logging carbohydrate information, but the database they use is not as robust as MyFitnessPal.

Until recently, widespread adoption of and long-term adherence to diabetes life-logging apps, such as mySugr and One Drop, were severely limited by the need for manual data entry. Because users previously needed to type in every glucose reading as well as time and date by hand, these apps historically were used only by the most engaged patients or during periods of special inspiration.

Wireless Glucose Meters Eliminate the Hassle of Manual Data Entry

For diabetes apps to thrive, there needed to be a way to automate the transfer of blood glucose measurements into the app without the need for manual entry. Advanced glucose meters with connectivity options ("connected glucose meters") provide an elegant solution to this dilemma by synchronizing data from glucose meters to smartphones or to an Internet-hosted platform ("the cloud"). Connected glucose meters come in a variety of forms: some plug in directly to the smartphone (e.g., Dario, iBG Star), others connect wirelessly via Bluetooth (e.g., iHealth, Accu-Chek Guide, Contour Next One), and some even connect directly to cellular networks without the need for a smartphone (e.g., Livongo, Telcare).

The number of connected glucose meters in use rose sharply when the major glucose meter manufacturers released their own Bluetooth-enabled connected meters, such as the OneTouch Verio Sync (2014) and Accu-Chek Aviva Connect (2015). The current crop of mainstream Bluetooth meters, such as the Accu-Chek Guide, Verio Flex, and the Contour Next One, followed soon after the first ones. With major manufacturer support and the corresponding widespread insurance coverage for testing supplies, many patients are now receiving wireless-enabled glucose meters at the time of diagnosis or when being prescribed a new meter.

Despite many patients now owning Bluetooth-enabled meters, many are not aware or do not know how to take advantage of this connectivity. The easiest way to teach a patient to learn how to pair their meter with their smartphone is to instruct them to download the official app made by the manufacturer of their meter (e.g., "OneTouch Reveal" for OneTouch meters, "Accu-Chek Connect" for Accu-Chek meters, "Contour Diabetes" for Contour meters). These manufacturer apps will walk them through the pairing process with specific instructions tailored to their meter. After the setup process is complete, individuals can continue using these apps to keep a glucose logbook or they can take advantage of data-sharing to take advantage of easy-to-use and visually appealing apps, such as mySugr or One Drop.

Apple Health, Google Fit, and S Health Share Health Data Across Apps

Coming alongside the development of connected glucose meters, Apple, Google, and Samsung each developed health-focused apps in Apple Health, Google Fit, and S Health, respectively. These apps serve as health data hubs, allowing users to seamlessly share health information like weight, glucose values, insulin doses, and step counts from one app to another. Without these sharing hubs, glucose meter vendors would have to customize their meter or app to be compatible with every individual single third-party app. Instead, by adding Apple Health connectivity to their meter, these vendors can automatically share data with all other Apple Health–enabled apps that currently exist, as well as those that will be developed in the future, without the need for additional updates.

Simplified data-sharing through these special hubs radically enhances the utility of third-party life-logging apps like mySugr and One Drop. Without the user having to manually enter in any information, mySugr and One Drop can automatically import a record from a patient's glucose meter measurements (via connected meter), activity record (via Fitbit or Apple Watch), and even insulin dosing (via connected insulin pens) through Apple Health. Although patients might not own every single one of these products, any reduction in manual data entry can be meaningful.

In addition to connecting to glucose meters, Apple Health can read and share data from continuous glucose monitors (CGM) like the Dexcom G5 and G6. Data are shared to Apple Health on a 3-h delay, however, at the request of the U.S. Food and Drug Administration (FDA).[6]

First-Party Apps for CGM and Insulin Pumps

The Dexcom G5 (and later, the G6) Mobile System introduced a ground-breaking advancement in diabetes devices by being the first CGM that allowed users to view their CGM data directly on their smartphone or smartwatch without the need to carry a dedicated receiver (Figure 5.2*A*). The G5 and G6 Mobile apps duplicate most of the functionality of the receiver by allowing users to input calibrations; view alerts for high, low, rising, or dropping glucose values; and modify alert settings.

In addition, the Dexcom Share feature within the Dexcom app allows users to share data with up to five "followers," who can remotely receive alerts and view real-time CGM data. The primary user can configure each follower to have different levels of visibility into their data (e.g., a college student can allow their parents to receive alerts only for extreme lows or highs and prevent their parents from seeing real-time blood glucose trends). To set this up, the primary user has to enable sharing within their Dexcom G5 or G6 app and the followers must install the Dexcom Follow app.

For clinicians, the Dexcom Clarity app proves extremely useful because it can instantly generate robust reports that provide meaningful data, such as the ambulatory glucose profile (AGP), time in range, average blood glucose, standard deviation, coefficient of variation, and daily graphs. Within the Dexcom Clarity app, the patient can generate a sharing code that clinicians can use to pull up CGM reports from any Internet-connected computer. This cloud-based sharing code conveniently eliminates the need for any cables or special software to be installed on a clinic computer, which can be especially challenging in larger institutions where clinicians are not allowed to install software or hardware drivers. Furthermore, the sharing codes can also facilitate telehealth and remote counseling because they allow clinicians to easily view Dexcom data without the need for an in-person handoff of data.

In my practice, I ask patients to install the Dexcom Clarity app as early in their care as possible, preferably as part of the CGM training process during initial startup. This allows the patient to have an easy way to generate reports for their own viewing, which is the easiest way for them to look back at their historical data. (The Dexcom G5 or G6 app that they use for real-time viewing goes back only 24 h.) Also, people tend to forget their App Store or Dexcom account passwords over time, so it's best to take advantage of the moment when their passwords are fresh in mind during setup.

For patients using the FreeStyle Libre, Abbott also offers a free, web-based reporting platform called LibreView, although the data download process still requires a software cable and driver installation process. (Unlike the Dexcom, the FreeStyle Libre is not compatible with smartphones in the U.S.) An advantage to the LibreView platform for clinics is that it can also download data from a modest number of glucose meters, so it's not limited to one single device. Although LibreView technically offers a way for clinicians to view their patients' data remotely, this process requires the patient to manually download their data on their home computer via a cable, which rarely takes place.

In Europe, Abbott FreeStyle Libre has an app (LibreLink) that enables iPhones and certain Android smartphones to scan and display flash glucose monitoring data, replacing many of the functions of the FreeStyle Libre Reader. There is not a clear timeline for when the LibreLink app will be available in the U.S.

In the second quarter of 2018, Insulet and Medtronic both announced FDA approval of options that enable smartphone viewing and data-sharing from an Omnipod Dash insulin pump and Guardian Mobile CGM, respectively. To view Omnipod pump data on the smartphone, the receiver still needs to be nearby. The Medtronic Guardian Mobile CGM can transmit data for viewing directly on the smartphone and smartwatch with the Guardian Connect app. Medtronic also partnered with IBM Watson to create Sugar.IQ, a patient-facing app that promises to use machine learning to identify patterns in blood glucose data, especially data related to certain foods and daily routines.

Third-Party CGM Apps Provide Improved Functionality and Configurability

The Dexcom apps for smartphones and smartwatches have been extremely well received; however, independent developers also have built their own apps that offer a different user interface and user experience.

Sugarmate (www.sugarmate.io) is a free Dexcom companion app for iOS, Mac, web, and Android (via web app). During initial setup, the user allows Sugarmate to become one of their five Dexcom "followers." Once fully configured, Sugarmate (Figure 5.2B) offers unique advantages, such as additional statistics (time in range, estimated A1C) and the ability to scroll back their glucose trend graph infinitely in time (the official Dexcom app can go back only 24 h). It also can call their phone when their blood glucose is running low or automatically text an emergency contact with their location in the event of a severely low blood glucose level. Furthermore, Sugarmate features a Mac-compatible app that allows users to easily view CGM data from a computer's status bar.

Sugarmate's Apple Watch app also goes beyond the official Dexcom app's functionality by displaying the exact time that the last blood glucose reading was measured and can be configured to display the exact difference (in mg/dL) between the last two measurements instead of a simplified trend arrow. Furthermore, Sugarmate even has an Alexa skill that allows users to ask Alexa-enabled speakers like the Echo to announce your blood glucose level and trend.

A caveat to third-party CGM apps is that the added functionality and configurability come at a cost in terms of complexity, especially during initial setup. Therefore, I recommend Sugarmate to more tech-savvy users who are willing to go the extra mile on their own and recommend the official Dexcom app for novice smartphone users.

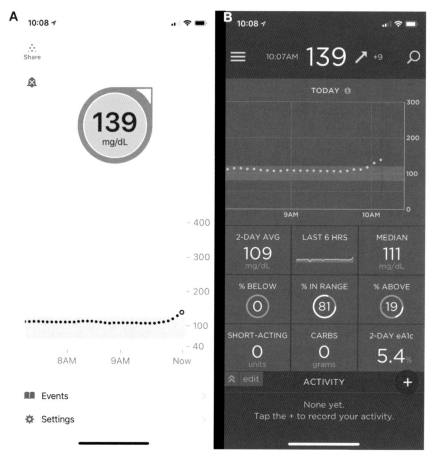

Figure 5.2. A: Dexcom G6 Mobile App. **B:** Sugarmate.

Third-Party Apps for Data Aggregation and Remote Health Management

Diabetes device manufacturers each create their own free software for downloading data from their own products, but this ultimately proves disadvantageous to patients and providers by creating data silos. For patients on an insulin pump, CGM, and a glucose meter, these data silos force providers to juggle multiple paper reports or view windows on their computer.

In response, companies like Glooko (which merged with Diasend) and Tidepool offer Health Insurance Portability and Accountability Act–compliant, web-based services that can download data from multiple diabetes devices and consolidate them into a single report. Glooko charges a subscription fee to clinics to utilize their software but offers the widest compatibility with devices. In addition, Glooko offers a smartphone app that enables remote health viewing and management, as long as patients also populate their Glooko smartphone app with data.

Tidepool is a not-for-profit, open-source company that offers a data downloading and aggregation service for free. Although they offer similar compatibility as Glooko for insulin pumps and CGM, Tidepool does not download as many glucose meters as Glooko. Tidepool also offers a free iOS app called Tidepool Mobile (or Blip Notes on Android phones) that allows users to upload glucose data and add relevant contextual notes to their data, either to review data remotely in real time or later at a clinic visit.

Unfortunately, at the time of publication, Medtronic's latest products were not compatible with any third-party data aggregation software, so the 630G, 670G, and Guardian Mobile CGM require the use of Medtronic CareLink software to download data and remain in the Medtronic data silo.

Apps and Remote Data-Sharing Enable Telehealth and Coaching

Smartphone-compatible CGMs, connected glucose meters, and diabetes logging apps allow diabetes data to be shared electronically, irrespective of location, eliminating a major hurdle to telemedicine. The bulk of a standard diabetes clinic visit is based on counseling and reviewing diabetes data, so a proper videoconferencing session paired with remote data-sharing can serve as a viable replacement for an in-person visit without the hassle of transportation or parking and possible health exposures of going into a clinic. Much like diabetes apps, telemedicine interventions require further clinical and economic validation, but the initial data are promising.[7,8]

For patients looking for a more casual interaction, the two previously discussed diabetes logbook apps, mySugr and One Drop, both offer monthly subscriptions that include remote certified diabetes educators (CDE) coaching and support. These text-based interactions with CDE coaches revolve around motivational support and behavioral counseling via in-app chat. These coaching services do not replace therapeutic interactions or medication changes under the guidance of a dedicated clinician, but they can help provide emotional encouragement and support at a reasonable cost.

Insulin Bolus Calculator Apps: Recommend with Caution

Thus far, all apps that have been mentioned have been largely used to monitor and log diabetes-related parameters. By avoiding therapeutic decisions or insulindosing suggestions, these app developers have mitigated the inherent risk of diabetes apps. Conversely, they also have missed out on the opportunity to provide solutions that have the potential to dramatically reduce the burden of diabetes management.

For patients who use multiple daily injections (MDIs) of insulin, a frequent challenge is to accurately calculate the appropriate dose of bolus insulin before meals or as a correction dose. Many of these individuals must perform a complex and time-consuming calculation with many inputs and variables, including insulin-to-carbohydrate ratios, insulin sensitivity factors (ISF), target glucose ranges, carbohydrates in their meal, and current blood glucose. These calculations prove especially challenging for people with deficits in literacy and numeracy, which are common among individuals with diabetes.[9]

Therefore, smartphone-based app calculators offer a convenient solution to eliminate mental math errors. We must proceed with caution, however, when recommending app bolus calculators to our patients. A 2015 study looked at 46 English-language bolus calculator apps in the iOS and Android App Stores. The authors found that only 14 (30%) provided documentation for the calculation formula, 42 (91%) lacked numeric input validation, and 27 (59%) allowed for a calculation when one or more inputs were missing (e.g., a correction bolus was calculated even though an ISF parameter was not provided).[10] By lacking these features, most of these bolus calculator apps did not protect against potentially harmful recommendations because of typos or configuration issues. Therefore, adding an extra zero to a blood glucose level (1,200 instead of 120 mg/dL) could lead to a potentially fatal dose of insulin when using some of the troublesome apps.

From this study, the only app that satisfied all of the investigators' criteria was an app named RapidCalc ($7.99 on the iOS App Store). Beyond the standard features one might expect in a bolus calculator app, RapidCalc offers insulin-on-board (IOB) tracking, six different schedules of insulin settings based on time of day, and input validation to reduce typos or erroneous entries. Disadvantages to using RapidCalc include an outdated user interface and laborious setup process. For example, the app requires you to type in parameters (e.g., ISF, target glucose level, and insulin-to-carbohydrate factors) for all six timing windows throughout the day, even if that individual will require only a single carbohydrate ratio and ISF at all times.

An alternative full-featured bolus calculator app named Diabetes:M is available for both Android and iOS platforms, using a freemium model (free to download, but $4.99/month for premium features including ad removal and reports). Although Diabetes:M has a much more modern interface than RapidCalc and includes some similar advanced features like IOB tracking, the app has minimal data entry validation—for example, I was able to configure it to suggest a bolus dose of 600 units.

The bottom line when it comes to recommending insulin bolus calculator apps is to proceed with caution and ensure that patients fully understand how to use these apps safely and effectively. Given the clunky user interfaces and complicated setup processes of even the best bolus calculator apps listed here, I strongly recommend that clinicians test and install these apps on their personal devices to familiarize themselves with each app's design language. Then, when recommending the app to their patients, the clinician or educator should walk the user closely through the installation and setup processes while the patient is still in the office. Although time-consuming and inconvenient, handholding patients through this process reduces the potential for incorrect parameters being used. Last, it is essential to remind patients that any dose calculation should be interpreted as a suggestion that requires clinical context, rather than as absolute authority.

Basal Insulin Titration Apps Offer FDA-Approved Approaches

A new, rapidly emerging app category for diabetes management is prescribed, automated insulin adjustment. Over the past 18 months, multiple companies have obtained FDA approval for basal insulin initiation and titration in type 2 diabetes, including Glooko's Mobile Insulin Dosing System, Amalgam's iSage Rx, and Voluntis' Insulia.

These apps guide individuals who are newly starting basal insulin or need assistance finding their appropriate dose. Instead of the traditional method, in which endocrinologists would send patients out with written instructions to increase their basal dose by a couple of units every few days until they reach a specific target blood glucose level, the clinician can "prescribe" an insulin titration app at the same time as the insulin, which can be configured with a clinician-selected algorithm for titration (e.g., increase/decrease by 2 units every morning to target a fasting glucose level between 80 and 120 mg/dL). Then, the patient will receive a personalized dose recommendation each day via the app according to the selected algorithm and the patient's blood glucose record.

Although a basal insulin titration app might feel unnecessary and simplistic in scope, I frequently find that my patients return to my office without having appropriately adjusted their dose and despite my lengthy efforts to provide them with detailed written instructions on how to adjust their dose. Furthermore, these companies are using basal insulin titration as a starting point for more advanced insulin titration, such as MDI, in the future.

Patient-facing, provider-prescribed insulin titration apps will play an increasing role in the management of diabetes. Widespread adoption by clinicians, however, will require seamless integration into the electronic medical record prescription-ordering workflows and additional algorithms that extend beyond basal insulin titration.

FUTURE DIRECTIONS FOR DIABETES APPS

People with diabetes are eager for apps that further reduce the burden of their chronic condition. In the same way that the device-connected glucose meters replaced the need for manual data entry of SMBG data, people with diabetes benefit greatly from tools that passively record other forms of diabetes data without user intervention. Connected insulin pens like Companion Medical's InPen utilizes an advanced app-based bolus calculator to help users determine their appropriate dose of mealtime insulin, and then automatically record the dose and time when it is administered, creating a digital record similar to an insulin pump.

Connected insulin pens are just now arriving to market, but the diabetes community still awaits a reliable solution that might automate nutrition and carbohydrate logging. App developers are actively working on app-based photo recognition software to help record nutrition information by simply snapping a photo of a meal, but reliably accurate and easy-to-use solutions are still a long way off.

When it comes to compelling decision support for patients, machine learning and artificial intelligence promise to improve diabetes management by offering glucose prediction algorithms and improved insulin dosing advice. In June 2018, One Drop announced an upcoming software update to their app that will provide a blood glucose "forecast" up to 12 h in the future and make behavioral change recommendations accordingly.[11] This feature eventually will grow beyond the initial population of individuals with type 2 diabetes who are not taking insulin. Furthermore, as previously discussed, companies like Glooko, AmalgamRx, and Voluntis hope to expand their insulin titration apps beyond basal insulin to include basal-bolus insulin dose recommendations.

An alternative strategy for increasing engagement and positive diabetes behaviors involves gamification (the use of game-like elements such as earning points or utilizing leaderboards) and incentivization (offering monetary or other rewards within the app). In spring 2018, Medtronic announced active development of an app called Inner Circle that will utilize gamification and incentivization to provide real-world rewards to individuals for maintaining their Guardian Mobile CGM data within a target range for as long as possible.[12] By offering tangible rewards, developers hope to reduce diabetes burnout and motivate patients to fully engage with their chronic condition in a positive way.

Ultimately, the Holy Grail for reducing the burden of diabetes is fully automated insulin delivery (AID), also known as the artificial pancreas or closed-loop systems. The majority of AID solutions in development plan to incorporate apps in some form or another, ranging from serving solely as a display to controlling settings or running the actual closed-loop algorithm.

CONCLUSION

As digital tools and telemedicine become increasingly prevalent and robust, smartphone apps will play a significant role in diabetes management and the interactions between patients and clinicians. We can serve our patients by staying informed and recommending specific diabetes apps that are best suited for their individualized needs. Just as a clinician might do for a patient requiring lifestyle counseling or starting insulin for the first time, I highly recommend walking patients through the app's initial setup process while they are still in the office. Installing and configuring the app during the visit is better than simply providing a list of resources. Although diabetes apps are definitely not suitable for every patient, they are underutilized by doctors and other members of the care team.

REFERENCES

1. Hou C, Carter B, Hewitt J, Francisa T, Mayor S. Do mobile phone applications improve glycemic control (HbA1c) in the self-management of diabetes? A systematic review, meta- analysis, and GRADE of 14 randomized trials. *Diabetes Care* 2016;39(11):2089–2095

2. Pew Research Center. Tech adoption climbs among older adults. Available from https://www.pewinternet.org/2017/05/17/tech-adoption-climbs-among-older-adults/. Accessed May 2017

3. Hard disk drive morph. Processing Power Compared. Available from https://pages.experts-exchange.com/processing-power-compared. Accessed 7 February 2019

4. Mazze RS, Shamoon H, Pasmantier R, Lucido D, Murphy J, Hartmann K, Kuykendall V, Lopatin W. Reliability of blood glucose monitoring by patients with diabetes mellitus. *Am J Med* 1984;77:211–217

5. Under Armour Notifies MyFitnessPal Users Of Data Security Issue. Available from http://www.uabiz.com/news-releases/news-release-details/under-armour-notifies-myfitnesspal-users-data-security-issue?ReleaseID=1062368

6. Frequently asked questions. Developer.dexcom. Available from https://developer. dexcom.com/content/frequently-asked-questions. Accessed 7 February 2019

7. Barjis J, Kolfschoten G, Maritz J. A sustainable and affordable support system for rural healthcare delivery. *Decis Support Syst* 2013;56:223–233

8. de la Torre-Díez I, López-Coronado M, Vaca C, et al. Cost-utility and cost-effectiveness studies of telemedicine, electronic, and mobile health systems in the literature: a systematic review. *Telemed J E Health* 2015;21:81–85

9. Cavanaugh K, Huizinga MM, Wallston KA, et al. Association of numeracy and diabetes control. *Ann Intern Med* 2008;148(10):737–746

10. Huckvale K, Adomaviciute S, Prieto JT, Leow MK, Car J. Smartphone apps for calculating insulin dose: a systematic assessment. *BMC Med* 2015;13:106

11. One drop announces blood glucose prediction and automated decision support, 23 June 2018. Cision PRNewswire. Available from www.prnewswire.com/news-releases/one-drop-announces-blood-glucose-prediction-and-automated-decision-support-300671187.html. Accessed 7 February 2019

12. Brown A, Levine B. What's new for Medtronics Diabetes? A look into CGM and pump pipeline, 8 June 2018. diaTribe Learn. Available from https://diatribe.org/whats-next-medtronic-diabetes-look-cgm-and-pump-pipeline. Accessed 7 February 2019

Chapter 6
Selecting Patients for Pumps and Continuous Glucose Monitoring: Who, Why, and Why Not?

Lauren Vincent, MD[1], and Steven V. Edelman, MD[2]

INTRODUCTION

When initiating insulin pump therapy, also known as continuous subcutaneous insulin infusion (CSII) and continuous glucose monitoring (CGM) devices, careful patient selection is of utmost importance. Devoting time and consideration to appropriate patient selection for these devices ultimately can conserve resources in the future, including provider time and effort. Patients who are less suitable for these devices are more likely to face frustration if inappropriately started on these therapies, which ultimately may lead to discontinuation. Thus, the decision to start an insulin pump or a CGM device should always involve a careful shared decision-making process between patient and provider.

Insulin Pump Therapy: Advantages and Disadvantages

When selecting patients to initiate insulin pump therapy, it is important to consider the benefits of CSII compared to a multiple daily injection (MDI) regimen. Of note, the Diabetes Control and Complications Trial study demonstrated the benefits of both MDI and CSII compared to the less intensive regimen of twice daily mixed insulin in terms of the primary prevention and secondary intervention of microvascular complications in type 1 diabetes (T1D), formerly referred to as insulin-dependent diabetes mellitus (IDDM).[1] Thus, in patients with T1D and insulin-requiring type 2 diabetes (T2D), both MDI and CSII are reasonable treatment options and patients can achieve treatment goals with either approach. Of note, CSII seems to be associated with slightly improved hemoglobin A_{1c} (A1C), and better diabetes-specific quality-of-life measures in adults with T1D.[2] Some studies also suggest an improvement in glucose variability and overall hypoglycemia events in patients with T1D on CSII compared to MDI.[3] Despite the higher upfront costs of CSII compared to MDI, studies have suggested that CSII is cost effective compared to MDI in patients with T1D when taking into account the improvements in A1C and hypoglycemia risk associated with CSII.[4] In patients with T2D, it also has been shown that CSII is associated with improved A1C, lower total daily insulin dosage, and increased treatment satisfaction compared to MDI.[5] In patients with poorly controlled T2D, CSII has been shown to be more cost effective when compared to MDI.[6] Thus, insulin pump therapy has

---

[1]Endocrinology Fellow, University of California, San Diego, CA.
[2]Professor of Medicine, University of California San Diego, CA; Veterans Affairs Medical Center; Founder and director, Taking Control of Your Diabetes.

many advantages over MDI and should be carefully considered as an option in patients both with T1D and insulin-requiring T2D.

The varied functionality of different insulin pumps is well suited to meet the specific needs of patients with diabetes. For example, insulin pumps allow much greater flexibility in basal rates. This is particularly useful in patients whose lifestyle involves varied activity levels. In such patients, different basal rates can be set to meet their different basal needs from day to day. Patients who exhibit the dawn phenomenon also benefit from the ability to increase their basal rates in the early hours of the morning. Insulin pumps are also more suited to patients who travel regularly between time zones, as they can simply adjust the time on their pump instead of having to retime their basal insulin injections. Certain insulin pumps that are integrated with CGM systems are equipped to suspend basal delivery in the setting of hypoglycemia and thus are particularly useful in patients with overnight hypoglycemia, which is especially important in those with hypoglycemia unawareness.

Insulin pumps are also beneficial in patients, particularly those with T1D, who have low total daily insulin requirements. Specifically, pumps allow for much lower and more precise bolus doses than can be achieved with MDI. Conversely, in patients on very high doses of insulin, including those with T2D, basal insulin delivery via continuous infusion may be superior to a large subcutaneous depot. This advantage must be weighed against the frequency with which the patient with high total daily insulin doses will need to change an infusion set, based on the size of the reservoir in a patient's pump. Use of concentrated rapid-acting insulin preparations in pumps has addressed this issue.

Pumps also allow patients more flexibility in terms of the timing of bolus delivery. Specifically, bolus doses can be given all at once or can be divided over a specified period of time, allowing for better coverage of more slowly absorbed foods. This option is also useful in patients who have the complication of gastroparesis. Most insulin pumps allow for easier calculation of bolus doses based on preset insulin-to-carbohydrate ratios and insulin sensitivity factors. Many pumps also take into account insulin on-board when calculating these boluses. Insulin pumps also facilitate quicker responses to changes in blood glucose levels without the need for additional injections. Although insulin pumps are equipped with many features capable of improving glycemic control and overall quality of life in patients with T1D and insulin-requiring T2D, many patients are not appropriate candidates and careful patient selection is critical for success.

Patient Selection for Insulin Pump Therapy

Specific criteria to evaluate patient appropriateness for insulin pump therapy as well as models to predict the success of insulin pump therapy are lacking, although studies have suggested screening protocols and mock trials as effective tools.[7] Characteristics of both ideal and inappropriate candidates for insulin pump therapy are presented in Table 6.1. In general, it is accepted that patients should be self-motivated, educated in how to use MDI, well-versed in self-monitoring of blood glucose (SMBG) or CGM, and also demonstrate a willingness to learn new insulin management strategies.[8] Patient education and shared decision-making responsibility are critical before initiating insulin pump therapy. Patient expectations should be carefully assessed, as some patients have misconceptions about insulin pump therapy. For example, some patients may think that an insulin pump is a way to simplify their diabetes management, when in actuality, insulin pump therapy often requires more complicated decision-making processes and troubleshooting. Furthermore, some patients incorrectly assume that all insulin pumps will serve as an artificial pancreas, with the ability to bolus insulin without the need to count carbohydrates. Currently, no insulin pumps offer this functionality. In addition, insulin pump therapy can be complicated by such factors as pump failure, infusion site issues, or infusion set blockages, necessitating that pump users demonstrate a basic capability to recognize and manage these issues. Some authors suggest implementing an online test when selecting patients for insulin pump therapy, not only to check a patient's knowledge base regarding insulin pump therapy but also to assess general motivation.[9]

Some patients do not like the concept of being continuously connected to a device. Specifically, tubing can get caught on clothing or other objects. This is especially troublesome during sexual activity. Patch pumps, such as the Omnipod, allow patients to avoid tubing, which some but not all patients prefer.[10] Patch pumps that are designed for insulin-requiring T2D are available, such as the V-Go, with several other pumps in development. These patch pumps typically are less complicated to use with limited unneeded functionality. A provider should also consider certain psychosocial and emotional characteristics when assessing a patient's readiness for insulin pump therapy. Some patients may be highly concerned about the appearance of an insulin pump or feel embarrassed about the pump being seen by others.[11] Other patients have fears about mechanical failure or question their ability to manage the technical aspects of an insulin pump and thus feel much more vulnerable with an insulin pump compared to MDI.[11] Thus, it is important to address a patient's concerns before initiating pump therapy. Finally, ongoing assessment of the appropriateness of insulin pump therapy is important, as patients who previously may not have seemed appropriate may become ideal candidates for insulin pump therapy in the future. Conversely, patients who seemed to be appropriate for insulin pump therapy in the past may no longer be benefiting from the therapy.

Table 6.1. Patient Selection for Insulin Pump Therapy

Appropriate candidate	Inappropriate candidate
• Self-motivated and willing to learn new insulin management strategies	• Resistant to learning new insulin management strategies
• Demonstrates appropriate expectations for insulin pump therapy	• Demonstrates unrealistic expectations for insulin pump therapy (e.g., considers insulin pump to be an artificial pancreas)
• Educated in how to appropriately use MDI	• Not properly using MDI
• Familiar with and correctly utilizing SMBG or CGM	• Inconsistently or incorrectly using SMBG or CGM
• Comfortable utilizing pump features	• Unable to utilize pump features
• Capable of troubleshooting pump issues	• Uncomfortable or incapable of troubleshooting pump issues
• Accepting of physical appearance of pump on body	• Unaccepting of physical appearance of pump on body

When initiating insulin pump therapy, it is important to consider a patient's practices regarding glucose monitoring. In the absence of frequent glucose monitoring, patients will not be able to maximize the benefits of their insulin pump.[8] Patients who infrequently perform SMBG are less likely to benefit from the clinical capabilities of insulin pump therapy.[8] As a result, insurance companies often require documentation of at least four blood glucose checks during the day to ensure better patient outcomes on insulin pumps. Infrequent SMBG actually can be more dangerous in patients on insulin pump compared to MDI. Specifically, if a patient is not checking blood glucose values while on an insulin pump, the patient may not realize that the pump has failed, potentially resulting in acute complications, such as diabetic ketoacidosis. Patients on an MDI regimen are less likely to suffer this consequence in the setting of infrequent SMBG because they are taking a basal insulin. Pump users do not have any circulating basal insulin, which means that any interruption in pump therapy will render the patient insulinopenic. Although not required, concurrent CGM therapy is extremely useful in terms of making treatment decisions for patients on insulin pump therapy and ensuring that patients are able to benefit fully from the functionality of their insulin pumps.

THE BENEFITS OF CGM

CGM devices have been shown to improve A1C without increasing the risk for severe hypoglycemia when compared to SMBG [2]. As such, it is generally accepted that most patients with T1D and insulin-requiring T2D on MDI or CSII should be offered a CGM device. CGM offers patients the significant benefit of seeing glucose trends rather than a single glucose value isolated in time, thus allowing more informed treatment decisions. Furthermore, CGM devices have alerts and alarms, which can be particularly useful in patients who have hypoglycemia unawareness or visual impairment. Alerts can be set at individualized high and low glucose values and also to notify the user when the glucose is rapidly rising or falling. CGM also may improve quality of life for certain patients. Specifically, it has been shown that patients on CGM had less fear of hypoglycemia and felt that they had increased control of their diabetes.[12] Despite the advantages of CGM, not all patients are ideal candidates for CGM therapy.

Patient Selection for CGM

Patients should be selected carefully before initiating CGM. Some characteristics of appropriate and inappropriate candidates for CGM are presented in Table 6.2. Assessing candidacy for CGM therapy is best achieved through a time-limited (e.g., 1- to 2-week) trial. Such a trial offers the patient a direct experience using the device and also will allow the provider to assess whether a patient is capable of deriving the maximum benefit from CGM by making appropriate self-adjustment decisions. Patients often are concerned about the inconvenience of wearing a sensor or having alarm fatigue, but after a 1-week trial they often realize that the benefits of CGM outweigh the inconveniences. Still, some patients do not utilize their CGM devices appropriately during a trial period. This presents the opportunity for additional education in the clinic setting and to reconsider whether the patient will fully benefit from CGM. Healthcare providers with CGM experience

Table 6.2. Patient Selection for CGM

Appropriate candidate	Inappropriate candidate
• Demonstrates ability to properly utilize CGM during a time-limited trial (not needed in most cases) • Capable of using CGM information, including trend arrows, to make treatment decisions • Able to appropriately react to CGM alarms and alerts • Willing to comply with the calibration requirements if needed by the CGM system being used • Comfortable wearing a CGM sensor	• Unable to properly utilize CGM during a time-limited trial • Not capable of using CGM information to make treatment decisions • Unable or unwilling to react to CGM alarms and alerts • Unwilling to calibrate the CGM device properly • Uncomfortable wearing CGM sensor

can often identify select patients who need and would utilize a CGM device successfully and therefore who can possibly bypass this trial period.

Some providers choose to use blinded-CGM devices in the office setting. Specifically, these CGM devices are blinded to the patient using them, but providers are able to download the data in the office setting. Because of their lack of alarms and the inability for a patient to interact with the device, blinded-CGM plays a limited role in managing patients with T1D. In select patients with T2D, blinded CGM might be useful for providers to establish glucose trends and make treatment decisions, especially in patients consistently lacking SMBG data. Recently, intermittently scanned or "flash" CGM devices have been developed (e.g., Abbot FreeStyle Libre). These devices provide glucose readings and trends only when the patient swipes a meter over the sensor. These devices are less useful in patients with T1D, specifically because they lack alert and alarm features. For patients with T2D, however, these devices offer a unique balance between the benefits of CGM without the potential for alarm fatigue. Finally, CGM devices are rapidly improving, so patients who may have decided against CGM in the past may be more inclined to try CGM now. Specifically, sensors are more accurate than prior generations and some CGM devices (e.g., Dexcom G6, Abbot FreeStyle Libre) do not require calibration. In addition, the Dexcom G6 does not suffer from acetaminophen interference. Finally, the Dexcom G5, G6, and Abbott FreeStyle Libre CGMs do not require confirmatory SMBG testing to make treatment decisions. As CGM technology continues to advance, it is likely that more patients will be suitable candidates for these devices.

CONCLUSION

Both insulin pumps and CGM offer many potential benefits to patients with T1D and patients with insulin-requiring T2D. As these technologies rapidly evolve, it is important for providers to carefully consider which patients might be appropriate for these devices. Patient selection for insulin pumps and CGM involves a multidisciplinary approach, including patient and family education sessions and possibly device trials. Proper patient selection is critical to ensure patient and provider satisfaction, proper resource allocation, and cost-effectiveness.

REFERENCES

1. Nathan DM, Genuth S, Lachin J, et al. The effect of intensive treatment of diabetes on the development and progression of long-term complications in insulin-dependent diabetes mellitus. *N Engl J Med* 1993;329(14):977–986

2. Yeh HC, Brown TT, Maruthur N, et al. Comparative effectiveness and safety of methods of insulin delivery and glucose monitoring for diabetes mellitus: a systematic review and meta-analysis. *Ann Intern Med* 2012;157(5):336–347

3. Maiorino MI, Bellastella G, Casciano O, et al. The effects of subcutaneous insulin infusion versus multiple insulin injections on glucose variability in young adults with type 1 diabetes: the 2-year follow-up of the observational METRO Study. *Diabetes Technol Ther* 2018;20(2):117–126

4. Roze S, Smith-Palmer J, Valentine W, et al. Cost-effectiveness of continuous subcutaneous insulin infusion versus multiple daily injections of insulin in Type 1 diabetes: a systematic review. *Diabetes Med* 2015;32(11):1415–1424

5. Vigersky RA, Huang S, Cordero TL, et al. Improved HBA1C, total daily insulin dose, and treatment satisfaction with insulin pump therapy compared to multiple daily insulin injections in patients with type 2 diabetes irrespective of baseline c-peptide levels. *Endocr Pract* 2018;24(5):446–452

6. Roze S, Duteil E, Smith-Palmer J, et al. Cost-effectiveness of continuous subcutaneous insulin infusion in people with type 2 diabetes in the Netherlands. *J Med Econ* 2016;19(8):742–749

7. Sanfield JA, Hegstad M, Hanna RS. Protocol for outpatient screening and initiation of continuous subcutaneous insulin infusion therapy: impact on cost and quality. *Diabetes Educ* 2002;28(4):599–607

8. Hirsch IB. Practical pearls in insulin pump therapy. *Diabetes Technol Ther* 2010;12(Suppl. 1):S23–S27

9. Stechova K, Vanis M, Tuhackova M, et al. Lessons learned from implementing a new testing/educational tool for patients using an insulin pump. *Diabetes Technol Ther* 2018, https://doi.org/10.1089/dia.2018.0095

10. Joshi M, Choudhary P. Multiple daily injections or insulin pump therapy: choosing the best option for your patient-an evidence-based approach. *Curr Diab Rep* 2015;15(10):81

11. Edelman, SV, Hirsch, IB, Pettus JH. *Practical Management of Type 1 Diabetes.* 2nd ed. West Islip, NY, Professional Communications, Inc., 2014, p. 168–169

12. Polonsky WH, Hessler D. What are the quality of life-related benefits and losses associated with real-time continuous glucose monitoring? A survey of current users. *Diabetes Technol Ther* 2013;15(4):295–301

Chapter 7

Starting Insulin Pump and Continuous Glucose Monitoring Therapy

Anne Peters, MD[1]

T echnology can be extremely helpful in the management of patients with diabetes. A patient's readiness to adopt technology can be highly variable, however, and it is vital that an individualized learning situation be created to optimize success. From a practical perspective, three basic patient types will begin using a new device:

1. Those who have never worn a pump or a sensor.
2. Those who are wearing one or the other (or who have successfully worn one in the past) and are learning a new device.
3. Those who wore a pump or sensor in the past, but stopped using it because of a negative experience.

In addition to historical experience with technology, learners come in all ages, all skill levels of numeracy and literacy, and a wide variety of learning styles. Some prefer group classes; others benefit from one-on-one training; some like learning on their own from educational videos and others like reading a manual. Ideally, all options are available to any given patient so that they can choose how to approach technology training.

Two elements are key to the success of initiating insulin pump and CGM therapy: *1)* education and *2)* expectation. Education is fairly straightforward and should be comprehensive, with specific instructions on troubleshooting. Expectation sets the stage for success—if a patient understands upfront exactly what a device will and will not do, it will make it much easier for the patient to adjust to the technology and feel that it is working appropriately.

CONTINUOUS GLUCOSE MONITORING

Continuous glucose monitoring (CGM) systems tend to come packaged with detailed instructions for initiation. Additionally, various websites and YouTube videos detail how to use them. Some of these videos are particularly good at showing how to place the CGM sensor in difficult-to-reach (and potentially off-label) locations. For some patient these teaching tools are adequate.

---

[1]Director, Clinical Diabetes Program, University of Southern California; Professor of Clinical Medicine, Keck School of Medicine, University of Southern California, Westside Clinic, Los Angeles, CA.

Many patients who are new to technology, however, are not comfortable getting started completely by themselves. Some need repeated sessions to learn how to operating the systems on their own. This is particularly true for older patients. For devices with a transmitter that needs to be placed on the sensor (and removed when done) education can be quite useful. Implanted sensors need to be inserted by someone trained in the technique, and the patient should be taught how to wear the transmitter.

In addition to the technical application of the CGM, setting alarms and alerts so that they are useful without over-alarming the patient initially is beneficial. This step is necessary for all CGM systems except for the FreeStyle Libre system. If too many alarms go off at first, it can frustrate the patient or their significant other. Therefore, when working with a patient who has never used of a CGM device, it is reasonable to set the following expectations and to set up the device as follows:

1. Tell the patient that the first time wearing a CGM will reveal many glucose patterns that they may never have been aware of before. The first patterns to look for are low glucose levels. It is important to warn the patient not to overreact to postprandial glucose levels and to avoid stacking (giving too many correction doses of insulin too often). Additionally, with the new use of a CGM, patients should be told to observe their glucose levels at first and not to make any major insulin dose adjustments without communicating with their diabetes care team.
2. Patients should turn on whichever alerts are the most meaningful with regards to detecting or predicting a low.
3. Patients should turn off or set very high the high alerts—these can be set once the typical glucose patterns have been documented and adjustments made.
4. Ensure that the patient knows who to contact (usually the device company) for failed sensors so they can get a replacement if one malfunctions.
5. At the first or second appointment (depending on the patient), set up some sort of data-sharing method so that the diabetes care team can remotely evaluate glucose levels, as needed.
6. In general, have the patient return to clinic within 2–4 weeks so an evaluation of the CGM data can be made, education given, and alerts adjusted or turned on. Additionally, at this follow-up visit, the concept of dose adjusting for trend arrows can be taught.[1]

Case Study 1

You see Sam for a clinic appointment. You would love to have him try a CGM, but he has not been interested in the past. He has had type 1 diabetes (T1D) for 16 years, since he was 18 years old. When he was in college, he was started on an insulin pump but did not like it. He felt uncomfortable having something attached to his body and often had infusion set issues. You point out the differences between a pump and a CGM, which you are recommending. In particular you point out that the CGM isn't infusing insulin and has no "tubing"; therefore, it isn't prone to infusion set issues. Additionally you tell him it is smaller and less obtrusive, results can be seen on his smartphone, and it can help him prevent low blood glucose reactions.

He is on multiple daily insulin injections (MDI) with a HbA$_{1c}$ of 7.6%. His variability data, based on self-monitoring of blood glucose (SMBG), are high, especially in the morning when his values range from 52 to 251 mg/dL. He notes episodes of mild hypoglycemia nearly daily. Based on what he has heard from others in the T1D community and your recommendation, he has become more interested in trying a CGM, particularly a Dexcom CGM G6, chosen because he is interested in having alerts at night to tell him whether his blood glucose levels are high or low. Therefore, you prescribe the CGM and provide charts notes, blood glucose logs, a Certificate of Medical Necessity, and everything else required for Sam to get the device. He says he would rather learn how to use it from an educator, given his prior experience with a pump, so you arrange for him to come back when the device arrives.

He returns to the office to be trained on the device by a certified diabetes educator (CDE) once he has received it. The CDE teaches him how to insert the sensor, perform calibrations if desired, and set up the device on his smartphone. Together they choose initial alerts, designed not to over-alert him but rather to start reducing his episodes of hypoglycemia. They agree to turn on the urgent "low soon" alert and the low-glucose alert set at 80 mg/dL. The high-glucose alert is set high initially (to 350 mg/dL) and the rise/fall alerts are turned to off. They discuss how alarms will be advanced and adjusted, and how different patterns may be helpful for different times of day. Troubleshooting the sensor and dealing with signal issues are also discussed, and he is reminded not to stack insulin after meals. Finally, the treatment of lows is reviewed. He is scheduled to return in a month to review data and settings and insulin dosing based on trend arrows.

INSULIN PUMP THERAPY

Starting insulin pump therapy requires comprehensive training before a patient begins to use the pump. Historically, this training was done in an inpatient setting, but now it is done in the outpatient clinic, either with a company-sponsored pump trainer or a pump trainer from the healthcare provider's office. Either way, the trainer needs to be well educated in terms of the pump they will be teaching. Organizations such as the American Association of Diabetes Educators offer courses for educators and each pump company offers resources for training trainers.

Patients should be encouraged to complete online training programs in advance of their in-person training. These tools prepare a user for the actual pump experience. Before starting use of the pump, however, it is helpful if patients learn or relearn the skills, such as carbohydrate counting, that are extremely valuable for successful pump use.

A summary of recommendations for pump education and training was published in the Endocrine Society Guidelines for Diabetes Devices (see Table 7.1).[2]

In terms of the initial pump settings, each pump company provides a form for calculating doses, generally according to one of two methods: a weight-based approach and an approach based on the current total daily dose (TDD) of insulin. In general, it is useful to calculate using both methods to ensure that there isn't some huge error in the calculations. One study concluded that using the TDD method worked best.[3]

Table 7.1. CSII—Considerations for Education and Testing

Patient
 Collaborate with HCP overseeing CSII use and/or the multidisciplinary diabetes team by returning for follow-up.
 Participate in using data management resources to make adjustments to therapy and evaluate self-care behaviors.

Provider
 Provide education as indicated to address deficiencies or when upgrading to new technology.
 Assess CSII use and evaluate for the loss of ability to operate insulin pump due to cognitive, physical, or age-related changes; changes in insurance coverage; or changes in healthcare-provider-managing CSII use.

Time periods to assess patient self-care behaviors and knowledge
 Before initiating CSII, assess:
  Glucose monitoring via SMBG frequency, and/or CGM use defined by HCP to meet individualized glycemic goals.
  Carbohydrate counting or another method of mealtime bolus determination.
  Ability to operate CSII and make setting changes due to factors such as dexterity, vision impairment, mental health, or cognition—independently or with assistance from a designated care provider.
  Infusion site health and selection.
  DKA prevention and treatment.
  Hypoglycemia—prevention, detection, and treatment.
  Emergency supplies.
  If using bolus calculator, assess these settings: insulin-to-carbohydrate ratio, insulin sensitivity factor, glucose targets, and active insulin time.

 Annually and/or when upgrading to a new CSII device, re-assess:
  Glucose monitoring via SMBG frequency and/or CGM use defined by HCP to meet individualized glycemic goals.
  Basal settings via basal rate testing across different time periods, adjust as indicated.
  Bolus calculator settings, if using feature, adjust as indicated.
  Infusion sites and type of infusion set, adjust as indicated.
  Ability to troubleshoot insulin pump malfunction.
  DKA prevention and treatment.
  Hypoglycemia prevention, detection, and treatment.
  Emergency supplies.
  Back-up plan for use of injected insulin should pump fail.

 When discontinuing CSII or transitioning to MDI, re-assess:
  Glucose monitoring via SMBG frequency and/or CGM use defined by HCP to meet individualized glycemic goals.
  New insulin plan for MDI.

The American Diabetes Association provides the following recommendations:[4]

1. Determine how much insulin to use in the insulin pump by averaging the total units of insulin you use per day for several days. (You may start with ~20% less if you are switching to rapid-acting insulin.)
2. Divide the total dosage into 40–50% for basal insulin and 50–60% for bolus insulin.

3. Divide the basal portion by 24 to determine a beginning hourly basal rate.
4. Then, adjust the hourly basal rate up or down for patterns of highs and lows, such as more insulin for dawn phenomenon and less for daily activity.
5. Determine a beginning carbohydrate dose (insulin-to-carbohydrate ratio) using the 450 (or 500) rule. Divide by the total units of insulin per day to get the number of grams of carbohydrate covered by 1 unit of insulin. This dose may be raised or lowered based on your history and how much fast-acting insulin you took in the past.
6. Determine the dose of insulin to correct high blood glucose using the 1,800 (or 1,500) rule. Divide 1,800 by the total units of insulin per day to see how much 1 unit of insulin lowers your blood glucose. This dose must be evaluated by your healthcare team. It is often too high for children or for people who have not had diabetes very long.

Case Study 2

Mary is a 48-year-old woman with a history of T1D since age 30. She has always been treated with MDI but has decided to switch to an insulin pump. She has been training for her first marathon, thinking she would be able to vary her basal rate to help her avoid lows while running. Her A1C has been well controlled—generally in the range of 6.6–6.8%.

She chooses a tethered pump and reviews the online tutorial before starting on the pump. You arrange a 2-h training session with a diabetes educator. In advance of this, she discusses her insulin doses with you. She is currently on 18 units of degludec (Tresiba), an insulin-to-carbohydrate ratio of 1:12 for breakfast and 1:15 for lunch and dinner. Her correction factor (sensitivity) is 1:40 (1 unit of insulin for blood glucose of 40 mg/dL) in the morning and 1:50 later in the day. Her total daily insulin dose ranges from 32 to 38 units. She weighs 72 kg. In addition to calculating her doses, you call in an order for vials of insulin at her pharmacy. Additionally, ketone test strips are ordered and her glucagon prescription renewed. Pump compatible test strips are ordered, as well.

To calculate her starting pump doses, several approaches can be used.[4] Her total daily dose of insulin can be reduced by 20–25%, especially if she is having frequent lows. Taking an average TDD of 36, this would be $36 \times 0.80 = 29$ units. That value is divided by 2, which equals 14.5 units (basal insulin dose) and then is divided by 24 to give the basal rate per hour. In this instance, it would be $14.5 \div 24 = 0.6$ unit/h.

Initially, the basal rate can be constant over 24 h, but it will need to be followed closely and adjusted over time.

A weight-based method can also be used, which can be helpful to validate the previous calculations. This is generally done by taking the patient's weight in kilograms and multiplying by 0.5 (0.5 unit/kg/day) for TDD of insulin. Her weight is 72 kg and $72 \times 0.5 = 36$ units as her estimated TDD. This can be used to calculate dosing as discussed earlier.

In terms of other settings, her carbohydrate and correction ratios can be set at what she has been using or can be calculated. To calculate her insulin-to-carbohydrate ratio, divide 450 by her TDD. This would be $450 \div 36 = 12$ or 1 unit of insulin for 12 g of carbohydrates. To calculate her correction dose, divide 1,800 by her TDD. This would be $1800 \div 36 = 50$. Her glycemic targets should probably be set as 100–140 mg/dL overnight and 90–130 mg/dL during the day. Her active insulin time should be set to 4 h (for analog insulins). All of these settings can be adjusted over time based on her responses—many individuals need more insulin for carbohydrates and corrections in the morning and less during the day. This underscores the importance of downloading devices and analyzing data at every visit.

It is important to review troubleshooting, explain how to call for assistance, and remind the patient that if all else fails, she can return to insulin injections until the pump issues are sorted out. She should learn to test for ketones and to inject insulin with a pen or syringe, if she has blood glucose levels that stay above 350 mg/dL 2–3 h after a correction dose is given through the pump.

She should be taught the basics of exercising with the pump, including reducing her basal in advance of and during exercise. Ideally, she would not do highly intense exercise for the first week or two, until she is used to wearing and troubleshooting the pump. Because this patients runs nearly daily and wants the pump to make her management easier during exercise, use of temporary basal rates could be helpful from the start.

CONCLUSION

Insulin pumps and sensors can help people with diabetes improve their health outcomes. Appropriate initiation, however, is a key factor to ensure success. Patients need support and education to succeed. For sensors, this means helping patients with the technical aspects of wearing the device—for instance making sure it adheres to the skin and transmits the signal effectively as well as aiding in real time and retrospective evaluation of glucose levels and trends.

Insulin pump therapy requires even more input. Proficiency in adjusting basal rates, calculating insulin-to-carbohydrate ratios, and determining correction doses and active insulin time all are necessary to fine-tune pump function. Additionally, troubleshooting techniques, including use of ketone testing and a pump failure backup plan, should be reviewed frequently. Patients using insulin pumps should have 24/7 access to a medical provider who can help in the event of pump failure or infusion set malfunction and always should have the capacity to give injected insulin, if necessary.

With appropriate expectation setting, education, and stepwise follow-up, most adherent patients with T1D can benefit hugely from the initiation of diabetes technology. These tools should be offered as part of routine diabetes care. Not every patient will embrace them, but all patients should be aware of the tools that exist. Various diabetes websites and bloggers can provide patients with peer-type experiences, and patients should be encouraged to explore their options as experienced by others with diabetes.

REFERENCES

1. Aleppo G, Laffel LM, Ahmann AJ, et al. Continuous glucose monitoring trend arrows in the management of adults with diabetes: a practical approach to using the Dexcom G5 CGM system. *J Endo Soc* 2017;12:1445–1460

2. Peters AL, Ahmann AJ, Battelino T, et al. Diabetes technology-continuous subcutaneous insulin infusion therapy and continuous glucose monitoring in adults: an Endocrine Society clinical practice guideline. *J Clin Endo Metab* 2016;101(11):3922–3937, PMID: 27588440

3. Chow N, Shearer D, Tildesley, et al. Determining starting basal rates of insulin infusion for insulin pump users: a comparison between methods. *BMJ Open Diabetes Res Care* 2016;4:e000145, doi:10.1136/bmjdrc-2015-000145

4. Getting started with an insulin pump. American Diabetes Association. Last modified 29 June 2015. Available from www.diabetes.org/living-with-diabetes/treatment-and-care/medication/insulin/getting-started.html. Accessed 12 July 2018

Chapter 8

Interpretation of Meters, Pumps, and Continuous Glucose Monitoring Downloads

KATHRYN WEAVER, MD,[1] AND IRL B. HIRSCH, MD[2]

INTRODUCTION

The ability to monitor blood glucose by a healthcare provider has been available since the 1960s[1] but on a limited scale. By the early 1980s, home monitoring of blood glucose became available. In the 1980s, the data could be stored in the meter and made available for patient and provider review. It was not until the mid-1990s, however, that patients and physicians were able to download results to a computer for a more facile and longitudinal view of the data.[1]

Since the development of self-monitoring of blood glucose (SMBG), interpretation of data has always been an important part of management of diabetes. Until the development of continuous glucose monitoring (CGM), data collection was significantly limited by patient adherence to finger-sticks. Even with excellent adherence, the gaps in data with SMBG are enormous. CGM offers the user updated point-of-care (POC) glucose data up to every 5 min, which is the equivalent of 288 finger-sticks per day. More recently, the manner in which we view and decipher CGM data also has changed, with greater focus given to the ambulatory glucose profile (AGP) and updated glucose metrics.

Continuous subcutaneous infusion of insulin (CSII) and the information available from the insulin pump also offer extensive data that requires download and interpretation. With integration of CSII and CGM, it has become possible for the provider to see the detailed impact that varying bolus and basal insulin amounts has on blood glucose.

This chapter describes the practicalities behind interpretation of information downloaded from blood glucose meters, CGMs, and insulin pumps. We provide examples of various available platforms and discuss developing technologies.

METERS

In endocrinology practices, the downloaded blood glucose and insulin data should be considered as important as the vital signs. Despite evolving technologies, the majority of patients with type 1 diabetes (T1D) continue to use multiple daily injections (MDI) and SMBG to manage diabetes. Approximately 25% of patients with T1D in the U.S. use CGM, but the number is growing quickly.[2] Because of

[1]Department of Medicine, Division of Metabolism, Endocrinology, and Nutrition, University of Washington, WA. [2]Professor of Medicine, School of Medicine, University of Washington, Seattle, WA.

this lag in acquiring the latest technologies, providers must continue to be adept at interpreting the data from finger-sticks and logbooks.

Unfortunately, software programs differ in terms of their statistical and graphic formats, making data interpretation at least slightly different for each patient. Efforts to standardize data across platforms has achieved limited success. As an example, in our practice, we use CliniPro (NuMedics, Inc.), which has the ability to download data from many popular diabetes devices. When this platform is used, the data are presented in a standardized fashion, with a Daily Hourly Summary on page 1, the Log Book on pages 2 and 3, Modal Day data on page 4, and BG Statistics on page 5 (Figure 8.1). The final page with the statistics provides the aggregate data on number of readings, average, minimum, and maximum blood glucose as well as a percent above range, percent in range, and percent below range. On download, most meters will provide some version of this listed data.

Several parameters must be considered when evaluating blood glucose meter downloads, including frequency of testing, blood glucose averages, and standard deviation (SD). This basic approach to interpretation of download was detailed by Hirsch in 2004.[3]. The frequency of testing is necessary to evaluate because it provides a simple and quick assessment of patient adherence. With a low number of blood glucose checks, all other data (average and SD) cannot be reliably interpreted. Furthermore, many insurance companies (and Medicare) are requiring a specific number of daily SMBG checks for patients to receive insurance coverage not only for ongoing use of their glucose testing but also for initiation of their CGM. The glucose average is potentially the most revealing question for a variety of reasons: Does the average glucose match the A1C and, if not, why does this discrepancy exist?[4] Is there an obvious trend emerging from the average glucose (e.g., consistent hyperglycemia or consistent hypoglycemia)? SD of the blood glucose values, or the square root of the variance, indicates whether glycemia is being controlled consistently or with drastic variations (indicative of high glycemic variability). A high SD also can be used as a clue of poor coordination between administration of prandial insulin and carbohydrate intake, either in errors of carbohydrate counting, frequent snacking, or poorly timed insulin. Most blood glucose meter downloads will provide the SD for specific blocks of day, which, along with average blood glucose, can help identify problem areas. The SD has

	NIGHT 12:00 AM	Breakfast 5:00 AM	MID-AM 9:00 AM	Lunch 11:00 AM	MID-AFTERN 2:00 PM	Dinner 5:00 PM	MID-EVENIN 8:00 PM	BED! 10:00 PM	Aggregate 12:00 AM	
# of Readings	5%	4 27%	23 15%	13 21%	18 15%	13 14%	12 1%	1 0%	0 100%	84
Readings Per Day									2 80	
Maximum mg/dL	201	180	190	250	267	223	102	0	267	
75th Percentile mg/dL	198.00	120 50	134.00	140 50	163.00	181.50	102.00	0.00	146.25	
Median mg/dL	164 00	99 00	116 00	130 50	137 00	124 50	102 00	0.00	119 50	
25th Percentile mg/dL	118.25	79.00	93.00	104 75	122.00	89.25	102.00	0.00	89.25	
Minimum mg/dL	80	71	72	82	58	56	102	0	56	
Mean mg/dL	152	106	117	131	135	135	102	0	124	
Std Dev mg/dL	50.13	32 65	32 56	37 32	53 94	53 97	0 00	0.00	43.87	
Events										
Hypo <=60	0	0	0	0	2	1	0	0	3	
Hyper >=180	2	1	1	1	2	4	0	0	11	
Above Target >=140	50%	2 17%	4 23%	3 28%	5 46%	6 42%	5 0%	0 0%	0 30%	25
On Target 101-139	25%	1 26%	6 38%	5 56%	10 31%	4 17%	2 100%	1 0%	0 35%	29
Below Target <=100	25%	1 57%	13 38%	5 17%	3 23%	3 42%	5 0%	0 0%	0 36%	30

Figure 8.1. Blood glucose data downloaded by CliniPro software (NuMedics, Inc). The "BG Statistics" shows blood glucose mean, standard deviation, median, and range as well as percent above, below, and in target. The data are divided into different time blocks and presented as in aggregate.

notable downsides, as it does not adjust for the mean glucose value. The coefficient of variation (CV), described in more detail in the following section, is arguably a much more accurate measure of glycemic variability. Before mainstream adaptation of the CV for glycemic variability, Hirsch[5] proposed the use of the following SD target to strive for as a marker of appropriate glycemic variability: SD × 3 < mean glucose, but only with a mean glucose between 120 and 180 mg/dL, which is equivalent to a CV of 33%. This suggestion was based initially on personal observations, with other groups later refining the data.

Despite advancing technology, most people with diabetes continue to use finger-stick blood glucose as the primary means to monitor their diabetes and to make insulin-dosing decisions. Blood glucose meters have become more sophisticated with data output and storage, transmission to phone apps, and passive uploading to the cloud. Download and interpretation of the data, regardless of the form, is essential in providing optimal care to patients with diabetes. As the field advances, more exciting devices are becoming available to our patients.

CGM

Until the routine use of CGM became attainable, A1C was used as the measure of average blood glucose. The A1C assay measures the percent of glycated hemoglobin, and thus measures the degree of chronic glycemia. It is typically used to evaluate the adequacy of diabetes treatment and to help guide therapy. Twenty-five years ago, landmark studies established glycated hemoglobin as the gold standard for estimating diabetes complications risk by showing that intensive insulin therapy in T1D, which resulted in lower levels of A1C, decreased the long-term incidence of vascular disease.[6]

In 2008, Nathan et al.,[7] as part of the A1C-Derived Average Glucose study group, published data on an international multicenter study that aimed to establish the relationship between average glucose assessed by CGM, SMBG, and A1C to determine the relationship among them. The results affirmed the performance of A1C on a population level. The results suggested unreliability when comparing individuals. Specifically, the 95% predictive interval, or range of corresponding average glucose, increased at each successive A1C level. The study highlighted the limited utility of glycated hemoglobin, especially when used as the sole marker of glycemic control.

Specifically, the A1C does not reflect the presence of glycemic excursions. Although controversial, much evidence suggests that acute excursions of glucose around a mean value constitutes a significant risk factor for diabetes complications.[8,9] These excursions around the mean are not detected by the A1C. Furthermore, an elevated A1C provides no information about when or why the blood glucose is elevated or low. Therefore, adjustment of a treatment regimen based on A1C alone is fraught with error. Additionally, the A1C is an unreliable marker in those with impaired erythrocyte life span, hemoglobin variants, iron deficiency anemia, and chronic kidney disease.[10] There is also significant biological variability with notable racial and ethnic differences in A1C[11,12] that limits the comparability between patients.

Consistent use of continuous glucose monitors has led to a reduction in A1C as demonstrated by several trials.[13] In 2000, MiniMed (later purchased by Medtronic) published data[14] on the performance of the first CGM. Since release of this first CGM tool, technology and accuracy has been improving. CGM quality, as measured with mean absolute relative difference (MARD), has evolved since initial release of glucose sensors. The MARD is the difference between laboratory (or occasionally finger-stick) glucose and sensor glucose. The lower the MARD, the more accurate the sensor. There are four companies with sensors on the market: Dexcom (San Diego, CA), Medtronic (Northridge, CA), Abbott Diabetes Care (Alameda, CA), and Senseonics (Germantown, MD). The accuracy of CGM continues to improve and MARD in the single digits is now standard.

With the improvement in the accuracy of CGM, the recognized limitations of A1C, and widespread coverage by insurance, use of CGM has become much more prevalent. CGM comes in three different forms: real-time CGM, intermittently viewed CGM (iCGM), and professional CGM. All CGM methods continuously monitor glucose concentrations in the interstitial fluid. In the case of professional CGM, the CGM is worn temporarily (typically for 2 weeks) and blood glucose is not assessed in real time but rather is viewed retrospectively by the provider. Intermittently viewed CGM provides current and retrospective glucose data upon "scanning" the transmitter with the receiving device.[15] Currently, the FreeStyle Libre (Abbott Diabetes Care) is the only intermittent CGM on the market. This is also known as "flash" monitoring. This sensor does not require calibrations with SMBG, but the receiver can act as a blood glucose meter with the correct strips.

The newest real-time continuous monitors currently on the market include the Dexcom G6 (Dexcom, San Diego, CA), the Guardian Connect (Medtronic, Northridge, CA), and the Eversense CGM system (Senseonics, Inc., Germantown, MD). These continuous glucose monitors provide real-time numeric and graphic information about glucose and the direction and rate of glucose change. Because these devices are monitoring in real time, they have the capability to alert users of high or low glucose. The Dexcom G6 CGM does not require SMBG calibration. Earlier versions of Dexcom sensors require at least two calibrations per day. The Medtronic Guardian Connect CGM is designed for people on MDI and can be used with the Sugar.IQ companion application. The Guardian Connect requires four calibrations per day to achieve its advertised MARD of 9.64%.[16] The Eversense CGM is an implantable sensor that was recently approved by the U.S. Food and Drug Administration (FDA) for 3 months of continuous wear. The MARD for this sensor is reported at 8.8% (when compared to YSI, Yellow Springs Instrument).[17]

As opposed to SMBG noted earlier, CGM offers the opportunity of the equivalent of 288 finger-sticks per day (monitoring of blood glucose every 5 min for 24 h, in the case of Dexcom). The amount of data offered is extraordinary when compared to SMBG. The strategy in which the data is viewed is also evolving. As discussed, the information from blood glucose meters typically is interpreted in the following context: mean, range, SD, and number of blood glucose checks. More granular data sometimes involve trends in values at different parts of the day (e.g., average at lunch versus average at dinner), but the availability of this information is highly dependent on patient adherence to finger-sticks. Conversely, CGM information output yields much more data. Until 2012, the reports generated by each CGM manufacturer were not standardized. In 2012, a panel of experts convened with the goal of formulating a universal software report, the AGP. Results of this meeting were published in 2013.[18] The AGP is a single-page report of glucose values and metrics (Figure 8.2). It is becoming standard for manufacturers to provide information on glucose statistics, such as glucose average, percent time in range (TIR, 70–180 mg/dL), time below range (TBR, <70 mg/dL), time above range (TAR, >180 mg/dL), and information of glycemic variability (GV, including the CV and SD). The graphic display of the average glucose is arguably the most useful picture, with the median blood glucose, the 25–75% interquartile range, and the blood glucose levels in the 10–90% percentile.

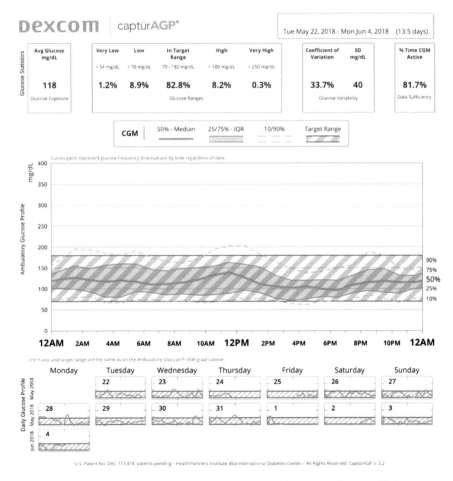

Figure 8.2. AGP report generated by Dexcom Clarity software. This standardized report encompasses glucose metrics, visual AGP with interquartile ranges, and daily views for the previous 2 weeks.

These data are overlayed on the target range. In 2017, Diabetes Care published *The International Consensus on Continuous Glucose Monitoring*[15] and recommended 14 key metrics that should be utilized to assess glycemic control. These include the following: mean glucose level, percentage of time with blood glucose <54 mg/dL, percentage of time with blood glucose <70–54 mg/dL, TIR (blood glucose 70–180 mg/dL), percentage of time with BG >180 mg/dL, percentage of time with BG >250 mg/dL, GV as reported by CV as a primary point and SD as a secondary point, estimated A1C, data for glucose metrics in three time blocks (sleep from 12 a.m. to 6 a.m., wake, 24 h), minimum 2 weeks of data, 70–80% of possible CGM readings over a 2-week period, episodes of hypoglycemia and hyperglycemia, area under the curve (for research purposes), and risk of both hyper- and hypoglycemia. Importantly, the term "estimated A1C" has recently been replaced with the phrase "glucose management indicator" (GMI).[19] Like the A1C, the GMI is reported in percentage points. The GMI is calculated from a standardized formula based on the CGM-derived mean glucose (www.jaeb.org/gmi).[20] In general, for every 25 mg/dL increase in mean glucose the GMI increases by 0.6%, with CGM-derived mean glucose of 100 mg/dL corresponding to a GMI of 5.7%. The most recent Dexcom AGP, generated by Dexcom Clarity (Figure 8.2) and Abbott Libre AGP (Figure 8.3) satisfy a majority of these requirements. In the newest versions of the AGP, the estimated A1C has been eliminated. Eversense has a cloud-based software program that yields an AGP similar to Dexcom and Abbott (Figure 8.4).

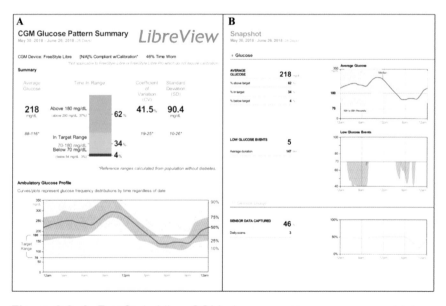

Figure 8.3. A: FreeStyle Libre CGM glucose pattern summary, which provides glucose metrics and visual AGP. **B:** The Snapshot provides visual data on low-glucose events and sensor wear.

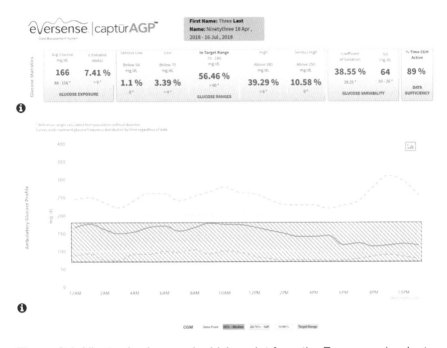

Figure 8.4. Ninety-day box-and-whisker plot from the Eversense implantable CGM by Senseonics.

Chronic hyperglycemia is the causative factor in the development of most complications from diabetes.[6] Monnier et al.[19] have described the "glucose triumvirate" as hyperglycemia, hypoglycemia, and GV. The second two components of this group are not as well studied regarding complications, but, as mentioned earlier, GV is a possible risk factor for complications.[8,9] Excess GV typically indicates that hypoglycemia is occurring more frequently. Although the Diabetes Control and Complications Trial did not find greater cognitive decline in those with a history of severe hypoglycemia,[21] other groups have shown that severe hypoglycemia is a risk factor for cognitive decline.[22] More recently, hypoglycemia has been documented as causing dangerous cardiac arrhythmias.[23] Undoubtedly, hypoglycemia needs to be minimized.

Assessment of variability has historically been done using the SD (around the mean glucose), as this typically is done with data from SMBG. The CV can be obtained using the following calculation: ([SD of glucose] ÷ [mean glucose]) × 100, According to Monnier et al., the CV is likely one of the most reliable markers of GV because it adjusts for the mean glucose value. In an elegant study with 376 patients with diabetes (both T1D and type 2 diabetes) wearing CGM, Monnier established that a CV of 36% is the most appropriate threshold that separates stable from labile glycemic control.[19] Although the use of CV in interpretation of blood glucose has become more widespread with the increasing use of CGM, it also can be applied to data downloaded from standard blood glucose meters using the equation stated earlier.

After the glucose has been downloaded from the CGM, the correct interpretation and use of the data by the provider is critical. All of the following metrics should be evaluated to adequately interpret the data: glucose control (TIR, TAR, TBR), glucose variability (with CV or SD), trends by time of day, and risk of both hyper- and hypoglycemia. The majority of this data is available on the single-page "dashboard" or "snapshot" described earlier. The daily view data are available if information is needed about trends or data points on a specific day. For patients on MDI and insulin pump therapy, assessment about the correctness of the basal insulin and the bolus insulin can be made by asking the patient to record 1 or 2 days of carbohydrates consumed and insulin given. In our practice, we frequently have our patients see the clinic certified diabetes educator (CDE) in between visits with the physician, with the explicit goal of honing either pump settings or insulin injection dosing.

INSULIN PUMPS

Devices designed to mimic pancreatic endocrine function have been under development since the 1970s. Since the 1980s, when MiniMed commercialized the first insulin pump, the 502, the field has been rapidly progressing. With the improving quality, data have shown improvements in glycemic control and decreased rate of hypoglycemia with use of CSII.[24] In 2013, the threshold suspend feature was approved by the FDA as part of the MiniMed 530G and Enlite sensor combination from Medtronic. This combined insulin pump-CGM was the first in the U.S. to allow the blood glucose readings on the sensor to control the function of the insulin infusion in the form of the Threshold Suspend feature, which stops the delivery of insulin when sensor glucose values reach a preset low limit. This technology known as a sensor-augmented pump (SAP) enables therapy management software to make decisions about insulin delivery based on blood glucose measured by the sensor. In 2017, Medtronic started marketing its most advanced CSII, the hybrid closed-loop (HCL) 670G insulin pump after Bergenstal et al. demonstrated safety of this device,[25] leading to rapid FDA approval. This insulin delivery system has the capacity for partially automated insulin delivery based on sensor glucose. The 670G insulin pump functions in two different modes: auto mode and manual mode. Manual mode is similar to previous CSII with linked CGM, with the added feature of stopping insulin before hypoglycemia occurs (known as Suspend Before Low). While in auto mode, the device responds to measured glucose levels and small adjustments are made in the basal insulin rate.

At the time this chapter was written, three companies were marketing insulin pumps in the U.S.: Tandem Diabetes Care (maker of the t:slim X2 and the t:flex insulin pumps), Medtronic (creator of the MiniMed series), and Insulet Corporation (which sells the Omnipod Insulin Management system). The manufacturers that currently have technology to augment insulin delivery based on sensor glucose are Medtronic (MiniMed 530G, 630G, and 670G) and Tandem Diabetes Care. Tandem received FDA approval of t:slim X2 insulin pump with Basal-IQ technology in June 2018. Basal-IQ is a predictive low-glucose suspend feature that will be integrated with the Dexcom G6 CGM.

The degree of automation changes the manner in which the pump and sensor data are reported in the download. All CSII delivery systems yield different reports, but data included are similar. All of the reports provide the following information: infusion set changes, average glucose (by sensor or meter), carbohydrate consumption, insulin use, information about individual bolus events with insulin, carbohydrates, blood glucose, and device settings (including basal and bolus insulin settings). In this discussion, given that the field is moving in the direction of exclusive use of SAP, we review strategies for interpreting sensor-augmented pump data, including the HCL insulin pump by Medtronic.

With improving and changing technologies, the requirements of the provider and the clinic are increasing. Without the appropriate system and clinic infrastructure, insulin pump management is extremely taxing on the provider, and patients are not likely to achieve optimal glycemic control without the necessary nucleus of CDE[26] who are essential in glycemic management in a large diabetes practice. Furthermore, data downloads require an additional point of staff involvement and resource utilization. Nonreimbursed time from our nonphysicians before the MiniMed 670G was ~$100,000 per year in our clinic.[27]

All providers will approach the downloaded CSII data differently, but the goals should be the same: *1*) assess the provided continuous glucose monitor snapshot as described to attain a high-level view of TIR, TAR, TBR, and GV; *2*) consider total daily dose (TDD) of insulin and the percent basal versus bolus, noting that many patients are "over-basalized" with >50% basal insulin; *3*) based on the daily blood glucose trends, evaluate the appropriateness of the basal insulin rates, paying special attention to overnight trends and presence of hypoglycemia; *4*) evaluate the individual bolus events (Figure 8.5), especially when blood glucose is noted to be <70mg/dL or >180mg/dL to determine correctness of insulin sensitivity factor (ISF) and insulin-to-carbohydrate ratio (ICR); and *5*) confirm the patient is changing the set and reservoir at suitable intervals. When patients are not using the built-in bolus calculator (which calculates insulin doses based on patient input of carbohydrate and blood glucose and takes into account "insulin on board"), it is extremely difficult to determine whether the ISF and ICR are correct. We encourage patients to use the bolus calculator even if they plan to deliver a different amount (override) of insulin. By doing this, we are able to understand whether the patient is thinking correctly about their diabetes. Additionally, a group out of Israel demonstrated that use of the bolus calculator is

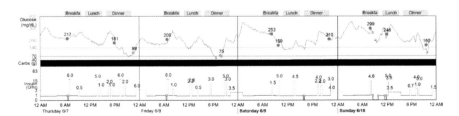

Figure 8.5. Data download of MiniMed 530G System (sensory augmented pump) by Medtronic. An excerpt from the "Sensor/Meter Overview," showing individual bolus events overlaid on sensor glucose.

associated with improved glycemic control with a reduction in A1C by 0.6% ($P = 0.008$) and a reduction in mean blood glucose by 25 mg/dL ($P = <0.0001$).[28]

The most recently released insulin pump, the MiniMed 670G system by Medtronic, is an HCL insulin delivery system. As mentioned earlier, when in auto mode, small adjustments are made to the basal rate of insulin delivery to keep blood glucose within a target range. When patients are in auto mode, only three settings can be changed: the active insulin time (AIT), ICR, and basal target glucose. Two prespecified blood glucose targets for basal insulin cannot be modified: 120 mg/dL and 150 mg/dL. The only way to bolus insulin in auto mode is at the time of a meal, by entering carbohydrate data into the pump. Despite the terminology of "auto mode" and the limited number of blood glucose targets, people have found ways to consistently decrease blood glucose levels below the target. This is achieved by the administration of "phantom carbohydrates"—that is, users inform the insulin pump that they are going to eat carbohydrates, when they are not going to eat anything. This practice can lead to hypoglycemia.

To effectively represent the way the HCL insulin delivery device functions, the CareLink (cloud-based data management system for Medtronic devices) reports also have changed. They contain all of the pertinent information mentioned earlier, with some changes. The "Assessments and Progress" page (Figure 8.6) has been updated to provide a high-level view of blood glucose control with the

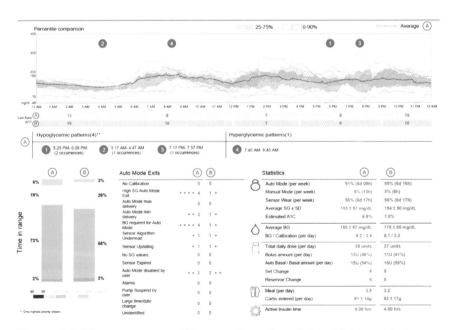

Figure 8.6. "Assessment and Progress" portion of CareLink reports from MiniMed 670G System by Medtronic. Information includes AGP with interquartile ranges, TIR, data on auto-mode exits, and statistics (see Figure 8.3).

aggregate sensor data. It contains a standard AGP, TIR, TAR, and TBR. Statistics are also included in this section, which shows the time the patient was in auto mode, the sensor wear, sensor glucose, total daily insulin, bolus insulin amount, and carbohydrates entered. The reasons for auto-mode "exits" also are given here. Automatic push to manual mode occurs for a variety of reasons, such as persistent hyperglycemia, sensor problems, and user problems (e.g., failure to calibrate). The "Weekly Review" portion of the report (Figure 8.7) shows individual bolus events paired with carbohydrate amount and denotes when the user was in auto mode versus manual mode. In future CareLink reports, the "Weekly Review" also will contain information previously noted in the "Daily Detail" from earlier versions of CareLink reports, including correction insulin given, override, and whether a dual or square-wave bolus was delivered. Importantly, this latter information on boluses is relevant only when the user is in manual mode. The "Meal Bolus Wizard" provides information on meal boluses timed by the meal with all glucose trends overlaid to provide a trend for the time of day.

The main objectives when evaluating the 670G reports are as follows: *1*) assess the AGP as described earlier; *2*) evaluate time in auto mode versus manual mode, average blood glucose, insulin statistics, and set changes; *3*) understand why auto-mode exits occurred; *4*) review the "Weekly Review" to assess bolus events and

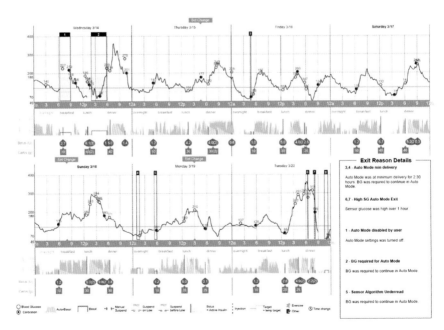

Figure 8.7. "Weekly Review" portion of CareLink reports from MiniMed 670G System by Medtronic. Visible in this portion are the CGM data with the basal rates (both while in auto mode and manual mode) and bolus events, including carbohydrates consumed.

specifically ask the patient about the use of phantom carbohydrates; and 5) make changes to the ICR, if needed. Once providers become savvy in their understanding of the functionality of the 670G and the updated CareLink reports, the data evaluation for people in auto mode will become easier than with a typical SAP because several settings are not adjustable—namely, the basal rate, the blood glucose target (outside of 120 mg/dL vs. 150 mg/dL), and the ISF. Settings for these variables exist when the patient is in manual mode, but they are obsolete in auto mode. For hyperglycemia, the insulin pump will suggest a correction based on a blood glucose target of 150 mg/dL, taking into account the provider-set AIT and the ISF that is calculated by the algorithm every 24 h. Thus, the AIT is the only way to adjust correction doses in auto mode. As care providers and patients become more comfortable with this device, we anticipate more efficient office visits.

The CSII and sensor data download is being refined continuously, which eventually will help with ease of interpretation and streamline our ability to make useful adjustments to insulin pump settings at each visit. Companies such as Glooko (Mountain View, CA), which recently merged with Diasend, and mySugr (Vienna, Austria), which was purchased by Roche in 2017, have created software that is compatible with several diabetes devices, although there have been some setbacks regarding the ability to download all brands of meters, sensors, and pumps.

Tidepool is a nonprofit, open-source effort that allows patients to upload and visualize data from different diabetes devices. The technology is supported by JDRF and is free to users. Tidepool has demonstrated feasibility[29] of this "device-agnostic" platform, and more recently, Wong et al.[30] demonstrated the usability of this platform by patients and caregivers. The Tidepool interface is user-friendly for both providers and patients, provides the standard data for CSII as discussed earlier, and works across all platforms. Data can be viewed in several different formats, including average blood glucose over 24 h with or without interquartile ranges (Figure 8.8). The daily view (Figure 8.9) shows sensor glucose trend, basal rates, and bolus events.

Despite the improving technology, the feasibility of achieving a detailed evaluation of the insulin pump data in a short office visit is questionable. We routinely utilize the skills of CDEs (nurses, nutritionists, and pharmacists) in our practice to see patients between visits with the physician and to continue evaluating the data and hone the insulin pump settings. Admittedly, the adjustment of insulin pump settings can be haphazard and involves quite a lot of trial and error.

To date, our practice does not have an effective way to track changes made in the past. With current cloud-based diabetes management technology (e.g., CareLink, Tidepool, Glooko) patients are able to download and interpret their own data. Few patients with T1D, however, download their own data,[31] and thus the burden continues to rest on the provider. The hope is that passive uploading to the cloud will continue to increase in use taking the burden off the providers. This will become even more critical when "smart insulin pens," which allow pen-dosing data to be transferred to a phone app, become the standard of care. This technology is a continued area for further development, especially as the demand for productivity increases.

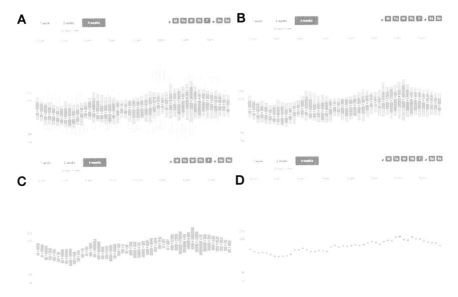

Figure 8.8. Download from Tidepool "Trends" view showing AGP based on 4 weeks of data and shown with **A:** 100% of the data, **B:** 80% of the data, **C:** 50% of the data, and **D:** median blood glucose.

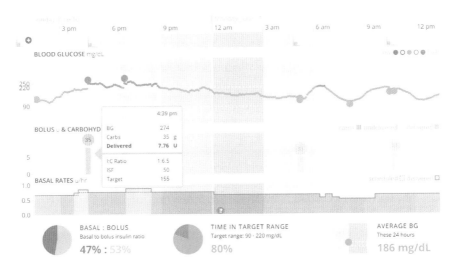

Figure 8.9. Download from Tidepool "Daily View" showing senor glucose, bolus events, basal rates, and glucose metrics (e.g., TIR, average blood glucose, and breakdown of percent basal and bolus).

CONCLUSION

The amount of diabetes technology has increased exponentially since SMBG was first introduced in the 1980s. With the introduction of CGM and eventually sensor-augmented CSII, and the increasing availability of these technologies to all patients with diabetes, the amount of data available for the care team and patient to utilize has risen steeply.

Historically, insulin and blood glucose data have not been standardized in the way they have been reported, leading to inconsistency in the way the information is downloaded and utilized. In the past several years, there has been a coordinated effort to standardized the reports of CGM by including an AGP with TIR, TBR, and TAR in addition to CV or SD. With the ability to streamline this reporting, the usefulness of the data has increased. At the same time, several groups have developed cloud-based platforms that provide a standard report regardless of the device. This advancement is an enormous step in the way diabetes technology can be used.

With the arrival of more novel technologies, such as the HCL MiniMed 670G by Medtronic, the field will continue to evolve in the way downloaded statistics are utilized. The expectation for the future is that as automation advances, the burden on the provider to painstakingly download, review, and act upon data from a CGM or CSII download will be lessened.

The downloaded data from all blood glucose management devices is essential to the optimal care of patients with diabetes. The glucose and insulin information should be considered as important as the vital signs in any clinical practice, but regularly acquiring and effectively interpreting this data is not a uniform practice. In our experience, the barriers to effective utilization of the downloaded data include *1*) inadequate infrastructure leading to inefficiency and high cost and *2*) the lack of training of care providers on how to efficiently and effectively interpret the downloaded data. Our goal in this review is to provide some basic strategies to help the provider efficiently assess the downloaded data and make changes to therapy that have a positive impact on blood glucose control.

REFERENCES

1. Clarke SF, Foster JR. A history of blood glucose meters and their role in self-monitoring of diabetes mellitus. *Br J Biomed Sci* 2012;69:83–93

2. The diaTribe Foundation. Available from https://diaTribe.org/CGM. Accessed 15 July 2018

3. Hirsch IB. Blood glucose monitoring technology: translating data into practice. *Endocr Pract* 2004;10:67–76

4. Rubinow KB, Hirsch IB. Reexamining metrics for glucose control. *JAMA* 2011;305:1132–1133

5. Hirsch IB. Glycemic variability: its not just about A1C anymore. *Diabetes Technol Ther* 2005;7:780–783

6. Nathan DM, Genuth S, Lachin J, Cleary P, Crofford O, Davis M, Rand L, Siebert C. The effect of intensive treatment of diabetes on the development and progression of long-term complications in insulin-dependent diabetes mellitus. *N Engl J Med* 1993;329:977–986

7. Nathan DM, Kuenen J, Borg R, Zheng H, Schoenfeld D, Heine RJ. Translating the A1C assay into estimated average glucose values. *Diabetes Care* 2008; 8:1473–1478

8. Sartore G, Chilelli NC, Brulina S, Lapolla A. Association between glucose variability as assessed by continuous glucose monitoring (CGM) and diabetic retinopathy in type 1 and type 2 diabetes. *Acta Diabetol* 2013;50:437–442

9. Hirsch IB. Glycemic variability and diabetes complications: does it matter? Of course it does! *Diabetes Care* 2015;38:1610–1614

10. Sacks DB. Hemoglobin A1C in diabetes: panacea or pointless. *Diabetes* 2013; 62:41–43

11. Saaddine JB, Fagot-Campagna A, Rolka D, Venkat Narayan KM, Geiss L, Eberhardt M, Flegal KM. Distribution of HbA1c levels for children and young adults in the U.S. *Diabetes Care* 2002;25:1326–1330

12. Bergenstal RM, Ga RL, Connor CG, Gubitosi-Klug R, Kruger D, Olson BA, Willi SM, Aleppo G, Weinstock RS, Wood J, Rickels M, DiMeglio LA, Bethin KE, Marcovina S, Tassopoulos A, Lee S, Massaro E, Bzdick S, Ichihara B, Markmann E, McGuigan P, Woerner S, Ecker M, Beck RW. Racial differences in the relationship of glucose concentrations and hemoglobin A1c levels. *Ann Intern Med* 2017;167:95–102

13. Klonoff DC, Ahn D, Drincic A. Continuous glucose monitoring: a review of the technology and clinical use. *Diabetes Res Clin Pract* 2017;133:178–192

14. Gross TM, Bode BW, Einhorn D, Kayne DM, Reed JH, White NH, Mastrototaro JJ. Performance evaluation of the MiniMed continuous glucose monitoring system during patient home use. *Diabetes Technol Ther* 2000;2:49–55

15. Danne T, Nimri R, Battelino T, Bergenstal RM, Close KL, DeVries JH, Garg S, Heinemann L, Hirsch I, Amiel SA, Beck R, Bosi E, Buckingham B, Cobelli C, Dassau E, Doyle FJ 3rd, Heller S, Hovorka R, Jia W, Jones T, Kordonouri O, Kovatchev B, Kowalski A, Laffel L, Maahs D, Murphy HR, Nørgaard K, Parkin CG, Renard E, Saboo B, Scharf M, Tamborlane WV, Weinzimer SA, Phillip M. International consensus on use of continuous glucose monitoring. *Diabetes Care* 2017;40:1631–1640

16. Christiansen MP, Garg SK, Brazg R, Bode BW, Bailey TS, Slover RH, Sullivan A, Huang S, Shin J, Lee SW, Kaufman FR. Accuracy of a fourth-generation subcutaneous continuous glucose sensor. *Diabetes Technol Ther* 2017;19:445–456

17. Christiansen MP, Klaff LJ, Brazg R, Chang AR, Levy CJ, Lam D, Denham DS, Atiee G, Bode BW, Walters SJ, Kelley L, Bailey TS. A Prospective Multicenter Evaluation of the Accuracy of a Novel Implanted Continuous Glucose Sensor: PRECISE II. *Diabetes Technol Ther* 2018;20:197–206

18. Bergenstal RM, Ahmann AJ, Bailey T, Beck RW, Bissen J, Buckingham B, Deeb L, Dolin RH, Garg SK, Goland R, Hirsch IB, Klonoff DC, Kruger DF, Matfin G, Mazze RS, Olson BA, Parkin C, Peters A, Powers MA, Rodriguez H, Southerland P, Strock ES, Tamborlane W, Wesley DM. Recommendations for standardizing glucose reporting and analysis to optimize clinical decision making in diabetes: the ambulatory glucose profile (AGP). *Diabetes Technol Ther* 2013;15:198–211

19. Monnier L, Colette C, Wojtusciszyn A, Dejager S, Renard E, Molinari N, Owens DR. Toward defining the threshold between low and high glucose variability in diabetes. *Diabetes Care* 2017;40:832–838

20. JAEB Center for Health and Research. Available from www.jaeb.org/gmi. Accessed 9 February 2019

21. Jacobson AM, Ryan CM, Cleary PA, Waberski BH, Weinger K, Musen G, Dahms W. Biomedical risk factors for decreased cognitive functioning in type 1 diabetes: an 18 year follow-up of the Diabetes Control and Complications Trial (DCCT) cohort. *Diabetologia* 2011;54:245–255

22. Ryan CM, Klein BEK, Cruickshanks KJ, Klein R. Associations between recent severe hypoglycemia, retinal vessel diameters, and cognition in adults with type 1 diabetes. *J Diabetes Complications* 2016;30:1513–1518

23. Riddle MC, Miller ME: Scientific exploration with continuous glucose monitoring systems: an early assessment of arrhythmias during hypoglycemia. *Diabetes Care* 2018;41:664–666

24. Pickup J, Keen H. Continuous subcutaneous insulin infusion at 25 years: evidence base for the expanding use of insulin pump therapy in type 1 diabetes. *Diabetes Care* 2002;25:593–598

25. Bergenstal RM, Garg S, Weinzimer SA, Buckingham BA, Bode BW, Tamborlane WV, Kaufman FR. Safety of a hybrid closed-loop insulin delivery system in patients with type 1 diabetes. *JAMA* 2016;316:1407–1408

26. Hirsch IB. Practical pearls in insulin pump therapy. *Diabetes Technol Ther* 2010;12:S23–S27

27. Huynh P, Toulouse A, Hirsch IB. One-year time analysis in an academic diabetes clinic: quantifying our burden. *Endocr Pract* 2018;24:489–491

28. Cukierman-Yaffe T, Konvalina N, Cohen O. Key elements for successful intensive insulin pump therapy in individuals with type 1 diabetes. *Diabetes Res Clin Pract* 2011;92:69–73

29. Neinstein A, Wong J, Look H, Arbiter B, Quirk K, McCanne S, Sun Y, Blum M, Adi S. A case study in open source innovation: developing the Tidepool Platform for interoperability in type 1 diabetes management. *J Am Med Inform Assoc* 2016;23:324–332

30. Wong JC, Neinstein AB, Look H, Arbiter B, Chokr N, Ross C, Adi S. Pilot Study of a Novel Application for Data Visualization in Type 1 Diabetes. *J Diabetes Sci Technol* 2017;11:800–807

31. Wong JC, Neinstein AB, Spindler M, Adi S. A minority of patients with type 1 diabetes routinely downloads and retrospectively reviews device data. *Diabetes Technol Ther* 2015;17:555–562

Chapter 9

Pumps and Continuous Glucose Monitoring in Children with Diabetes

Jenise C. Wong, MD, PhD;[1] Gina Capodanno, MD;[1] and Saleh Adi, MD[1]

All people with type 1 diabetes (T1D) and an increasing number of people with type 2 diabetes (T2D) require life-long insulin therapy. The central task in insulin replacement therapy is to mimic the normal pattern of insulin secretion and controlling blood glucose (BG) levels in a range that is close to normal—that is, between 70 and 140 mg/dL.[1] Achieving such tight control with exogenous insulin is nearly impossible, however. In normal physiology, tight glucose control is achieved by virtue of continuous sensing of BG levels in the pancreatic islet cells and other glands, and by immediately responding to changes in BG levels by secreting a number of hormones that decrease (insulin) or increase BG (glucagon, cortisol, growth hormone, adrenaline). The effectiveness of this system relies on the fact that it is a bidirectional control system (up and down), with an inherent ability to respond instantaneously and continuously and that the responses are quick and short-lived, allowing the system to adjust its response and change direction within seconds to minutes. This is possible because glucose sensing is continuous and in real time, measuring glucose concentrations directly in the blood, and insulin and other hormones are secreted directly into the blood stream where they exert an immediate but short-lived effect.

Therefore, some fundamental differences exist between normal physiology and the way we manage diabetes with exogenous insulin, namely that we attempt to control BG in one direction (insulin *lowers* BG), and that we deliver insulin not into the blood stream but in the subcutaneous space where it takes time (up to 3–4 h) for it to travel through the interstitial space before reaching the blood stream. Another important issue is that the sensitivity of the human body to insulin can vary from day to day and hour to hour, making insulin requirements somewhat different throughout the day. This is especially true in children whose insulin requirements can vary dramatically at different times of the day. For these reasons, traditional regimens of once-a-day long-acting insulin and frequent doses of rapid-acting insulin with meals cannot mimic the normal pattern of insulin secretion, resulting in suboptimal control of BG levels.

Findings from the seminal Diabetes Control and Complications Trial (DCCT)[1,2] provided evidence for the need for tighter control, which required more frequent dosing for all carbohydrate intake. Although the introduction of rapid-acting insulin (lispro in 1996 and aspart soon after) made it more practical

---

[1]Department of Pediatrics and Madison Clinic for Pediatric Diabetes, University of California, San Francisco, CA.

to dose frequently, because doses can be taken immediately before a meal or snack, it was still burdensome to take multiple injections each day. Additionally, it still was not possible to titrate basal insulin delivery to meet variable needs throughout the day because it was delivered as once- or twice-a-day injections of long-acting insulin. This led to greater interest in advancing the development of insulin pumps that can deliver rapid-acting insulin continuously based on a preset variable hourly or even half-hourly rates. This continuous "basal rate" infusion of rapid-acting insulin is more favorable to long-acting insulin, because it can be customized to meet the variable insulin requirements throughout the day. In addition, basal rate infusion can be quickly interrupted, temporarily increased, or temporarily decreased to match insulin requirements, which are influenced by a multitude of factors, such as exercise, illness, stress, allergic reactions, and hormonal changes.

The second important feature of insulin pumps is their ability to calculate and deliver more precise doses of insulin as frequently as desired, without the need for additional injections using a syringe or a pen. A pump dose calculator can be programmed with different parameters and thresholds for different times of the day, and even for different days of the week, and can accurately calculate and deliver doses to the tenth of a unit. This is of paramount importance in children whose activity and eating patterns may not be easily predicted.

More recently, continuous glucose monitoring (CGM), another important technology for the management of diabetes, has witnessed an accelerated advancement.[3] Traditionally, patients and clinicians relied on measurements of BG levels using fairly accurate and easy-to-use glucose meters. Glucometer readings were done only periodically each day, before each meal, at bedtime, and before exercise, which provided an incomplete view of true glucose levels and missed a lot of valuable information and opportunities to act on BG levels in between meals and especially at night. Advancements in glucose-sensing technology and software development have led to the emergence of a few CGM devices that are easy to use, fairly accurate, and reliable.

Currently, most CGM devices consist of a sensor probe that is inserted through the skin where it can remain for 7–10 days. The probe measures glucose concentrations in the subcutaneous interstitial fluid, which reflects the glucose concentration in the blood after several minutes of lag time. Sensor probes are connected to an external small hardware device that is taped to the outside of the skin, which is referred to as the transmitter because it transmits glucose concentration readings wirelessly to a separate receiving device, an insulin pump, or a smartphone through a Bluetooth connection. Most current CGMs do not require calibration, thus completely replacing traditional finger-stick BG readings.

The following sections provide practical guidance on use of insulin pumps and CGMs, which are drawn primarily from our clinical experiences over the past decade. Although our practice focuses primarily on children with T1D, we believe that most practical issues, obstacles, and benefits of technology are relevant across all ages. In addition, we provide guidance on optimizing the use of the data generated by pumps and CGMs, an area that can have significant benefits.

PUMPS IN CHILDREN WITH DIABETES

Pump therapy has become increasingly the preferred mode of intensified insulin delivery in children and adolescents with T1D. It allows for precise tailoring of insulin dosing at very small increments with the option to temporarily override settings and adjust insulin delivery based on needs,[4,5] which are all important to consider for the active, growing child whose insulin needs are continually changing.[6] Although debated, the majority of large-center studies, meta-analyses, and guidelines suggest that pump therapy improves on several clinical factors over MDI, including lowering total daily insulin dose, decreasing frequency of severe hypoglycemia, and improving glycemic control, especially in those of younger age.[7–10]

Pump therapy also offers practical benefits, such as being able to minimize skin punctures, autocalculate insulin doses, decrease the time spent on daily tasks, and remotely deliver insulin via smart technologies, which all simplify the routine of insulin administration to improve quality of life.[11]

Who Should Get an Insulin Pump?

Every child and young adult with T1D or with T2D on intensive insulin therapy should be offered the option of starting pump therapy. Very few exceptions can be made, such as children with severe developmental issues that will render them likely to not tolerate or accept a device to be permanently placed on their skin or to dislodge the pump without the parent's knowledge. Even children with severe autism, however, can successfully use an insulin pump. It is our experience that most children and parents, when presented with the rationale for pump use, are always eager to start pump therapy as soon as possible. Children in their mid-teens, especially girls who dislike the idea of being "connected" to a device, are the most likely to disagree with pump therapy. It is best to not argue with adolescents and respect their wishes, but also to keep bringing up the topic of pump therapy at every visit. Most youth eventually will see the benefits and order a pump, especially around the time they prepare for transitioning out of high school.

A persistent debate is whether patients with T1D who seem to be "unengaged" and choose to perform a minimal amount of diabetes management tasks, such as skipping BG measurements and dosing for most meals, should not be offered an insulin pump. It is arguable that using a pump may in fact ease the burden of diabetes management and facilitate more dosing for meals. In addition, we find that, especially in adolescents, having a pump download provides a more accurate history of whether the patient is measuring BG and dosing insulin and how much, instead of relying on self-reported information.

Another common debate is whether pump therapy should be even offered in the first 6 months after diagnosis of T1D. Insurance carriers often use this argument to deny coverage of an insulin pump. To our knowledge, there is no real basis for such recommendation. On the contrary, increasing evidence, supported by our own experience, indicates that very early implementation of intensive insulin therapy with a pump (and CGM) may be beneficial for the health of β-cells resulting in prolongation of the honeymoon stage,[12] with the benefits of tighter BG control, lower hemoglobin A_{1c} (A1C), and reduced incidence of hypoglycemia.

Choosing an Insulin Pump

Because an insulin pump is worn and operated all the time, and because children and parents must interact with their pump several times a day, there must be a high level of acceptability and trust in this new hardware that quickly becomes an extension of their body. Therefore, the choice of which pump to use must be made by the children and their caregivers in collaboration with their clinical providers, after receiving complete information about all the available pumps and their differentiating features.

Although the same principles underlie pump technology as a whole, individual pumps have their differences, and providers should share their thoughts on the pros and cons on these differences from experience that may suggest one more suitable than another for a certain patient. Standard "tethered" pumps make use of a thin tube attached on one end to an infusion set that is taped to the skin and on the other end to the pump reservoir. Patch pumps are typically smaller, but the entire pump is attached directly to the body without tubes and is operated discretely by a remote handheld device or a smartphone. Although the idea of not having any tubing attached may be appealing, especially for young children and athletes, other features must be weighed, such as the ability to deliver very low rates of hourly infusion for infants and toddlers, and the maximum amount of insulin that can be loaded into the pump (for adolescents who consume large amounts of insulin). Conversely, tethered pumps can be easily disconnected during highly physical sports or swimming, or for bathing, whereas patch pumps may not be disconnected. Patch pumps also may be a good choice for patients with special needs as well as for patients with certain behavioral issues and for whom having tubing could be a liability and operating the pump remotely is highly desirable.

Another key factor in pump choice is the user-interface. Children and their caregivers must be adept and confident at operating the pump without frustrations and uncertainty. Therefore, the user-interface must be intuitive and accurate and should convey a high level of confidence. It is not uncommon that adolescents skip an entire insulin dose simply because "it takes too long to bolus." No single design, however, is universally agreeable to all patients, and our recommendation is for patients to be presented with all of the options and be allowed to interact with and operate demonstration pumps before making a final decision. Following are important features that should be considered when selecting a pump.

- Patch or tube pump
- Size and weight of pump
- Water-resistance versus waterproof (the latter can be submerged in water)
- Minimum rates of hourly basal rate infusion (especially in infants and toddlers who may require rates as low as 0.025 unit/h)
- Maximum capacity of insulin reservoir (ideally should hold enough for 3 days)
- User interface
- Alarm features
- Connectivity to a CGM
- Ability to upgrade to newer models
- Insurance coverage (some insurance plans cover only certain pumps)
- Software for uploading pump data and integrating with CGM data
- Company customer support
- Future pipeline and development of closed-loop systems

Most diabetes centers conduct extensive educational classes to review the pros and cons of pump therapy and the different features of each pump, and some centers even invite representatives from each pump company to interact directly with the patients. Clinicians who operate smaller clinics and care for a smaller number of patients on insulin may find it more efficient to encourage their patients to attend these classes at the nearest diabetes center.

Starting Pump Therapy

Pump therapy should be initiated as early as possible after diagnosis of T1D or after starting intensive insulin therapy in children with T2D. Once a pump is chosen and ordered, there will a lag of a few weeks before insurance processing and shipping to the patient. This presents an ideal period for patients to get accustomed to using individual multiple daily injections (MDI) by syringes or pens and to become familiar with the concepts of long- versus rapid-acting insulin, because they likely will need to intermittently revert to using MDI during times of pump failure or pump vacation (discussed in the section "Taking a Pump Vacation"). Once the pump is approved and received, it is important to set clear and reasonable expectations and to ensure that patients understand that to successfully transition to using a pump, they need to follow a process rather than a single event. The child must have a positive initial experience with the pump. The following initial three-step process for starting pump therapy is generally successful:

1. Initial training: This training can be done at home by a company-designated certified pump trainer or by a diabetes educator in the clinic. We recommend that this training be done no longer than 7–10 days before the anticipated actual pump start to ensure that the information and training remain fresh.
2. Pump with saline: Once the initial training is completed successfully, the pump can be filled with saline and worn and operated for 7–10 days. This allows the family to practice infusion set insertions and changes and even to try different types of infusion sets. The child can get used to having the sets and pump physically attached while performing their normal daily routine and activities, including sports, sleeping, and bathing.
3. Pump start with insulin: This step should be done in clinic with a diabetes educator who is familiar with pump features and operation. These visits are typically lengthy, up to 2–3 h, during which time the educator will review all of the training on infusion set insertions and pump operation. At this point, an individual decision should be made whether to review all of the advanced pump features, including use of temporary basal rates and the different types of boluses for meals, or to keep things simple to avoid overwhelming the family with too much information and options.

At this point, it is essential that families are receiving training on how to upload their pump data (and CGM if they already have one) from home, allowing the clinic providers the opportunity to review the data and make frequent adjustments in the insulin regimen. The shift from MDI of long- and rapid-acting insulin to continuous administration of rapid-acting insulin represents a change in insulin delivery dynamics, which adds to the rapidly changing dynamics of endogenous insulin production during the honeymoon phase in newly diagnosed children. Because of this, frequent reviews of glucose and pump data should be performed every 1–3 days in the first 2–4 weeks after insulin pump starts, both in newly diagnosed patients and in patients transitioning to pump therapy after long-term use of MDI.

Pump Settings

It is debatable whether initial pump settings should be optimized from the start. Because of the previously mentioned dynamic adjustment period, it may be more practical to start with simple settings with the goal of adjusting them quickly based on the child's responses and data reviews. Pump settings include basal rates, insulin-to-carbohydrate ratios (ICR), and insulin sensitivity factor (ISF) or high BG correction factor. All insulin pumps include a "smart bolus calculator," which calculates a suggested insulin dose based on either the current BG value, carbohydrate amount to be eaten, or both. The calculator also takes into account any potential residual activity from the last insulin bolus.

- Basal rates: One of the most essential functions of an insulin pump is the continuous delivery of small doses of rapid acting insulin every few minutes. This basal insulin provides for the requirements of basal metabolism and energy production, aside from the insulin required to cover food-derived carbohydrates. Thus, an ideal basal insulin regimen would maintain BG levels steady in the absence of carbohydrate intake or excessive physical activity. The challenge is that basal insulin requirements are quite variable from hour to hour and are highly individualized. Many providers start with a single hourly rate throughout the day and adjust it progressively, whereas others begin with a more variable rate that follows a certain expected pattern based on the age, weight, and pubertal developmental stage of the child. Figure 9.1*A* represents a typical basal rate pattern for a young preschool child and Figure 9.1*B* represents a typical pattern for a pubertal midteen patient. These patterns illustrate the daily variability and the timing and magnitudes of the peaks and valleys and are not necessarily indicative of the absolute values of each hourly basal rate. These settings must be individualized to each patient's actual needs and adjusted for their bedtime and wake-up time; both patterns assume a wake-up time around 7:00 A.M. and a bedtime around 7:00 P.M. for the preschool child (Figure 9.1*A*) and 11:00 P.M. for the adolescent (Figure 9.1*B*).

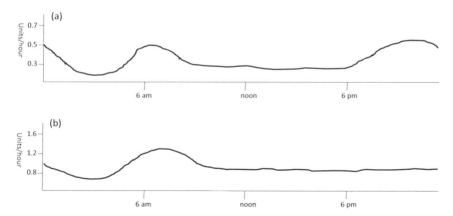

Figure 9.1. Schematic representation of insulin pump basal rate pattern in a) pre-pubertal children, and b) post-pubertal children.

Another important consideration in optimizing basal rates is the ratio of basal insulin to the total daily dose (TDD) of insulin, which includes all boluses for all meals. In a typical young adult with long-standing T1D, total basal insulin represents 40–50% of TDD, whereas in a typical infant with T1D, the basal insulin may be as low as 20–25% of TDD. These ratios progressively change throughout childhood, with a gradually increasing percentage of basal insulin before reaching the typical 45% of TDD in young adults. Once again, individual goals must take into account any exceptions in lifestyle; illnesses; concomitant medications; and, importantly, dietary restrictions, such as low carbohydrate diets, which significantly increase the basal insulin ratio to 60% or higher. The opposite is often true in midteen adolescents during their peak growth spurt when they consume relatively large amounts of carbohydrates rendering the ratio of basal to TDD insulin much lower in these individuals.

- ICR: This value represents the estimated amount of insulin required to cover a certain amount of carbohydrates consumed. A typical ratio is 1 unit of insulin for every 10–15 g of carbohydrates. There is generally a higher requirement of insulin for carbohydrates in the mornings, because of the relative resistance to insulin during the early morning hours. This is true for most children who have an ICR of 1:10 for breakfast and 1:15 for the rest of the day. Interestingly, it has been our experience that ICRs change very little across all ages of children with diabetes, averaging around 1:10 to 1:25, with the exception of midpubertal children who may require much higher doses of insulin with ratios as low as 1:3 and 1:5 g of carbohydrates.
- ISF: Also referred to as the high BG correction factor, this represents the predicted decrease in BG level by a dose of 1 unit of insulin (on top of the basal rate being delivered). This setting is used by the bolus calculator and must be individualized for each patient. Unlike the ICR which is somewhat constant across all ages, the ISF varies dramatically for each age-group, with the youngest infants being most sensitive, having an ISF of up to 500 (1 unit of insulin can decrease BG levels by 500 mg/dL) or more, whereas the most resistant midteen adolescents having an ISF of 20–30 (1 unit of insulin decreases BG levels by only 20–30 mg/dL) or even less in extremely obese individuals. An important consideration, especially in young children, is the fact that their sensitivity can vary at different times of the day, with their highest sensitivity occurring at ~1–3 A.M. (which correlates with the lower basal requirements at that time), making it necessary to set different ISF for nighttime versus daytime.
- Insulin duration time or insulin action time: This is an arbitrary setting that is programmed in the pump settings by the users, which allows the bolus calculator to anticipate any potential further decrease in BG because of a residual effect from the last bolus of insulin given within the estimated action time. Most rapid-acting insulins have an action duration time of 3–4 h, with higher doses lasting longer, and very small doses such as 0.5–1 units having a duration time of 2–2.5 h. Note that different pumps use different algorithms to calculate the estimated residual insulin action from the last bolus dose; therefore, this setting must be individualized and adjusted if a patient changes pumps and as they grow and require much larger doses of insulin.

Following these initial steps, we recommend that families return to clinic at 2 weeks then at 4–6 weeks after their pump start, before returning to their routine visit schedule every 2–3 months. It is highly encouraged that pump and CGM data be uploaded for review by the family and by their clinicians on a monthly basis.

Taking a "Pump Vacation"

It is not unusual for children of any age who are using an insulin pump to request a vacation from their pump, either because they're just tired of having a pump, or to accommodate for vacation and travel time, especially if it involves prolonged water activities. In these cases, it is good to set a time limit after which the child is expected to return to pump use. There are two different ways to manage diabetes while disconnected from the pump: *1*) return to using MDI for all insulin doses, or *2*) use one or two injections of long-acting insulin to replace the basal insulin infusion, while still using the pump to deliver boluses of insulin by intermittently connecting the pump back for a few minutes at a time. The latter approach is more favorable because it takes advantage of using the pump calculator for more precise dosing. In either scenario, the dose of long-acting insulin to be taken by injections is equivalent to the amount of missed basal insulin that would have been delivered via the pump.

CGM IN CHILDREN WITH DIABETES

The past 5 years have brought significant advances in CGM technology. Currently available CGM devices measure interstitial glucose concentrations every 1–5-min, mostly without interference by concomitant medications or substances and without the need for calibration. Glucose readings can be transmitted in real time or can be collected for retrospective review and analysis (blinded CGM, also referred to as professional CGM). Real-time CGMs display BG values every 5 min and can sound an alarm when glucose levels reach predefined thresholds to alert for hypoglycemia and hyperglycemia as well as for rapid glycemic excursions. In contrast, a flash glucose monitor provides a glucose reading to a reader or a smartphone when the user desires to see the BG value. Flash glucose monitors do not currently provide any alerts.

One implantable sensor that lasts up to 6 months (3 months in the U.S.) has been recently developed. It transmits data to a dedicated receiver that must be worn over the skin in proximity to the implanted sensor. Implantation and removal of the sensor require a minor surgical procedure by trained clinical staff.

With these advances, CGM use is rapidly becoming a standard of care and must be offered to all people with diabetes, and some argue, even for children with T2D who are not yet on insulin therapy. In fact, most insurance plans currently provide coverage for CGM in children, and many get their CGM devices before they get their pumps approved. Despite this, it is estimated that only about half of the children with T1D in the U.S. use a CGM.

Unlike pump training and initiation, CGM sensors can be easily self-applied by most people, after viewing provided instructional videos. The data provided by CGM often can be overwhelming to the patients, however, resulting in increased anxiety, too many alarms, and a negative initial experience, particularly during school time. It is highly advisable that patients and families discuss the use of the CGM with their healthcare providers (HCPs) before they start. This opportunity lets families set conservative parameters and thresholds for the alarms and reasonable expectations for the benefits from CGM. It is our experience that the learning curve for optimal use of CGM data may take several months and should be done with guidance from the diabetes healthcare team.

In addition to the use of real-time data to guide insulin dosing for patients, the data collected by CGM devices provides crucial opportunities for patients and clinicians to optimize insulin therapy and pump settings, to reduce A1C and to increase time spent in the ideal BG target range, while also reducing hypoglycemia. The following sections discuss the value of a retrospective data review and provide practical recommendations based on our clinical experience.

RETROSPECTIVE USE OF DIABETES DEVICE DATA

Purpose of a Retrospective Data Review

Although the real-time uses of information presented by insulin pump and CGM are important for moment-to-moment diabetes management decisions, a retrospective review of data patterns and trends is essential for understanding the big picture, planning to avoid extremes in glucose levels, and optimize care and health outcomes. This process of data review can be done by the HCP or the person with diabetes. A few studies have suggested that data review is related to improved outcomes in children with T1D. In one study of children using insulin pumps, those whose parents uploaded their data to a software program at home, which was then reviewed remotely by the healthcare team, had improvement in HbA_{1c}, as compared to those who did not have access to or did not use the software.[13] In a randomized controlled study of both children and adults who were pump users, those who used data-uploading software had a decrease in average HbA_{1c}, whereas those who did not use the software had no change.[14] In both of these studies, data were reviewed by the healthcare team, and it is not known whether the patients or their parents reviewed the glucose data after uploading. Prior studies of participants in the DCCT showed that those who reviewed their own data and made self-adjustments based on glucose patterns had lower HbA_{1c}.[15] We have also shown that average HbA_{1c} is lower in people with diabetes who report uploading and reviewing their diabetes data routinely at home.[16] The importance of retrospectively reviewing data from insulin pumps and CGM has been recognized by experts and professional societies and should be a critical part of diabetes management.[17,18]

What can be done with the information obtained from insulin pumps and CGM systems? First, review of glucose data patterns can help with adjustment of insulin regimens (basal insulin or basal rates, ICRs, ISFs, or glucose targets). Second, data review can help the HCP and patient understand the impact of different food choices, exercise, illness, or other stresses on glucose levels and sensitivity to insulin. For CGM users, data review will reveal overnight glucose patterns, including previously unrecognized hypoglycemia, or evidence of an inadequately treated dawn phenomenon. In addition, although it may seem that retrospective data review may not be necessary with hybrid closed-loop (HCL) systems, in fact, data review is just as important with these systems to understand insulin needs and to troubleshoot problems, such as the ability to stay in auto mode. The rest of this chapter will provide a guide to approaching diabetes device data and using it to perform these essential tasks.

The Data: How to Get It and What to Do with It

Many pediatric diabetes practices review device data as a part of a standard diabetes patient visit. To do this, the diabetes HCP or office staff uploads the data from glucose meters, insulin pumps, and CGM devices to data visualization software at the clinic. In some cases, the clinic may request that the family upload data at home and provide the clinic with access to the data or bring printed downloaded data to the visit. Historically, and in many practices today, uploading has been done using data management software designed by the device manufacturer, which is only compatible with that manufacturer's devices. HCPs and patients alike, however, are challenged by the need to use and learn to understand a different software program for each of their different brands of devices, which in many cases prevent the data from being viewed together in an integrated fashion. To simplify this process, a few tools have been developed to integrate diabetes device data from multiple, discrete sources. These tools include the Glooko clinician platform and patient mobile application[19] and the Tidepool platform for the uploading and visualization of diabetes data.[20] These software tools help address the need for interoperability of diabetes device software, which can help HCPs overcome obstacles to data review, including the need to become familiar with one uploading system and one unified software interface.[21,22]

Insulin Pump Data

Regardless of brand or management software that is used, there is a rich, and initially seemingly complex, set of data that can be reviewed from insulin pumps. These data include information on current insulin pump settings; frequency and timing of insulin boluses and carbohydrates entered; amount of insulin used for basal rates and boluses; and use of advanced features, such as using alternate basal rate profiles, temporary basal rates, or extended or split boluses. The following are some examples of how these data may be used to gain insight on current diabetes management and assist the provider in making recommendations for the future.

- Total daily dose (TDD): For pediatric patients, review and trending of the total daily dose (in units/kg/day) is important in understanding insulin needs and insulin sensitivity. For children who are recently diagnosed with T1D, a significant increase in TDD may indicate the end of the honeymoon period and the need to be more aggressive with insulin dosing. Similarly, as a child approaches and progresses through puberty, their TDD will increase as insulin needs increase (up to 2 units/kg/day). Reviewing TDD in a growing preadolescent or adolescent can enable providers to be proactive about anticipating increased needs, guiding conversations with the family to expect higher glucose values and recommending more frequent data review and insulin adjustments. This has the potential to lessen the typical rise in HbA_{1c} seen during the teen years.
- Percent basal/bolus: In general, the amount of the total basal insulin required by most children is around 30–50% of their TDD,[8] as discussed above.[17] If the proportion of basal insulin is much greater than 50%, this may be an indicator of *1*) basal rates that are too high, *2*) ICR or ISFs that are not strong enough, or *3*) missed boluses for carbohydrates or high

glucose corrections, the latter of which is not uncommon in adolescents or children transitioning to more independent management who may be receiving most of their insulin through basal rates because of missed boluses.

- Frequency of glucose checks and correction boluses: The pump history will include any glucose data manually entered from a glucose meter or CGM reading, and any glucose data automatically transferred from a connected meter. Whether from a meter or a CGM device, entry of glucose values into the pump shows that the child and family are aware of glucose levels, and if most glucose entries are followed by use of pump bolus calculators and delivery of insulin boluses, this is a sign that they are responding to the information. If there are very few glucose entries per day, or in total, this might initiate a conversation about the obstacles or barriers to either checking a glucose level with the meter or using the CGM device and may help guide management strategies to increase monitoring and delivery of bolus insulin to avoid hyperglycemia. The provider might note the frequency of insulin boluses delivered without a glucose entry or without using the pump bolus calculator (i.e., frequency of using manual boluses). The glucose patterns following the manual bolus should also be noted: Is the patient "over-bolusing," resulting in hypoglycemia, or "under-bolusing," resulting in persistent hyperglycemia? This information may help direct the conversation about whether use of manual boluses is appropriate for this patient in the particular scenario.
- Carbohydrates: The amount and frequency of carbohydrates entered into the pump is incredibly helpful. From a nutritional perspective, reviewing the typical amount of carbohydrates per meal and the average amount of carbohydrates per day can indicate whether the child is receiving an appropriate amount of carbohydrates. Too few carbohydrates entered might suggest that the child or family is restricting necessary carbohydrates or that the child is missing boluses for actual carbohydrates eaten (in which case, glucose patterns would reveal frequent hyperglycemia). A large excess of carbohydrates may indicate overnutrition. Further discussion with the child, however, may reveal that they have noticed that their glucose levels have been higher or that their glucose levels are not decreasing appropriately in response to the current regimen. The child then may be reacting by entering in "fake carbohydrates" to bolus and receive more insulin.
- Frequency of set changes: Depending on the type of infusion set used, most pump users should be changing their infusion set (or patch pump) every 2–3 days. Each pump brand has a different way of indicating a change in their uploaded data. If the child has too many days between set changes, this might initiate a conversation about why and the benefits of changing the site. If the family is changing the set too frequently (every 1–2 days), this could result in a discussion about ways to troubleshoot getting the set or patch pump to stay in place.
- Pump suspensions: The frequency and duration of pump suspensions should be reviewed with pump users during their visits. Providers should take note of short suspensions for bathing or showering or for short activities

or sports. Longer suspensions (for >60 min) for sports and activities should be reviewed carefully, and any hyperglycemia that follows suspensions should prompt discussions about proper management. This might include encouraging the child to briefly check glucose levels and to reconnect the pump to give a bolus, if needed, during the suspension period. It might also lead to the recommendation to give a small dose of basal insulin by injection to cover basal needs during the time at which the pump is suspended for an extended period of time.

- Temporary basal rates: Families of children with T1D may use temporary basal rates for a number of different reasons. They may increase their basal rates in the case of fever or illness, during growth spurts, or in relation to menstrual periods. Basal rates can be decreased with, or after, rigorous physical activity, with gastrointestinal illness and poor carbohydrate intake or absorption, or with changes in the overall activity level. Frequent use of temporary basal rates may indicate that programmed basal rates or other ratios need to be adjusted.

CGM Data

Families living with children with T1D tend to highly value the real-time functions of CGM, including high or low alerts, the decreased number of finger-stick glucose checks with nonadjunctive use with certain sensors, and the use of features that allow parents to remotely view their child's CGM data in real time. Reviewing and understanding retrospective CGM data with the HCP, however, is just as important as adjusting insulin regimens and making management decisions. Typically, a review of 10–14 days of recent CGM data is needed to identify overall patterns and trends, along with a detailed review of 5–7 days to look at the effects of specific meals, activity, or insulin doses on glucose levels. Decisions should not be made on just 1 day of data or on just a single occurrence of a particular glucose pattern. Essential elements of CGM data to review include the amount of time spent in, above, and below target range as well as trends and patterns overnight, after meals, after correction boluses, and after treatment of low glucose values.

- Time in target, hyperglycemic, and hypoglycemic ranges: The time in various ranges can be described as a percentage of glucose readings or in terms of hours per day. The "target" range has been proposed to be 70–180 mg/dL.[23] Although time in target range is becoming more widely accepted as an outcome measure, no studies have correlated time in range with long-term outcomes.[18,23] Nevertheless, review of time in range, time in hyperglycemic range, and time in hypoglycemic range can provide an understanding of the fluctuations in glucose levels better than the average glucose or A1C. A larger percentage of time in hyperglycemic range (i.e., greater than the time in target range) may indicate fear of hypoglycemia, inadequate insulin doses (basal or bolus), or missed boluses. If the CGM data show a large percentage of time (>10%) in hypoglycemic range, this might suggest that the patient has hypoglycemia unawareness, insulin treatment is too aggressive, or plans need to be made to adjust for physical activity.

- Overnight trends: The period of time between when the child goes to bed and wakes up is a critical time in which to evaluate CGM data. Rise in glucose levels after bedtime may result from inadequate basal rates; some children experience increased insulin resistance and increased needs due to nocturnal surges in growth hormone that can occur a couple hours after going to sleep), which may explain the dawn phenomenon.[24] Alternatively, families may be inadequately bolusing for high glucose levels at bedtime—for fear of overnight hypoglycemia—by giving smaller correction doses, underriding recommended pump boluses, or setting ISFs that are too weak. Similarly, they may be allowing the child to eat extra carbohydrates at bedtime without adequate insulin coverage, leading to rises in glucose levels overnight. Another common cause of nighttime hyperglycemia is delayed absorption of heavier dinner meals, such as pizza or pasta, which may take several hours to completely digest and require a long extended bolus at dinner time.

The opposite also may be true, in which review of overnight CGM data reveals frequent hypoglycemia, which may be due to basal rates that are too strong or overcorrecting for high glucoses or carbohydrates at bedtime. In addition, overnight hypoglycemia may be due to higher levels of activity earlier in the day. The effects of physical activity may last many hours after the activity has concluded, often increasing insulin sensitivity well into the evening and overnight period. CGM patterns of overnight hypoglycemia may prompt a discussion about exercise and physical activity and lead to preexercise management recommendations (i.e., using temporary basal rates during and for a number of hours after exercise).

- Patterns after meals: Postprandial CGM patterns can help determine whether mealtime boluses are adequate. Postmeal rises in glucose levels can be due to ICRs that are not strong enough; inaccurate carbohydrate counting and entry; or bolusing for carbohydrates after, instead of before, the meal. Postprandial hyperglycemia should prompt a discussion about carbohydrate counting, how doses are determined, and the timing of the insulin bolus in relation to the meal. Discussion should include if and when the patient has higher fat meals (i.e., pizza) and review of the CGM patterns after these types of meals. Immediate postprandial hypoglycemia followed by hyperglycemia may indicate the need for extended or square-wave boluses or combo or split boluses.
- Patterns after correction boluses (no carbohydrates): CGM patterns that occur after insulin boluses given for a high glucose, in the absence of carbohydrates, should be reviewed to discern whether boluses given are appropriate. Patterns of high glucoses after correction boluses suggest that ISFs are inadequate or perhaps that the patient may be giving less insulin than recommended due to their fear of hypoglycemia. Conversely, CGM patterns may reveal dramatic drops in glucose levels after correction boluses, perhaps even to the hypoglycemic range. This should prompt discussion about whether the family is giving more insulin than recommended (possibly to try to make the high glucose level go down more quickly) or potentially to weaken ISFs. A rapid response and hypoglycemia following a correction bolus might also be due to the effects of exercise earlier in the

day, and a pattern of low glucoses after correction boluses should include a discussion of physical activity before the hypoglycemic episodes. Another benefit of reviewing CGM data after high BG correction doses at night (in the absence of any food) is the ability to calculate the average decrease in BG after each bolus, which can lead to a more accurate determination of the true ISF for each patient.

- Response to treatment of low glucose: In children, it is not at all unusual to find patterns of glucoses higher than target range, following episodes of hypoglycemia. This may be due to the caregiver's concern (and possible fear) of hypoglycemia, and the instinct to treat the low glucose with more fast-acting carbohydrates than necessary to rapidly bring the glucose level into the normal range. Many children then "inherit" these behavioral tendencies from their caregivers, because that is how they are used to treating hypoglycemia. It is important to review the CGM patterns following episodes of hypoglycemia to determine if the family is overtreating low glucose levels. Discussion should focus on the appropriate actions in response to a low glucose, including the amount of carbohydrates to give (based on both the actual glucose level and the direction of the trend arrows) and the use of temporary basal rates when glucose levels trend downward. Another important benefit of reviewing response to treatment of low BG is the ability to estimate the typical rise in BG after consumption of each gram of fast-acting carbohydrate, which can help the family estimate how much juice or glucose tablets they should use to treat a typical episode of hypoglycemia. It is not uncommon for parents to overtreat low BG in a toddler with 10–15 g of juice, while 2–4 g may be sufficient to increase the BG >150 mg/dL.

In general, we find that when pump and CGM data are integrated into a single display, the review process is much more effective because of the visual impact of the CGM tracings, which make the information more intuitive than abstract discussions of numbers and hypothetical scenarios.

CONCLUSION

This chapter provides general recommendations based on data in the literature and on our own experience in a large pediatric diabetes center where we promote a higher rate of technology use in our patients. We strongly emphasize the need for individualization of diabetes management for every child and family affected by diabetes, and the importance of reviewing and analyzing diabetes device data to optimize insulin regimen for each individual patient.

REFERENCES

1.   White NH, Cleary PA, Dahms W, et al. Diabetes Control and Complications Trial (DCCT)/Epidemiology of Diabetes Interventions and Complications (EDIC) Research Group. Beneficial effects of intensive therapy of diabetes during adolescence: outcomes after the conclusion of the Diabetes Control and Complications Trial (DCCT). *J Pediatr* 2001;139(6):804–812

2. The Diabetes Control and Complications Trial Research Group. The effect of intensive therapy of diabetes on the development and progression of long-term complications in insulin-dependent diabetes mellitus. *N Engl J Med* 1993;329:977–986

3. Danne T, Nimri R, Battelino T, et al. International consensus on use of continuous glucose monitoring. *Diabetes Care* 2017;40(12):1631–1640

4. Fuld K, Conrad B, Buckingham B, Wilson DM. Insulin pumps in young children. *Diabetes Technol Ther* 2010;12(Suppl 1.):S67–S71

5. Bode BW, Kaufman FR, Vint N. An expert opinion on advanced insulin pump use in youth with type 1 diabetes. *Diabetes Technol Ther* 2017;19(3):145–154

6. Adi S. Type 1 diabetes mellitus in adolescents. *Adolesc Med State Art Rev* 2010; 21(1):86–102

7. Eugster EA, Francis G. Position statement: Continuous subcutaneous insulin infusion in very young children with type 1 diabetes. *Pediatrics* 2006;118(4): e1244–1249

8. Phillip M, Battelino T, Rodriguez H, et al. Use of insulin pump therapy in the pediatric age-group: consensus statement from the European Society for Paediatric Endocrinology, the Lawson Wilkins Pediatric Endocrine Society, and the International Society for Pediatric and Adolescent Diabetes, endorsed by the American Diabetes Association and the European Association for the Study of Diabetes. *Diabetes Care* 2007;30(6):1653–1662

9. Sherr J, Tamborlane WV. Past, present, and future of insulin pump therapy: better shot at diabetes control. *Mt Sinai J Med NY* 2008;75(4):352–361

10. Grunberger G, Abelseth JM, Bailey TS, et al. Consensus Statement by the American Association of Clinical Endocrinologists/American College of Endocrinology Insulin Pump Management Task Force. *Endocr Pract Off J Am Coll Endocrinol Am Assoc Clin Endocrinol* 2014;20(5):463–489

11. Barnard KD, Lloyd CE, Skinner TC. Systematic literature review: quality of life associated with insulin pump use in type 1 diabetes. *Diabet Med J Br Diabet Assoc* 2007;24(6):607–617

12. Brancato D, Fleres M, Aiello V, et al. The effectiveness and durability of an early insulin pump therapy in children and adolescents with type 1 diabetes mellitus. *Diabetes Technol Ther* 2014;16(11):735–741

13. Corriveau EA, Durso PJ, Kaufman ED, et al. Effect of CareLink, an internet-based insulin pump monitoring system, on glycemic control in rural and urban children with type 1 diabetes mellitus. *Pediatr Diabetes* 2008;9(4 Pt. 2):360–366

14. Shalitin S, Ben-Ari T, Yackobovitch-Gavan M, et al. Using the Internet-based upload blood glucose monitoring and therapy management system in patients with type 1 diabetes. *Acta Diabetol* 2014;51(2):247–256

15. Pearson J, Bergenstal R. Fine-tuning control: pattern management versus supplementation: View 1: pattern management: an essential component of effective insulin management. *Diabetes Spectr* 2001;14(2):75–78

16. Wong JC, Neinstein AB, Spindler M, Adi S. A minority of patients with type 1 diabetes routinely downloads and retrospectively reviews device data. *Diabetes Technol Ther* 2015;17(8):555–562

17. Scheiner G. CGM retrospective data analysis. *Diabetes Technol Ther* 2016; 18(S2):S2-14-22

18. Fonseca VA, Grunberger G, Anhalt H, et al. Continuous glucose monitoring: a consensus conference of the American Association of Clinical Endocrinologists and American College of Endocrinology. *Endocr Pract Off J Am Coll Endocrinol Am Assoc Clin Endocrinol* 2016;22(8):1008–1021

19. Clements MA, Staggs VS. A mobile app for synchronizing glucometer data: impact on adherence and glycemic control among youths with type 1 diabetes in routine care. *J Diabetes Sci Technol* 2017;11(3):461–467

20. Neinstein A, Wong J, Look H, et al. A case study in open source innovation: developing the Tidepool Platform for interoperability in type 1 diabetes management. *J Am Med Inform Assoc* 2016;23(2):324–332

21. Picton PE, Yeung M, Hamming N, et al. Advancement of the artificial pancreas through the development of interoperability standards. *J Diabetes Sci Technol* 2013;7(4):1066–1070

22. Silk AD. Diabetes device interoperability for improved diabetes management. *J Diabetes Sci Technol* 2016;10(1):175–177

23. Agiostratidou G, Anhalt H, Ball D, et al. Standardizing clinically meaningful outcome measures beyond HbA$_{1c}$ for type 1 diabetes: a consensus report of the American Association of Clinical Endocrinologists, the American Association of Diabetes Educators, the American Diabetes Association, the Endocrine Society, JDRF International, The Leona M. and Harry B. Helmsley Charitable Trust, the Pediatric Endocrine Society, and the T1D Exchange. *Diabetes Care* 2017;40(12):1622–1630

24. Edge JA, Matthews DR, Dunger DB. The dawn phenomenon is related to overnight growth hormone release in adolescent diabetics. *Clin Endocrinol (Oxf)* 1990;33(6):729–737

Chapter 10

Physical Activity, Sport, and Recreation with Insulin Pumps and Continuous Glucose Monitoring

Sheri R. Colberg, PhD, FACSM,[1] and Gary Scheiner, MS, CDE[2]

INTRODUCTION

It is well established that most people with type 1 diabetes (T1D)—whether they are youth or adults—can benefit physically and mentally from engaging in regular physical activities, including planned exercise, sports, and other recreation.[1,2] In fact, most of the health benefits that are available to all individuals also arise from being active with diabetes of any type, including an improved cardiovascular disease risk profile, body composition, functional capacity, and quality of life.

Managing blood glucose, particularly in individuals who use insulin, is highly complex. Although population studies yield inconsistent results in terms of the glycemic benefits of exercise in individuals with T1D, it is generally accepted that physical activity improves insulin sensitivity and leads to lower insulin requirements.[3] Furthermore, properly *timed* exercise can reduce postprandial glycemic excursions.

For those who take exogenous insulin, it is critical that physical activities are balanced with appropriate adjustments to food, insulin, or both. Managing blood glucose levels during exercise is essential for personal safety as well as for optimal physical performance. Of course, keeping blood glucose at or near optimal levels with physical activity is an added variable that frequently is easier said than done. The good news is that some of the latest diabetes management technologies can help guide people in making more informed and effective regimen change decisions.[4] Thus, the purpose of this chapter is to discuss how the body responds to various forms of physical activity; which adjustments must be made to keep blood glucose in balance; and how diabetes technologies may be used to enhance blood glucose management before, during, and after physical activities.

MANAGING BLOOD GLUCOSE WITH PHYSICAL ACTIVITY

It is no small feat to keep blood glucose at normal or close to normal levels when physical activity itself can exert effects on glycemic balance. During exercise, the body's normal physiological response is to reduce levels of circulating insulin. Unfortunately, injected insulin is only delivered peripherally instead of into the portal vein (as would be the case in someone without T1D), and its absorption from the skin may be enhanced during exercise, raising peripheral levels. Given that

[1]Professor Emerita, Old Dominion University, Norfolk, VA. [2]Owner and Clinical Director, Integrated Diabetes Services, LLC, Wynnewood, PA.

insulin and muscle contractions induce uptake of blood glucose into muscles through separate but additive mechanisms, the inability to lower circulating insulin during exercise is a leading cause of hypoglycemia.

Factors Affecting Glycemic Responses to Activity

Many different factors can potentially affect how blood glucose levels respond when someone with T1D is physically active (Figure 10.1). These factors include the intensity, duration, and timing of exercise as well as other bodily and environmental concerns. For example, vigorous activities may lead to a rise in blood glucose levels because of an immediate, exaggerated release of glucoregulatory hormones like epinephrine, norepinephrine, and glucagon, along with a later release of cortisol and growth hormone during more intense workouts. Duration has an effect as well, particularly given that longer activities typically lead to a greater reliance on blood glucose as a fuel and a decrease in blood glucose over time during the activity.

Furthermore, the timing of activities can be impactful. Aerobic exercise usually decreases blood glucose levels,[5] especially when exercise coincides with peak insulin activity or for long periods of time.[6,7] Conversely, doing physical activity during fasting conditions in the early morning typically results in more stable glycemia, with less of a decline or even a small increase in overall levels.[8] Thus, it is likely that different sports and activities will require individualized adjustments to food intake and insulin dosing during and after exercise.

General Recommendations for Managing Glycemia during Activities

The responses to physical activity are so individualized and variable that making uniform recommendations for regimen changes is nearly impossible. Limited studies, however, have attempted to do so, and their recommendations follow:

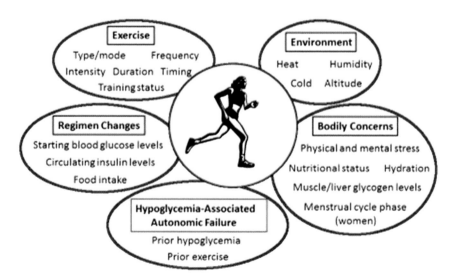

Figure 10.1. Factors affecting exercise blood glucose responses.

- In general, individuals will need to increase their carbohydrate intake or reduce circulating insulin levels for aerobic activities.[9]
- For low- to moderate-intensity aerobic activities lasting 30–60 min during fasting or with only basal insulin on board, individuals may need only 10–15 g of carbohydrate to prevent hypoglycemia.[4]
- When active after taking a bolus insulin dose, they may need more in the range of 30–60 g of carbohydrate per hour.[10,11]
- In some cases, it may be possible for exercisers to reduce their insulin dosing by 25–75% and either reduce or completely eliminate their need to take in additional food or carbohydrate to prevent hypoglycemia during exercise.[12]

Preventing Exercise-Induced Hypoglycemia and Hyperglycemia

One of the biggest deterrents to engaging in physical activity, particularly insulin users, is fear of hypoglycemia.[13] A number of strategies can lower the risk of delayed-onset hypoglycemia, such as lowering basal insulin doses, eating a slowly digesting snack, and frequent monitoring of blood glucose levels. In addition, a variety of low-technology techniques have been undertaken to lower the risk of its occurrence, such as using short sprints to raise blood glucose, performing resistance exercise before aerobic exercise done in the same workout, and exercising when insulin levels are at their lowest.[14–16] Delayed-onset hypoglycemia, however—frequently occurring during the night following exhaustive daytime exercise—remains a major concern.[17] Most hypoglycemia happens within 6–15 h after a workout,[18] but the risk can last up to 48 h.

On the flipside, intense activities like sprinting,[15] brief but intense aerobic exercise,[19] and heavy powerlifting[20] may promote an abrupt rise in glycemia. It may be possible to better manage or prevent exercise-induced hyperglycemia with dosing of additional insulin, along with interspersing moderate aerobic activity between intense bouts, or doing a low-intensity cooldown following more vigorous workouts.[21]

TECHNOLOGIES AND STRATEGIES TO ASSIST GLYCEMIC MANAGEMENT

Managing glucose levels during and after exercise requires cutting-edge tools, utilized in a skillful manner. For example, the ability to fine-tune basal and bolus insulin places patients in a position to achieve greater success. Having more frequent feedback on glycemic levels and trends also may lead to better exercise management.

Insulin Pump Features and Exercise Strategies

Insulin pumps give their users the opportunity to reduce basal insulin levels or bolus doses in desired amounts and for desired durations. As a result, pump use may reduce exercise-induced hypoglycemia risk compared to multiple daily injections.[22] The following strategies using pump features may be helpful, based on the purpose and timing of insulin dosing:

- Bolus doses: Meal and correction doses of rapid- or short-acting insulin may be adjusted with a high degree of accuracy to accommodate for exercise. In most cases, it is best to calculate boluses as usual (entering the actual carbohydrates and blood glucose), and then to adjust the pump's recommendation by a percentage. For postmeal activity (i.e., taking place starting when bolus insulin is still at peak levels, such as within 2 h after administration), the bolus is commonly reduced by 25%, 33%, or 50%, depending on the nature of the exercise. Users need to make this adjustment on their own as current pumps sold in the U.S. do not offer this feature. (The Accu-Chek Combo pump by Roche, marketed primarily in Europe, does offer this feature.)

- Use of temporary basal rates: Reductions in basal rates of pump insulin delivery can prevent hypoglycemia and reduce the quantity or frequency of supplemental carbohydrates, particularly during prolonged physical activities lasting ≥2 h. This feature is available in all insulin pumps, although it may be necessary to specify that the adjustments be made in percentages rather than in units per hour. It is important that the temporary basal reduction be made in advance (1–2 h) of the onset of activity so that the insulin active in the bloodstream is reduced during early stages of exercise. A reduction of 50% is a common starting point, although intense or prolonged exercise may require a greater percentage (as much as 80%).

- Post-exercise temporary basal reductions: Lowering basal insulin following physical activity can be useful for preventing delayed-onset hypoglycemia. These types of events are common following prolonged or intense exercise during which muscle glycogen is largely depleted. The exact amount and timing of basal reductions will vary from person to person and by situation. A common starting point is to reduce the basal rate by 25% for 6–8 h whenever delayed hypoglycemia is anticipated.

- Alternate basal patterns (or insulin delivery profiles): Altered delivery patterns can be used whenever full-day activity is expected, such as during summer camp, engaging in intense sports conditioning, or while completing major projects around the home. In cases like these, the user may switch to a basal pattern that is entirely different from the usual one. Rates can be reduced significantly during periods of peak physical activity, and more modestly during postactivity recovery periods. With pumps that allow the user to alter bolus calculation formulas along with basal settings (insulin delivery profiles), such as the Tandem pump, it may be prudent to use a reduced hyperglycemia correction factor to decrease the insulin-to-carbohydrate ratio, and raise the target glucose level during times of enhanced insulin sensitivity.

Case Study 1: Kelly Uses an Insulin Pump. Kelly, age 11 and T1D since age 8, just completed her second summer at gymnastics camp. During the first summer, she experienced frequent bouts of hypoglycemia during the day and a severe episode overnight that required the camp nurse to administer glucagon. Her hypoglycemic events often were followed by rebound hyperglycemia that took several hours to correct. To avoid a repeat of those experiences, Kelly utilized a secondary basal insulin program on her pump to help prevent hypoglycemia during the second summer. Her daytime settings (during peak activity times) were reduced by 50%, and her overnight settings were reduced by 25% to compensate for heightened insulin sensitivity that followed a full day of physical activity, as shown in Table 10.1.

Table 10.1. Case Study 1

	Usual basal rates (u/h)	Camp basal rates (u/h)
12 A.M.–5 A.M.	0.40	0.30
5 A.M.–8 A.M.	0.35	0.25
8 A.M.–8 P.M.	0.30	0.15
8 P.M.–12 A.M.	0.60	0.45

Kelly was also taught to reduce her meal boluses before intense conditioning exercises. As a result, her second summer at camp was a huge success with regard to her diabetes management. During the 3-week camp, she experienced only two mild bouts of hypoglycemia, which were easily corrected with a small amount of carbohydrate, and she had no overnight events. She reported feeling more energetic and "in control," and is eager to return to camp next summer.

Challenges Associated with Insulin Pump during Exercise

Insulin pump use presents its own set of challenges related to physical activity and sports. For instance, some athletes have issues with getting infusion sets to stay in place during certain activities or with excessive sweating. Others have complained that the pump or tubing simply gets in the way during exercise, and they may prefer to remove the pump entirely while active. Given that pumps deliver rapid-acting insulins only, removal of the pump for an excessive length of time (typically >1 h) can result in severe hyperglycemia and ketone formation, potentially leading to diabetic ketoacidosis. Exposing pumps to water and extreme weather conditions can also threaten the integrity of the pump, as well as the insulin contained therein. Table 10.2 contains some strategies that can minimize these types of issues.

Continuous Glucose Monitoring Devices

A number of different real-time continuous glucose monitoring (CGM) systems now have approval from the U.S. Food and Drug Administration (see Table 10.3) and may be covered by insurance providers (at least for insulin users with T1D). Over time, these devices have increased in accuracy and some have been approved for use in place of finger-stick glucose monitoring when determining appropriate regimen changes. Providing nearly continuous feedback (every 5 min) on blood glucose before starting activities, as well as during and after participation, CGM devices may lower the risk of developing exercise-induced hypoglycemia and track patterns that allow users to optimize glucose control during and after physical activity.[23,24]

"Flash" glucose monitoring is a recent development, possessing some but not all of the features of traditional CGM. Flash monitors provide instantaneous glucose values and recent trending information, but they lack the alerts that notify users when glucose levels may be heading high or low. CGM and flash monitors can be used to enhance the exercise experience in a variety of ways:

Table 10.2. Insulin Pump Challenges and Potential Solutions

Challenge	Potential solutions
Water damage	• Use a fully waterproof pump • Disconnect from pump while in the water • Switch to injection plan for the day

Extreme temperatures	• In frigid weather, keep pump close to body
	• In extreme heat:
	   ○ Place pump in cooling pouch (Frio)
	   ○ Keep pump out of direct sunlight
	   ○ Change insulin reservoir frequently
	   ○ Switch to injection plan for the day

Inadequate adhesion	• Use overtape on infusion set • Place infusion set on less-susceptible area (buttocks, lower back) • Use adhesive aid prior to insertion (skin prep, mastisol)
Inconvenience	• Use tubeless patch pump (Omnipod) • Disconnect during activity, but reconnect hourly to replace missed basal insulin via bolus • Switch to injection plan for the day

- Glucose values before exercise can let the user know if extra carbohydrates or boluses are needed.
- Trending information before exercise can help the user make a more informed decision regarding the need for carbohydrate or insulin.
- High and low alerts during and after exercise can help the user avoid dangerous glucose extremes, particularly when alerts are set at preemptive or conservative levels.
- Reviewing downloaded trend graph reports can allow the user to detect patterns of dysglycemia during and after exercise, particularly when individuals use event markers or keep workout logs.

Case Study 2: Jessie Takes Multiple Daily Injections and Uses CGM. Jessie, age 33, T1D since age 15, uses the gym at her worksite for a 30-min workout on the elliptical machine on weekdays before eating lunch. This morning, her glucose level was unusually high after breakfast, so she took a correction dose of rapid-acting insulin.

Before her workout (at around 12:30 p.m.), she checked her blood glucose level on her meter, and it read 95 mg/dL. Her CGM, however, showed a higher reading with a rapid decline (the discrepancy likely the result of the lag time between CGM and finger-stick values, with CGM following behind). Ordinarily, with a glucose level of 95 mg/dL, she would consume 15 g of carbohydrate in the form of a granola bar before her workout. Because of the rapid decline, she consumed 30 g of carbohydrate in the form of juice instead and waited 15 min to give the juice a chance to reverse the downward trend in her blood glucose before beginning exercise (Figure 10.2).

Table 10.3. Available CGM Systems and Features

System	Features	Connections/Display Options
Dexcom G5 and G6	• Glucose values every 5 min • Rise and fall trending information • High- and low-glucose alerts • Data and alerts can be shared via phone app in real time • Integrated into open APS hybrid closed-loop system for automated basal insulin delivery (using Medtronic paradigm pump) • Sensors last 7 or 10 days • G5 requires calibration every 12 h; G6 model requires no calibration • Downloadable to multiple software options and web-based platforms	• Handheld receiver • Android and iOS smartphones • iPads • iWatch • Tandem X2 insulin pump • Animas Vibe insulin pump (older G4 model only)
Medtronic Guardian Connect	• Glucose values every 5 min • Rise and fall trending information • High and low alerts • Integrated into hybrid closed-loop system for automated basal insulin delivery (using Medtronic 670G pump) • Sensors last up to 7 days • Requires calibration every 12 h • Downloadable to Carelink software • Sugar.IQ program provides pattern recognition and feedback	• Guardian Connect smartphone app • Medtronic 670G insulin pump • Medtronic 630, 530, Revel pumps (Enlite sensor only)
FreeStyle Libre	• Glucose values every minute • Rise and fall trending information, but no real-time alerts available • 10-h warmup period • Sensors last for 14 days • Requires no calibration • Downloadable to LibreView software and LibreLink cellular phone app	• Handheld scanner • "Flash" monitoring by passing scanner over monitor • Readings on phone every 5 min using Ambrosia BluCon device with app
Senseonics Eversense	• Real-time glucose readings • Implanted fluorescence-based sensor (the size of a headphone connector) • Sensors last for 90 days (XL version approved for 180 days in Europe) • Sensor insertion and removal done by a physician • Rise and fall trending information • High- and low-glucose alerts • Day-long initial warmup period • Requires calibration every 12 h • Data easily transmittable to medical team via mobile app	• Smart transmitter worn on skin over implanted sensor • Mobile app (iOS or Android) for displaying glucose values, trends, and alerts on phone or other mobile device • App charts by day, week, 2 weeks, month, or quarter • Ability to enter events (food, insulin, activity, etc.) via app • On-body vibratory alerts as well as on-screen alerts • Bluetooth transmitter can be removed and recharged without discarding the sensor

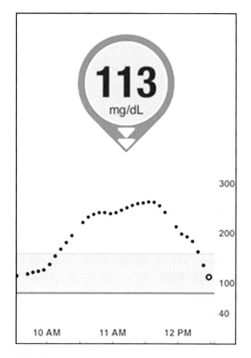

Figure 10.2. Case Study 2.

By taking the CGM's rate of change into account, Jessie was able to make a better preworkout decision and circumvent potential hypoglycemia during her exercise session. She finished her workout with a glucose level of 105 mg/dL and in a stable state going into lunch.

CGM CHALLENGES

CGM technology is not infallible. During exercise, CGM devices provide glucose readings that lag behind actual blood glucose values, simply because they measure interstitial levels of glucose in the subcutaneous fat rather than levels in the blood. CGM users may experience adhesion issues similar to those experienced by pump users. Other reported problems include accuracy issues,[25] sensor filament breakage, carrying the sensor display (using a watch to display sensor values can mitigate this problem), inability to calibrate during exercise,[24] and variable sensor performance. Anecdotally, exercisers have reported a "compression effect" when wearing the CGM sensor under compression shorts. This results in a greater lag time, presumably because of a reduced blood flow to skin in compressed areas.

Case Study 3: Rick Uses an Insulin Pump and CGM. Rick, age 64, T1 since age 21, is a self-employed realtor who enjoys bodybuilding. He performs intense strength training three mornings a week and lighter cardiovascular workouts the rest of the week, and he consumes a protein drink containing 30 g protein, 10 g carbohydrates, and 15 g fat before his weightlifting workouts with no insulin bolus. His blood glucose is usually in-range going into his workouts but often rises very high by the end. He feels that this is affecting his strength and wonders whether he should skip the protein drink. The printout in Figure 10.3 shows the CGM trend graphs from Rick's weight lifting days last week.

Rick has clearly been experiencing a sharp and significant glucose rise during his weightlifting workouts. His preworkout snack probably has little to do with this change given that its carbohydrate content is modest, and the absorption of the protein and fat would likely be delayed until well after the workout ended. He appears to be experiencing an adrenaline-induced glucose rise. To counter this, he was advised to bolus a small dose* of rapid-acting insulin 30 min before the onset of his workout and to titrate the dose upward until achieving satisfactory glucose levels during and after his workouts.

*Given his average glucose rise of 150 mg/dL and his usual correction factor of 50 mg/dL per unit, he was advised to begin with a 1.5-U bolus, which was 50% of the amount he usually needed to offset such a rise.

Hybrid Closed-Loop Systems

CGM devices currently are being paired with insulin pumps into closed-loop systems run by algorithms. They work most effectively when metabolic conditions are relatively stable, such as overnight during sleep. Effective use of a hybrid closed-loop system has the potential to produce more stable glucose control leading up to exercise than can be achieved with traditional means. The technological issues with CGM during exercise (such as the time lag and rapid changes in blood glucose) make these systems less helpful for managing glycemia during physical activities. Closed-loop systems have limited ability to prevent hypoglycemia during exercise because of their ability to make only miniscule adjustments to basal insulin. Users must continue to make their own food and bolus insulin adjustments before and during exercise. It is also necessary to actually wear the pump

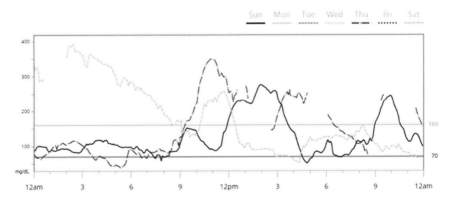

Figure 10.3. Case Study 3.

(without disconnecting) for the closed-loop algorithm to work during physical activity.

A number of strategies can be adopted that will enhance the use of such hybrid systems during physical activity. Effective strategies to manage such systems may include the following:

- If available, apply the temporary rise in blood glucose target at least 1 h before the scheduled activity: It takes at least this long for a change in basal delivery to effectively raise the glucose level. Consider switching the system to "manual" mode (i.e., turn off the self-adjustment algorithm) before and during exercise to allow full use of temporary basal rates and manual bolus overrides. When switching to manual mode during exercise, activate low-threshold suspend features to prevent hypoglycemia. Users must do this each time when switching from auto mode to manual mode.
- Override the pump's bolus recommendation prior to exercise: If the pump does not allow manual adjustment of recommended doses, consider entering fewer carbohydrates than what actually are consumed; likewise, if snacking during exercise for prevention of hypoglycemia, do not enter these carbohydrates into the pump's bolus calculator.
- Allow the closed-loop algorithm to function after exercise as a tool to prevent delayed-onset hypoglycemia.

Use of Other Exercise-Related Technologies

Some individuals have benefited from use of newer technologies that allow them to monitor their heart rate, blood pressure, steps, sedentary time, exercise intensity, and other variables in real time. For instance, heart rate monitors are good for achieving and maintaining appropriate exercise intensity. Target heart rates, however, must be individualized based on health status and use of medication that may limit heart rate. Step counters can be effective for motivating patients to seek activity throughout the day, and not just during exercise times. A daily log of step counts can be used to show the correlation between physical activity and glucose control. Apps for tracking workout progress—analyzing glucose patterns related to different forms of exercise—can also supply needed feedback for making regimen adjustments in real time.

CONCLUSION

Given the challenges present when people with diabetes exercise, use of the latest technologies can be beneficial for managing blood glucose and maximizing the benefits of physical activity. Insulin pumps offer the ability to regulate basal insulin levels and carefully fine-tune bolus doses. CGM devices provide an added level of safety and offer the opportunity for improved decision making in real time and in a retrospective manner. Hybrid closed-loop systems have the potential to improve glycemic control leading up to exercise and may allow users to avoid undesired increases and decreases following workouts. All forms of technology have inherent drawbacks and limitations, but these issues can be mostly resolved through strategic planning.

REFERENCES

1. Manohar C, Levine JA, Nandy DK, Saad A, Dalla Man C, McCrady-Spitzer SK, Basu R, Cobelli C, Carter RE, Basu A, Kudva YC. The effect of walking on postprandial glycemic excursion in patients with type 1 diabetes and healthy people. *Diabetes Care* 2012;35:2493–2499. doi: 2410.2337/dc2411-2381. Epub 2012 Aug 2498

2. Piercy KL, Troiano RP, Ballard RM, Carlson SA, Fulton JE, Galuska DA, George SM, Olson RD. The Physical Activity Guidelines for Americans. *JAMA* 2018;320:2020–2028

3. MacMillan F, Kirk A, Mutrie N, Matthews L, Robertson K, Saunders DH. A systematic review of physical activity and sedentary behavior intervention studies in youth with type 1 diabetes: study characteristics, intervention design, and efficacy. *Pediatr Diabetes* 2014;15:175–189

4. Riddell MC, Milliken J. Preventing exercise-induced hypoglycemia in type 1 diabetes using real-time continuous glucose monitoring and a new carbohydrate intake algorithm: an observational field study. *Diabetes Technol Ther* 2011;13:819–825

5. Tansey MJ, Tsalikian E, Beck RW, Mauras N, Buckingham BA, Weinzimer SA, Janz KF, Kollman C, Xing D, Ruedy KJ, Steffes MW, Borland TM, Singh RJ, Tamborlane WV. The effects of aerobic exercise on glucose and counter-regulatory hormone concentrations in children with type 1 diabetes. *Diabetes Care* 2006;29:20–25

6. Mallad A, Hinshaw L, Schiavon M, Dalla Man C, Dadlani V, Basu R, Lingineni R, Cobelli C, Johnson ML, Carter R, Kudva YC, Basu A. Exercise effects on postprandial glucose metabolism in type 1 diabetes: a triple-tracer approach. *Am J Physiol Endocrinol Metab* 2015;308:E1106–1115

7. Manohar C, Levine JA, Nandy DK, Saad A, Dalla Man C, McCrady-Spitzer SK, Basu R, Cobelli C, Carter RE, Basu A, Kudva YC. The effect of walking on postprandial glycemic excursion in patients with type 1 diabetes and healthy people. *Diabetes Care* 2012;35:2493–2499

8. Turner D, Luzio S, Gray BJ, Bain SC, Hanley S, Richards A, Rhydderch DC, Martin R, Campbell MD, Kilduff LP, West DJ, Bracken RM. Algorithm that delivers an individualized rapid-acting insulin dose after morning resistance exercise counters post-exercise hyperglycaemia in people with type 1 diabetes. *Diabet Med* 2016;33:506–510

9. Colberg SR, Sigal RJ, Yardley JE, Riddell MC, Dunstan DW, Dempsey PC, Horton ES, Castorino K, Tate DF: Physical activity/exercise and diabetes: a position statement of the American Diabetes Association. *Diabetes Care* 2016;39:2065–2079

10. Francescato MP, Stel G, Stenner E, Geat M. Prolonged exercise in type 1 diabetes: performance of a customizable algorithm to estimate the carbohydrate supplements to minimize glycemic imbalances. *PLoS One* 2015;10:e0125220

11. Adolfsson P, Mattsson S, Jendle J. Evaluation of glucose control when a new strategy of increased carbohydrate supply is implemented during prolonged physical exercise in type 1 diabetes. *Eur J Appl Physiol* 2015;115:2599–2607

12. Campbell MD, Walker M, Bracken RM, Turner D, Stevenson EJ, Gonzalez JT, Shaw JA, West DJ. Insulin therapy and dietary adjustments to normalize glycemia and prevent nocturnal hypoglycemia after evening exercise in type 1 diabetes: a randomized controlled trial. *BMJ Open Diabetes Res Care* 2015; 3:e000085

13. Brazeau AS, Rabasa-Lhoret R, Strychar I, Mircescu H. Barriers to physical activity among patients with type 1 diabetes. *Diabetes Care* 2008;31:2108–2109

14. Bussau VA, Ferreira LD, Jones TW, Fournier PA. The 10-s maximal sprint: a novel approach to counter an exercise-mediated fall in glycemia in individuals with type 1 diabetes. *Diabetes Care* 2006;29:601–606

15. Fahey AJ, Paramalingam N, Davey RJ, Davis EA, Jones TW, Fournier PA. The effect of a short sprint on postexercise whole-body glucose production and utilization rates in individuals with type 1 diabetes mellitus. *J Clin Endocrinol Metab* 2012;97:4193–4200

16. Campbell MD, West DJ, Bain SC, Kingsley MI, Foley P, Kilduff L, Turner D, Gray B, Stephens JW, Bracken RM. Simulated games activity vs continuous running exercise: a novel comparison of the glycemic and metabolic responses in T1DM patients. *Scan J Med Sci Sports* 2015;25:216–222

17. Frier BM. Hypoglycaemia in diabetes mellitus: epidemiology and clinical implications. *Nat Rev Endocrinol* 2014;10:711–722

18. Tsalikian E, Mauras N, Beck RW, Tamborlane WV, Janz KF, Chase HP, Wysocki T, Weinzimer SA, Buckingham BA, Kollman C, Xing D, Ruedy KJ, Diabetes Research in Children Network Direcnet Study Group. Impact of exercise on overnight glycemic control in children with type 1 diabetes mellitus. *J Pediatr* 2005;147:528–534

19. Marliss EB, Vranic M. Intense exercise has unique effects on both insulin release and its roles in glucoregulation: implications for diabetes. *Diabetes* 2002;51(Suppl. 1):S271–S283

20. Turner D, Luzio S, Gray BJ, Dunseath G, Rees ED, Kilduff LP, Campbell MD, West DJ, Bain SC, Bracken RM. Impact of single and multiple sets of resistance exercise in type 1 diabetes. *Scan J Med Sci Sports* 2015;25: e99–109

21. Guelfi KJ, Jones TW, Fournier PA. The decline in blood glucose levels is less with intermittent high-intensity compared with moderate exercise in individuals with type 1 diabetes. *Diabetes Care* 2005;28:1289–1294

22. Heinemann L, Nosek L, Kapitza C, Schweitzer MA, Krinelke L. Changes in basal insulin infusion rates with subcutaneous insulin infusion: time until a change in metabolic effect is induced in patients with type 1 diabetes. *Diabetes Care* 2009;32:1437–1439

23. Yardley JE, Sigal RJ, Kenny GP, Riddell MC, Lovblom LE, Perkins BA. Point accuracy of interstitial continuous glucose monitoring during exercise in type 1 diabetes. *Diabetes Technol Ther* 2013;15:46–49

24. Bally L, Zueger T, Pasi N, Carlos C, Paganini D, Stettler C. Accuracy of continuous glucose monitoring during differing exercise conditions. *Diabetes Res Clin Pract* 2016;112:1–5

25. Herrington SJ, Gee DL, Dow SD, Monosky KA, Davis E, Pritchett KL. Comparison of glucose monitoring methods during steady-state exercise in women. *Nutrients* 2012;4:1282–1292

Chapter 11

Continuous Glucose Monitoring and Insulin Pumps in the Management of Diabetes in Pregnancy

Jennifer M. Yamamoto[1] and Helen R. Murphy[2]

INTRODUCTION

Diabetes is among the most common complications in pregnancy, affecting more than 20 million live births per year globally.[1] Gestational diabetes accounts for the majority (85%) of instances of diabetes in pregnancy, and preexisting diabetes (type 1, type 2, and other) accounts for the remaining 15%.[1] The prevalence of all forms of diabetes is rising. This includes a 44% increase in type 1 diabetes (T1D) and a 90% increase in type 2 diabetes (T2D) over the past 15 years.[2] With the high and increasing prevalence of diabetes in pregnancy, it is essential to continually develop improved management strategies.

Despite the many advances in the treatment of diabetes, there has been little improvement in the risk of adverse pregnancy outcomes over the past 15 years.[3] Unfortunately, preexisting diabetes remains associated with serious complications, including a fourfold increased risk of stillbirth and a one-in-two chance of neonatal complications directly related to maternal hyperglycemia, such as neonatal hypoglycemia and being large for gestational age.[4,5]

The importance of tight glycemic control before and throughout pregnancy for improving neonatal and maternal outcomes is undisputed; however, these targets are difficult to achieve. A nationwide cohort study in the U.K. found that only 14% of women with T1D and 37% with T2D achieve target HbA_{1c} levels of <6.5% (48 mmol/mol) in early pregnancy.[3] Even with the help of specialized interdisciplinary diabetes teams, only 40% of women with T1D achieved HbA_{1c} <6.5% (48 mmol/mol) in late pregnancy.[3]

Pregnancy is a time of substantial physiologic shifts, including changes in insulin sensitivity and pharmacokinetics, as well as changes in glucose absorption and disposal. Early pregnancy is a high-risk period for severe hypoglycemia. Thereafter, paralleling the dramatic increase in insulin resistance in midpregnancy, there is an increase in insulin requirements. Among women with preexisting T1D, this translates to twice- or three-times their prepregnancy prandial insulin doses. Immediately postpartum, there is a sudden decrease in insulin resistance following the delivery of the placenta, thus requiring a concomitant decrease in insulin

[1]Department of Medicine, Division of Endocrinology and Metabolism, University of Calgary, Alberta, Canada. [2]Cambridge University Hospitals NHS Foundation Trust, Cambridge, U.K.; Women's Health Academic Centre, Division of Women's and Children's Health, King's College London, London, U.K.; Norwich Medical School, Bob Champion Research and Education Building, University of East Anglia, Norwich, U.K.

doses. In addition, circumstances in pregnancy, such as hyperemesis gravidarum, antenatal steroid administration, and the peripartum period, represent unique glycemic challenges. These changes throughout pregnancy require close clinical follow-up, meticulous attention to dietary intake, physical activity, and insulin dose adjustment—all of which can cause a considerable emotional burden.

Diabetes technologies, such as continuous glucose monitoring (CGM), insulin pumps, and closed-loop insulin delivery, are promising tools. Outside of pregnancy, they have been shown to improve glycemic control in selected individuals. During pregnancy, they have the potential to reduce obstetric and neonatal complications closer to those of the general obstetric population. With the fast-paced improvements in these technologies, they also have the potential to reduce diabetes distress and emotional burden, and potentially to improve quality of life in women with diabetes pregnancies.

This chapter discusses the current evidence and the role of CGM, insulin pumps, and closed-loop insulin delivery in the management of women with diabetes in pregnancy.

GLUCOSE MONITORING IN PREGNANCY

Glucose monitoring is the cornerstone of the management of diabetes. Although this is true of all people with diabetes, the dramatic physiologic changes and unique gestational challenges throughout pregnancy make frequent glucose testing especially important. Traditionally, this is in the form of capillary glucose monitoring and HbA_{1c} measurement. Both methods of glucose testing have benefits and drawbacks.

Capillary glucose monitoring is recommended at least 7–10 times per day and includes fasting, premeal, postmeal, and overnight measurements, depending on the clinical scenario. Many women with T1D perform >10 tests per day to safely titrate insulin doses to the very tight pregnancy targets. Capillary glucose testing is onerous and still inadequate for optimal glucose control after meals and overnight, providing only snapshots of day-to-day glycemia. Furthermore, capillary glucose testing likely underestimates glucose variability and is impractical overnight. HbA_{1c} is inexpensive, widely available, and can be measured in the nonfasting state. An above-target HbA_{1c} is a well-established marker of adverse obstetric and neonatal outcomes across many studies.[4,5] However, it is a limited marker of day-to-day glycemic excursions. In pregnancy, HbA_{1c} concentration is affected by changes in red cell turnover and fasting glucose, as well as iron deficiency anemia and iron supplementation, which are commonplace. HbA_{1c} is a surrogate measure of average glycemic control and therefore does not assist women and their healthcare teams with daily insulin treatment decisions.

Using a subcutaneously inserted sensor, CGM records interstitial glucose concentrations every few minutes, resulting in 288 measurements per day. This gives women with diabetes, and their clinicians, detailed information about glycemic patterns and variability that can allow tailored dietary and insulin.

Clinical Insights Using Continuous Glucose Monitoring

CGM has given us important insight into the physiology and management of diabetes pregnancies. Despite close follow-up and specialized guidance, masked

CGM has demonstrated that pregnant women with T1D using intensive insulin therapy (either pumps or multiple daily injections [MDI]) spend only 50% of the day (12 h) with glucoses in target.[6,7] This highlights that there remains much room for improvement in day-to-day glucose management.

The use of CGM has allowed researchers to better understand the relationship of HbA_{1c} to maternal glucose in pregnancy. We have shown that the decline in maternal HbA_{1c} precedes any change in mean glucose using real-world clinical data.[8] Using trial data from two CGM randomized intervention trial,[9,10] researchers have demonstrated that the relationship between HbA_{1c} and estimated average glucose is different during pregnancy compared with outside of pregnancy.[11] Specifically, for a given change in HbA_{1c}, there is smaller change in estimated average glucose during pregnancy. This translates the National Institute for Health and Care Excellence (NICE) recommended HbA_{1c} targets of <6.5% to a target estimated average glucose of 115–121 mg/dL (6.4–6.7 mmol/L).

CGM also may be used to identify specific glucose patterns associated with various neonatal outcomes. Specific glycemic patterns have been identified in relation to large-for-gestational-age neonates. Using 1.68 million CGM glucose measurements, researchers demonstrated that mothers of large-for-gestational-age neonates had lower mean glucose in the first trimester and higher mean glucose in the second and third trimesters.[12] Additionally, certain patterns throughout the day (lower mid-morning and early evening glucose levels in the first trimester, higher early morning and afternoon glucose levels in the second trimester, and higher evening glucose levels in the third trimester) were associated with large-for-gestational-age neonates. Insight from these CGM data sets may lead to more personalized diabetes therapy in the future.

Clinical Trials of CGM in Pregnancy

There are two contemporary randomized trials of CGM in pregnancy.[6,13] The Continuous Glucose Monitoring during Diabetic Pregnancy (GlucoMOMs) study was a multicenter randomized controlled trial.[13] GlucoMOMs included women with T1D (n = 109), T2D (n = 82), and gestational diabetes requiring insulin (n = 109). Participants were randomized to intermittent masked CGM (use of the sensor for 5–7 days every 6 weeks) versus a control group. Authors did not find any significant difference in the primary outcome, macrosomia (defined as adjusted birth weight >90th percentile), between the two groups (31% in the intermittent CGM group vs. 28.4% in the control group). They did note less preeclampsia in women randomized to CGM (3.5%) versus the control group (18.4%). Importantly, 44 of the 143 women randomized to the masked CGM group did not adhere to the study protocol and seven participants with T1D switched to real-time CGM during the study. The trial was substantially underpowered to detect between-group differences in maternal glycemia or neonatal outcomes in T1D.

Continuous glucose monitoring in women with T1D in pregnancy trial (CONCEPTT) was a multicenter, international, open-label, randomized controlled trial of real-time CGM used throughout pregnancy.[6] Participants in the pregnancy trial (n = 225) were randomized to either CGM plus capillary glucose monitoring or capillary glucose monitoring alone. The authors found that pregnant women randomized to CGM had significantly tighter glycemic control, including a larger decrease in HbA_{1c} from baseline (mean difference of –0.2%; p = 0.021) and a higher time spent in target range (100 min more per day; $p = 0.003$) compared to the control group. More important, CGM was associated with significantly fewer large-for-gestational-age neonates (odds ratio [OR] 0.51; $p = 0.021$), neonatal hypoglycemia requiring treatment with intravenous dextrose (OR 0.45; $p = 0.025$), neonatal intensive care unit admission (OR 0.48; $p = 0.016$), and a 1-day-shorter hospital stay ($p = 0.009$). These improvements in neonatal outcomes were attributed to the improved maternal glycemic control and were present across all 31 study sites, regardless of method of insulin delivery (pump or MDI). Overall, adherence was quite high compared to earlier CGM pregnancy trials with 70% of pregnant women using CGM for >75% of the time likely owing, at least in part, to the run-in phase allowing women to opt out before randomization.

When examining the available evidence, it is important to recognize that these trials tested completely different technologies; GlucoMOMs assessed intermittent masked CGM, whereas CONCEPTT examined real-time CGM used continuously throughout pregnancy (Table 11.1). In addition, other important elements of trial design likely explain the difference in outcomes. First, GlucoMOMs was underpowered to show a difference in primary outcome macrosomia. The power calculation performed assumed a baseline macrosomia rate of 45% in all participants, regardless of whether they had T1D, T2D, or gestational diabetes. This is accurate in T1D but represents a very large overestimation both in T2D and in gestational diabetes participants, whose rates approximate 25% and 10%, respectively.[3,14] Furthermore, the trial was powered to detect only a large 30% relative decrease in macrosomia, which seems optimistic in this diverse patient population. The interpretation of the GlucoMOMs results is also limited by the high number of women who did not adhere to the study protocol ($n = 44$ in the CGM group) and the women who switched to real-time CGM ($n = 7$ with T1D).

Taken overall, there are definitive data to recommend only continuous use of real-time CGM in pregnant women with T1D. It is unclear whether intermittent masked or intermittent use of real-time CGM is effective in improving glycemic control or neonatal outcomes.[9,13]

On-Demand Glucose Monitoring in Pregnancy

On-demand glucose monitoring uses a sensor (the FreeStyle Libre) inserted into the back of the arm, which can be worn for up to 14 days. The user scans a receiver over the sensor to display glucose measurements. Unlike earlier generation CGM, flash glucose monitoring is designed to replace capillary blood glucose measurements and does not require capillary glucose calibration. The extended sensor life span, lack of user calibration, and competitive cost compared to 7–10 daily capillary glucose tests make it a potentially attractive option in pregnancy. A recent commercially sponsored study including 74 women with diabetes (T1D, T2D, and gestational diabetes) suggested that the FreeStyle Libre is accurate, safe, and acceptable to pregnant users. Specifically, the overall mean absolute difference was 11.8%.[15] With glucose concentration <100 mg/dL (5.6 mmol/L), the mean absolute difference was 9.6 mg/dL (0.53 mmol/L), so care should be taken when interpreting glucoses in the lower range. To date, there are no randomized, controlled trial data to examine its effectiveness on obstetric and neonatal outcomes.

Table 11.1. Real-Time versus Intermittent CGM in Pregnancy

	Clinical Trials	Benefits	Drawbacks
Real-time CGM worn *continuously*	CONCEPTT[6]	- Immediate feedback regarding glycemic control - Frequent adjustments to insulin, diet, and exercise made throughout the day - Hypo- and hyperglycemic excursions can be avoided with alerts and real-time information on glucose trends	- Large amount of data can be overwhelming - Cost (this may be offset by improvement in costly neonatal outcomes)
Intermittent real-time CGM	Secher et. al.[10]	- Periods of time without CGM may be less overwhelming	- Gives information only during discrete time periods - Real-time changes limited to only the period in which it is worn
Intermittent masked CGM	GlucoMOMs[13] Murphy et al.[9]	- Information can be reviewed with healthcare team, which may be less overwhelming - Can be helpful for bigger picture pattern recognition - No alerts, which can be frustrating for users	- Gives information only during discrete time periods - Women cannot make real-time changes to insulin, diet, and exercise - Can be difficult for women to remember possible causes of glycemic excursions

Practical Tips for CGM in Pregnancy

The amount of information provided by CGM can be overwhelming for some; however, comfort with the technology and the information it provides as well as instruction on how to use the information provided will help teams to use CGM effectively. Some practical tips for the use of CGM as a tool in pregnancy are provided in Tables 11.2–11.4.

Conclusions and Future Directions of CGM in Pregnancy

There have been substantial improvements in CGM technologies over the recent past. Improvements in sensor accuracy and user acceptability have allowed for increased uptake in clinical practice. Thus far, trials in pregnancy have used older-generation, real-time CGM devices, which were bulky and required capil-

Table 11.2. Using CGM Rate of Change to Adjust Insulin in Real Time*

	At Meals	At Times Other Than Meals
↑↑ (glucose rising >1 mmol every 10 min)	Increase dose by 20%, bolus at least 15 min before eating	Increase dose by 20%
↑ (glucose rising by 0.5–1 mmol every 10 min)	Increase dose by 10%, bolus at least 15 min before eating	Increase dose by 10%
→ (glucose stable)	No change in dose	No change in dose
↓ (glucose falling by 0.5–1 mmol every 10 min)	Decrease dose by 10%, bolus and eat immediately	Decrease dose by 10%
↓↓ (glucose falling by >1 mmol every 10 min)	Decrease dose by 20%, bolus and eat immediately	Decrease dose by 20%

* All suggestions must be tailored to clinical scenario.
Source: Adapted from CONCEPTT.[6]

Table 11.3. Quick Guide to CGM Downloads*

Step 1	Clear the hypoglycemia if 2–3 hypoglycemic episodes a week or time below target <10%
Step 2	Get the basal rates right before adjusting insulin to carbohydrate ratios
Step 3	Examine for patterns that occur on 2–3 days at the same time of day:
	Look at the insulin-to-carbohydrate ratios (only for meals <70 g of carbohydrate)
	Look at corrections factors (ideally corrections outside of meal insulin dosing)
	Review accuracy of carbohydrate counting
	Consider the practical tips for additional guidance in Table 11.4

* All suggestions must be tailored to clinical scenario.

Table 11.4. Practical Tips for Using CGM Parameters to Adjust Insulin, Diet, and Exercise

CGM Element	Practical Tips
Time in target	Aim for a time in target of >65% with a 5% improvement each 1–2 weeks as required.
Time below target	If >10% time below target, adjust insulin to avoid lows.
Time above target	Aim for small improvements week to week, every little bit helps.
Patterns that occur on 2–3 days at the same time of day:	
Before breakfast	If glucose before breakfast is out of target, check before-bed glucose to ensure that it is in target before changing overnight insulin dosing.
After meal highs	Assess carbohydrate type and count with the aim to include low glycemic index carbohydrates and, if needed, limit the number of carbohydrates with each meal (20–30 g with breakfast, 50–60 g with lunch, 50–60 g with dinner).
	Assess insulin dose (insulin-to-carbohydrate ratio and insulin sensitivity factor) taking into account before meal glucose.
	Change insulin time to 30–60 min before eating.
After meal lows	Assess carbohydrate type and count with the aim to include low glycemic index carbohydrates and, if needed, limit the number of carbohydrates with each meal. Assess insulin dose (insulin-to-carbohydrate ratio and insulin sensitivity factor) taking into account before-meal glucose.

* All suggestions must be tailored to clinical scenario.

lary glucose calibration as well as meticulous attention to skin care. Newer CGM devices are smaller, are cheaper, and have longer sensor life spans; some models (specifically the Dexcom G6) are calibration free and accurate enough for premeal insulin dosing, which will further CGM use in pregnancy.

There remain, however, limitations and barriers to the widespread use of CGM in pregnancy. The first is that the cost of CGM remains prohibitive for many women with diabetes in pregnancy. CGM also requires additional teaching and clinic time. Cost-effectiveness studies are required to see whether the potential cost savings reflected by improved neonatal outcomes will offset the cost of CGM. Although on-demand glucose monitoring is currently much less expensive and does not require additional teaching, it is not clear whether it will be as effective as real-time CGM in improving maternal glycemic control or neonatal outcomes. There are also frustrations associated with CGM use. In CONCEPTT, 80% of women reported frustrations with the CGM device.[6] These frustrations were most commonly in the form of skin reactions (48% of participants using CGM). With new-generations sensors, this may improve but likely will not be eliminated.

INSULIN PUMPS IN PREGNANCY

The insulin pump, also known as continuous subcutaneous insulin infusion, is a desirable option in pregnancy for variety of reasons. Unlike MDI, basal insulin delivery by the insulin pump is achieved by giving frequent small amounts of basal insulin throughout the day. This allows for flexible and fine-tuned basal rates. This is especially important in pregnancy, where the amount of basal insulin requirement increases disproportionally in the early morning (2:00 to 4:00 A.M.) compared with later in the day as pregnancy progresses. The different bolus pattern options available with the pump may help to manage postprandial glucose excursions, and the bolus calculator facilitates meal- and correction-insulin delivery. Also, the lack of an additional injection required for correction doses between meals may facilitate corrections and insulin delivery with between-meal snacks.

Despite these theoretical advantages, the literature regarding the effectiveness of insulin pumps compared to MDI in achieving glycemic targets is discordant. Previous randomized trials were small and of variable quality, and used older pump models. Therefore, they can no longer be used to inform clinical practice. Observational studies of pumps versus MDI are more contemporary, although they are confounded by the fact that women using the pump differ at baseline from women using MDI. Women using the insulin pump are more likely to access prepregnancy care, have lower baseline HbA_{1c} levels, be older, and have a longer duration of diabetes.[16] The largest study of insulin pumps versus MDI in pregnancy found that insulin pump use was associated with a lower HbA_{1c}, even after adjustment for potential confounders.[16] When the literature is taken as a whole, however, there is no clear evidence for one mode of insulin delivery over the other in terms of glycemic control or neonatal outcomes.

Studies suggest that the insulin pump is safe in pregnancy. Adverse outcomes, such as diabetic ketoacidosis and severe hypoglycemia, are relatively uncommon, however, so studies are likely underpowered to show any existing difference in these outcomes. Therefore, the risk of diabetic ketoacidosis with pump failure must be discussed with all pregnant women. Strategies to avoid unrecognized pump failure overnight, such as overnight testing, must be reviewed.

Pump Initiation in Pregnancy

Ideally, patients who use insulin pumps should be initiated prepregnancy to establish appropriate insulin dosing, should achieve prepregnancy targets, and should develop comfort and expertise with pump use. It is likely safe, however, to change the mode of insulin delivery during pregnancy in select women who have the guidance and close follow-up of a specialized interdisciplinary team.

Pump Titration in Pregnancy

As pregnancy progresses, there are substantial changes insulin requirements and strategies for insulin delivery. Early in pregnancy, women often require less insulin and are at increased risk of hypoglycemia. Some women may experience substantial nausea or vomiting. If this is a concern, women may give 50% of their bolus insulin before eating and the remaining 50% postmeal. After ~18 weeks gestation, there is a steady increase in insulin resistance, leading to substantial increases in insulin doses. This increase tends to be most pronounced in bolus insulin, which may account for 70–80% of their total daily dose in late gestation.[17] Because of changes in glucose absorption and insulin pharmacokinetics, by the end of pregnancy, the mealtime insulin dose is best given 30–60 min before eating.

Pump Use Postpartum

Immediately postpartum, insulin resistance drops dramatically. This requires an immediate change in insulin dosing. These doses are often variable and difficult to predict; therefore, frequent glucose testing and insulin titration is required. A starting place for most pump settings is a basal rate of 0.5 units/h, an insulin-to-carbohydrate ratio of 1:15, and insulin sensitivity factor of 40, although this will need to be tailored to the individual clinical scenario. It is essential to change the glucose targets on the pump (generally 108–144 mg/dL [6–8 mmol/L]) to reflect the relaxed targets postpartum (108–180 mg/dL [6–10 mmol/L]) and to minimize the risk of maternal severe hypoglycemia.

Conclusions and Future Directions of Pumps in Pregnancy

It remains unclear whether insulin pump use is superior to MDI in pregnancy, but it is likely safe and appropriate for selected women with T1D. No trials or studies have examined newer insulin pump models with features such as predictive low-glucose suspend. The insulin pump allows for fine-tuning of insulin doses that reflect physiologic changes throughout pregnancy. Large, high-quality, prospective randomized trials of the newer insulin pump models versus MDI are required.

CLOSED-LOOP INSULIN DELIVERY IN PREGNANCY

Women with T1D in pregnancy who are on intensive insulin therapy and using CGM still spend >7 h/day out of target.[6] Therefore, even with more widespread adoption of diabetes technologies, much room for improvement remains. Closed-loop insulin delivery, also known as the artificial pancreas and sensor-integrated insulin delivery, is composed of a hormonal pump, CGM, and a computer algorithm. Hybrid closed-loop doses basal insulin uses a computer algorithm in response to real-time glucose measurements every 10–15 min, but still requires manual premeal insulin boluses. Given the tight glycemic control required and the consistently changing insulin doses in pregnancy, automated insulin delivery is an enticing tool.

Two randomized crossover studies of home, closed-loop insulin delivery have been performed.[18,19] Both included 16 pregnant women with T1D who were randomized to start with either 4 weeks of closed-loop or sensor-augmented pump therapy. After a washout period, women crossed over to complete an additional 4 weeks of therapy in the other arm. The first study examined overnight closed-loop insulin delivery.[18] It found that participants using closed-loop insulin delivery spent 15% more time in target overnight compared to those on sensor-augmented pump therapy. The second study evaluated day and night closed-loop insulin delivery.[19] When compared to sensor-augmented pump therapy, participants using closed-loop insulin delivery spent a similar time in target (62% vs. 60% respectively; $p = 0.47$). There was less hypoglycemia, however, while using closed-loop insulin delivery, both in terms of number of episodes (8 vs. 12.5 over a 28-day period; $p = 0.04$) and time spent <63 mg/dL (3.5 mmol/L) (1.6 vs. 2.7%; $p = 0.02$).

Both trials included a continuation phase in which participants could choose to continue closed-loop day-and-night insulin delivery. This demonstrated that a closed-loop system worn throughout pregnancy was feasible and effective in achieving good glycemic control (~70% median time in target), despite the dramatic changes in insulin requirements as pregnancy progressed and unique circumstances, such as antenatal steroids, hospital admissions, and labor and delivery, rose. Although these studies were small, they included women with a long duration of diabetes (23.6±7.2 and 19.4±10.2 years for the overnight and day-and-night studies, respectively), complicated obstetrical histories, varying experience with diabetes technologies (40% pump naïve), and variable control before pregnancy. Importantly, participants described closed-loop insulin delivery as exciting and empowering, allowing the women to feel more "normal" and "less diabetic," although they also expressed such concerns as device visibility, alarms, glitches, and potential for deskilling.[20]

Conclusions and Future Directions for Closed-Loop in Pregnancy

Although these studies are promising, larger randomized trials comparing closed-loop insulin delivery to the current standard of care in a more diverse population are required. This would allow for an assessment of closed-loop insulin delivery beyond short-term glycemic outcomes to include obstetric and neonatal outcomes. Economic studies also will be required to evaluate whether this technology is cost effective.

TECHNOLOGY IN THE MANAGEMENT OF LABOR AND DELIVERY

Labor and delivery is a period of dynamic changes in glucose utilization, hormonal profiles, and insulin sensitivity. This can make achieving glucose targets during this time especially challenging. Maternal intrapartum glycemic control has been variably associated with risk of neonatal hypoglycemia; therefore, most guidelines recommend tight glycemic targets during this time.[21] Given the tight glycemic control required (typically 72–126 mg/dL [4–7 mmol/L]), hypoglycemia is common and can occur in up to half of women during or before delivery.[21] Technologies, including CGM, insulin pumps, and closed-loop insulin delivery, have been studied in the management of T1D during labor and delivery.

Continuous Glucose Monitoring

The detailed glucose measurements provided using CGM may provide useful information to achieve these tight targets. With the possible distractions of labor and delivery, it is unclear whether this information can be used to its full potential. One observational study suggested that glucose control could be improved with the use of CGM; however, these women were self-selected and had a significantly lower third trimester HbA_{1c} than women not using CMG (5.2±0.4 vs. 6.2±1.7%; $p <0.01$).[22] Another study included women who participated in a randomized control of CGM in pregnancy who agreed to use CGM during labor and delivery.[23] Women using CGM achieved comparable glycemic control in the 8 h before delivery compared with women who only used self-monitored plasma glucoses during this time.

Insulin Pump

Women on MDI typically are switched to an intravenous insulin infusion for labor, whereas women on an insulin pump may choose to continue pumping through labor and delivery. Using the insulin pump throughout labor and delivery has benefits and drawbacks. Subcutaneous insulin delivery using the pump is less invasive than intravenous therapy. Also, these women are experts in their own diabetes management and are likely more knowledgeable in diabetes management than the obstetric-ward staff. Furthermore, women may be reluctant to give up control of their management to members of the inpatient team who may have many competing interests. Caution must be taken to ensure that women who are laboring can effectively self-manage their diabetes. If there is persistent hypo- or hyperglycemia, or concerns with which the demands of labor or the influence of medications are interfering, women should be quickly switched to intravenous insulin.

The literature on the use of insulin pump therapy during labor and delivery is limited and consists of retrospective observational studies. Two studies (one in Italy and the other in Canada) with a total of 96 women who used the insulin pump during labor and delivery suggested that it is safe in selected patients.[22,24] Only 1 of the 96 women in the two studies intending to use pump therapy during labor and delivery was switched to intravenous insulin. Drever et al.[24] compared the glycemic control achieved by pump therapy to that achieved by intravenous insulin and found that pump use was associated with a lower mean glucose (99 vs. 115 mg/dL [5.5 vs. 6.4 mmol/L]; $p = 0.01$). The cost of tight glycemic control during labor and delivery in this cohort was frequent hypoglycemia, however, with 30% of women experiencing at least one hypoglycemic episode during this time.

Closed-Loop Insulin Delivery

The efficacy of closed-loop insulin delivery in labor and delivery was evaluated in a recent cohort study.[25] This was a secondary analysis of participants included in the two randomized crossover studies of home closed-loop insulin delivery who chose to continue closed-loop delivery in pregnancy.[18,19] The study found that closed-loop insulin delivery performed well during labor and delivery, achieving an 82% time in target (target range 63–140 mg/dL [3.5–7.8 mmol/L]) with no cues to the system indicating the onset of labor.[25] Similarly, the closed-loop system performed well immediately postpartum, achieving an 83% time in target (target range 70–180 mg/dL [3.9–10.0 mmol/L]). There was minimal hypoglycemia during both periods. Additional studies are required to compare closed-loop systems to conventional therapy (typically intravenous insulin infusion or insulin pumps). Additionally, qualitative studies that assess the acceptability of closed-loop insulin delivery to women with diabetes and their obstetrical ward team should be performed.

CONCLUSIONS AND FUTURE DIRECTIONS

The use of technologies, such as CGM, insulin pumps, and closed-loop systems, in the management of women with diabetes in pregnancy may help improve glycemic control and, ultimately, obstetric and neonatal outcomes. Technology has already shown great promise in improving glycemic control and outcomes in women with diabetes. CONCEPTT demonstrated women using CGM spent

100 min/day longer in target, leading to a decreased risk of large-for-gestational-age neonates, neonatal hypoglycemia, and neonatal intensive care–unit admission.[6] Closed-loop insulin delivery has shown improvement in overnight time in target and decreased hypoglycemia.[18,19] These technologies also may have the potential to reduce the burden of diabetes self-management for women with diabetes in pregnancy, as well as reduce substantial clinic-to-clinic variations in diabetes control.[3,20] Future directions in the use of technology in the management of diabetes pregnancies include virtual clinics and telemedicine, as well as device technologies. The use of these technologies, however, must be evidence-based, person-centered, and cost-effective.

Even with the use of more sophisticated technology, optimal glycemic control cannot be achieved without using the full diabetes armamentarium. Furthermore, without an insulin with the sufficient absorption and fast action to match that of glucose, target glucose may remain elusive for many women in pregnancy. It is essential that women receive close interdisciplinary follow-up by specialized healthcare teams; basics and diet and exercise are understood and utilized; care in the timing of insulin dosing be taken; and that women with diabetes continue their hard work before and throughout pregnancy.

REFERENCES

1. Guariguata L, Linnenkamp U, Beagley J, Whiting DR, Cho NH. Global estimates of the prevalence of hyperglycaemia in pregnancy. *Diabetes Res Clin Pract* 2014;103:176–185

2. Mackin ST, Nelson SM, Kerssens JJ, Wood R, Wild S, Colhoun HM, Leese GP, Philip S, Lindsay RS, Group SE. Diabetes and pregnancy: national trends over a 15 year period. *Diabetologia* 2018;61:1081–1088

3. Murphy HR, Bell R, Cartwright C, Curnow P, Maresh M, Morgan M, Sylvester C, Young B, Lewis-Barned N. Improved pregnancy outcomes in women with type 1 and type 2 diabetes but substantial clinic-to-clinic variations: a prospective nationwide study. *Diabetologia* 2017;60:1668–1677

4. Tennant PW, Glinianaia SV, Bilous RW, Rankin J, Bell R. Pre-existing diabetes, maternal glycated haemoglobin, and the risks of fetal and infant death: a population-based study. *Diabetologia* 2014;57:285–294

5. Maresh MJ, Holmes VA, Patterson CC, Young IS, Pearson DW, Walker JD, McCance DR, Diabetes, Pre-eclampsia Intervention Trial Study Group. Glycemic targets in the second and third trimester of pregnancy for women with type 1 diabetes. *Diabetes Care* 2015;38:34–42

6. Feig DS, Donovan LE, Corcoy R, Murphy KE, Amiel SA, Hunt KF, Asztalos E, Barrett JFR, Sanchez JJ, de Leiva A, Hod M, Jovanovic L, Keely E, McManus R, Hutton EK, Meek CL, Stewart ZA, Wysocki T, O'Brien R, Ruedy K, Kollman C, Tomlinson G, Murphy HR, Group CC. Continuous glucose monitoring in pregnant women with type 1 diabetes (CONCEPTT): a multicentre international randomised controlled trial. *Lancet* 2017;390:2347–2359

7. Murphy HR, Rayman G, Duffield K, Lewis KS, Kelly S, Johal B, Fowler D, Temple RC. Changes in the glycemic profiles of women with type 1 and type 2 diabetes during pregnancy. *Diabetes Care* 2007;30:2785–2791

8. Murphy HR. Intensive glycemic treatment during type 1 diabetes pregnancy: a story of (mostly) sweet success! *Diabetes Care* 2018;41(80):1563–1571

9. Murphy HR, Rayman G, Lewis K, Kelly S, Johal B, Duffield K, Fowler D, Campbell PJ, Temple RC. Effectiveness of continuous glucose monitoring in pregnant women with diabetes: randomised clinical trial. *BMJ* 2008;337:a1680

10. Secher AL, Ringholm L, Andersen HU, Damm P, Mathiesen ER. The effect of real-time continuous glucose monitoring in pregnant women with diabetes: a randomized controlled trial. *Diabetes Care* 2013;36:1877–1883

11. Law GR, Gilthorpe MS, Secher AL, Temple R, Bilous R, Mathiesen ER, Murphy HR, Scott EM. Translating HbA1c measurements into estimated average glucose values in pregnant women with diabetes. *Diabetologia* 2017;60:618–624

12. Law GR, Ellison GT, Secher AL, Damm P, Mathiesen ER, Temple R, Murphy HR, Scott EM. Analysis of continuous glucose monitoring in pregnant women with diabetes: distinct temporal patterns of glucose associated with large-for-gestational-age infants. *Diabetes Care* 2015;38:1319–1325

13. Voormolen DN, DeVries JH, Sanson RME, Heringa MP, de Valk HW, Kok M, van Loon AJ, Hoogenberg K, Bekedam DJ, Brouwer TCB, Porath M, Erdtsieck RJ, NijBijvank B, Kip H, van der Heijden OWH, Elving LD, Hermsen BB, Potter van Loon BJ, Rijnders RJP, Jansen HJ, Langenveld J, Akerboom BMC, Kiewiet RM, Naaktgeboren CA, Mol BWJ, Franx A, Evers IM. Continuous glucose monitoring during diabetic pregnancy (Gluco-MOMS): a multicentre randomized controlled trial. *Diabetes Obes Metab* 2018;20(8):1894–1902

14. Crowther CA, Hiller JE, Moss JR, McPhee AJ, Jeffries WS, Robinson JS, Australian Carbohydrate Intolerance Study in Pregnant Women Trial Group. Effect of treatment of gestational diabetes mellitus on pregnancy outcomes. *N Engl J Med* 2005;352:2477–2486

15. Scott EM, Bilous RW, Kautzky-Willer A. Accuracy, user acceptability, and safety evaluation for the FreeStyle Libre flash glucose monitoring system when used by pregnant women with diabetes. *Diabetes Technol Ther* 2018;20(3):180–188

16. Kallas-Koeman MM, Kong JM, Klinke JA, Butalia S, Lodha AK, Lim KI, Duan QM, Donovan LE. Insulin pump use in pregnancy is associated with lower HbA1c without increasing the rate of severe hypoglycaemia or diabetic ketoacidosis in women with type 1 diabetes. *Diabetologia* 2014;57:681–689

17. Mathiesen JM, Secher AL, Ringholm L, Norgaard K, Hommel E, Andersen HU, Damm P, Mathiesen ER. Changes in basal rates and bolus calculator settings in insulin pumps during pregnancy in women with type 1 diabetes. *J Matern Fetal Neonatal Med* 2014;27:724–728

18. Stewart ZA, Wilinska ME, Hartnell S, Temple RC, Rayman G, Stanley KP, Simmons D, Law GR, Scott EM, Hovorka R, Murphy HR. Closed-loop insulin delivery during pregnancy in women with type 1 diabetes. *N Engl J Med* 2016;375:644–654

19. Stewart ZA, Wilinska ME, Hartnell S, O'Neil LK, Rayman G, Scott EM, Barnard K, Farrington C, Hovorka R, Murphy HR. Day-and-night closed-loop insulin delivery in a broad population of pregnant women with type 1 diabetes: a randomized controlled crossover trial. *Diabetes Care* 2018;41(7):1391–1399

20. Farrington C, Stewart ZA, Barnard K, Hovorka R, Murphy HR. Experiences of closed-loop insulin delivery among pregnant women with Type 1 diabetes. *Diabet Med* 2017;34(10):1461–1469

21. Yamamoto JM, Benham J, Mohammad K, Donovan LE, Wood S. Intrapartum glycaemic control and neonatal hypoglycaemia in pregnancies complicated by diabetes mellitus: a systematic review. *Diabet Med* 2018;35(2):173–183

22. Fresa R, Visalli N, Di Blasi V, Cavallaro V, Ansaldi E, Trifoglio O, Abbruzzese S, Bongiovanni M, Agrusta M, Napoli A. Experiences of continuous subcutaneous insulin infusion in pregnant women with type 1 diabetes during delivery from four Italian centers: a retrospective observational study. *Diabetes Technol Ther* 2013;15:328–334

23. Cordua S, Secher AL, Ringholm L, Damm P, Mathiesen ER. Real-time continuous glucose monitoring during labour and delivery in women with Type 1 diabetes—observations from a randomized controlled trial. *Diabet Med* 2013;30:1374–1381

24. Drever E, Tomlinson G, Bai AD, Feig DS. Insulin pump use compared with intravenous insulin during labour and delivery: the INSPIRED observational cohort study. *Diabet Med* 2016;33:1253–1259

25. Stewart ZA, Yamamoto JM, Wilinska ME, Hartnell S, Farrington C, Hovorka R, Murphy HR: Adaptability of closed loop during labor, delivery, and postpartum: a secondary analysis of data from two randomized crossover trials in type 1 diabetes pregnancy. *Diabetes Technol Ther* 2018;20(7):501–505

Chapter 12
Practical Use of Insulin Pumps and Continuous Glucose Monitoring in the Hospital

Kristen Kulasa, MD;[1] Patricia Juang, MD;[1] and Robert J. Rushakoff, MD[2]

INTRODUCTION

Insulin pumps, also called continuous subcutaneous insulin infusion (CSII), and continuous glucose monitoring (CGM) devices are becoming more prevalent in the management of diabetes. It has been estimated that up to 30–40% of patients with type 1 diabetes (T1D) and a growing number of patients with type 2 diabetes (T2D) are using insulin pumps and CGM devices in the outpatient setting.[1] Patients with diabetes have a two- to six-fold greater chance of hospitalization and longer hospital stays compared to those without diabetes.[2-6] About 25–35% of hospitalized patients have diabetes or hyperglycemia.[7] Therefore, it is increasingly more likely that hospital providers will encounter patients using these technologies. The American Diabetes Association supports the use of CSII pump therapy in the hospital in a select group of patients, but the Association recommends appropriate hospital policies and procedures outlining guidelines to support the safe use of CSII in the inpatient setting.[8]

INSULIN PUMPS IN THE HOSPITAL

When patients using CSII are admitted to the hospital, a decision must be made as to whether they can continue their insulin pump during hospitalization. Insulin pumps are a complex piece of technology with which most hospital staff and providers are unfamiliar. The various insulin pumps on the market, each with their individual nuances, make it impractical to train staff and providers on all the pumps and their functions. Insulin itself is a high-risk medication, and combined with the unfamiliarity of insulin pumps, can lead to errors in insulin dosing and mismanagement that can be extremely dangerous in the hospital setting. Patients on insulin pumps, however, are used to self-management of their diabetes and relinquishing control of insulin dosing during hospitalizations may cause significant stress and anxiety. There is high patient satisfaction when insulin pumps are allowed to be continued during hospitalization.[9,10]

Studies have shown decreased rates of hypoglycemia with CSII with comparable average glucose levels.[11] Severe hyperglycemia (glucose >300 mg/dL) and hypoglycemia (glucose <40 mg/dL) were also significantly less common among

[1]Division of Endocrinology, Diabetes, and Metabolism, University of California, San Diego, San Diego, CA. [2]Division of Endocrinology and Metabolism, University of California, San Francisco, San Francisco, CA.

insulin pump users.[12] Although CSII users may be comfortable with and adept at managing their diabetes in the outpatient setting, variables specific to the inpatient setting often can make self-management challenging, including stress, glucocorticoids, varying renal function, NPO periods, dextrose-containing intravenous (IV) fluids or medications, pain, and pain medications.[13] In addition, some CSII users may have only rudimentary knowledge about how to manage their pumps, may only be able to give themselves meal boluses, and may rely on their outpatient healthcare providers to make all programing adjustments. Thus, using CSII during hospitalizations can be done, but it requires a joint effort with good communication between patients and providers, and clear hospital policies and procedures to maximize safety and meet regulatory requirements. Nurses and providers also need to be educated on the basic function of insulin pumps and a diabetes or endocrinology consult should be placed to assist with any pump adjustments that might be required during the hospitalization. Patients on insulin pumps need to be carefully evaluated not only for their basic pump management skills but also for their physical and mental ability to self-manage the insulin pump during their hospitalization. A temporary transition to subcutaneous basal-bolus therapy or intravenous (IV) insulin infusion may be necessary for those patients who cannot self-manage or in situations in which use of an insulin pump is unsafe.

Insulin Pump Overview

Insulin pumps are devices that deliver a continuous infusion of insulin subcutaneously. They are preprogrammed to continuously deliver varying doses of insulin to cover basal needs. Insulin pumps also have preprogrammed insulin-to-carbohydrate ratios (ICR) and insulin sensitivity factors (ISF) to cover nutritional and correctional insulin needs. Patients input their carbohydrate intake and blood glucose values into the insulin pump, and calculators within the pump use the preprogrammed rates to calculate and administer insulin boluses throughout the day.

Some insulin pumps are paired with a continuous glucose monitoring system (CGMS) that provides real-time glucose data, and the CGM device can communicate the blood glucose values wirelessly to the insulin pump. Most insulin pumps connect to the patient using flexible tubing with a fine-bore cannula placed in the subcutaneous tissue. The Omnipod is the only insulin pump on the market at the time of this publication that does not use tubing. Instead, it has an insulin-containing pod with a built-in cannula that is controlled wirelessly with a handheld device called a personal diabetes manager. The MiniMed 670G is the only hybrid closed-loop pump on the market at the time of this publication. It allows automatic adjustment of the basal rate based on real-time CGMS glucose data. The Tandem insulin pumps have color touch screens. Table 12.1 summarizes the insulin pumps available on the market at the time of this publication.[14]

Terminology and Basics

Insulin Type. Insulin pumps infuse rapid-acting insulins (lispro, aspart, glulisine) or short-acting insulin (regular). Patients who are extremely insulin resistant may use regular U-500 insulin in the pump as well.

Basal Rate. This is the amount of insulin needed to keep blood glucose levels stable during periods of fasting, such as between meals and overnight. In the fasting state, the liver is continuously secreting glucose, known as gluconeogenesis.

Table 12.1. Currently Available Insulin Pumps

Company	Product	Battery	Reservoir	Basal range	Bolus range	Special features	Website
Insulet Corp.	Omnipod	POD: battery integrated PDM: 2AAA	200 units	0.05-30 units/hr 0.05 unit increments	0.05 to 30 units 0.05, 0.1, 0.5 or 1 unit increments I:CHO in whole units only	No tubing Waterproof pod at 25 feet for 1 hour Personal diabetes manager (PDM) controls function with built in glucose meter PDM needs to be within 5 feet to deliver bolus doses	www.omnipoddelivery.com
Medtronic Diabetes	MiniMed 530G System	1 AAA	300 units	0.025 to 35 units/hr 0.025 unit increments up to 0.975 units 0.05 unit increments between 1 and 9.95 units 0.1 unit increments for >10 units	0.025 to 25 units 0.1 unit increments I:CHO allows for fraction of grams	Pump-CGM combo uses SmartGuard technology and can stop insulin delivery for up to 2 hours if glucose reaches preset low level and user not reacting to low-glucose alarm	www.medtronicdiabetes.com/products/minimed-530g-diabetes-system-with-enlite

(continued)

Table 12.1. Currently Available Insulin Pumps *(continued)*

Medtronic Diabetes	MiniMed 630G System	1 AA	300 units	0.025 to 35 units/hr	0.025 unit increments up to 0.975 0.05 unit increments between 1 and 9.95 units 0.1 unit increment for >10 units	0.025 to 25 units	0.025 unit increments I:CHO allows for fraction of grams	Pump-CGM combo uses SmartGuard technology and can stop insulin delivery for up to 2 hours if glucose reaches preset low level and user not reacting to low-glucose alarm Waterproof at 12 feet for 24 hours Full color screen	www.medtronicdiabetes.com/products/minimed-630g-insulin-pump-system
Medtronic Diabetes	MiniMed 670G System	1 AA	300 units	0.025 to 35 units/hr	0.025 unit increments up to 0.975 0.05 unit increments between 1 and 9.95 units	0.025 to 25 units	0.025, 0.05 and 0.1 unit increments I:CHO allows for fraction of grams	Hybrid closed-loop pump Auto mode automatically adjusts basal insulin delivery based on CGM sensor glucose readings and insulin delivery Pump-CGM combo uses SmartGuard technology and can stop insulin delivery for up to 2 hours if glucose reaches preset low level and user not reacting to low-glucose alarm	www.medtronicdiabetes.com/products/minimed-670g-insulin-pump-system

(continued)

Manufacturer	Pump	Power source	Reservoir	Basal increments	Bolus increments	Other features	Website
Medtronic Diabetes	MiniMed Paradigm Revel	1 AAA	300 units	0.025 to 35 units/hr; 0.025 unit increments up to 0.975; 0.05 unit increments between 1 and 9.95 units; 0.1 unit increment for >10 units	0.025 to 25 units; 0.1 unit increments; 0.1 unit increment for >10 units; I:CHO allows for fraction of grams	Waterproof at 12 feet for 24 hours; Optional CGM capabilities; Customizable "skins"	www.medtronicdiabetes.com/products/minimed-revel-insulin-pump
Sooil Development	Dana Diabecare IIS	3.6 volt DC lithium	300 units	0.04 to 16 units/hr; 0.01 or 0.1 unit increments	0.1 to 80 units; 0.1, 0.5, 1 unit increments; I:CHO in whole units only	Icons instead of works in menu; Five color choices; Waterproof at 3.3 feet for 1 hour	www.sooil.com/eng/product/insulin-iis.php
Tandem Diabetes Care	T:slim X2 Pump	Rechargeable lithium polymer battery	300 units	0.1 to 15 units/hr; 0.001 unit increments	0.05 to 25 units; 0.01 unit increments with option for up to additional 25 units; I:CHO allows for fraction of grams	Color touch screen; Watertight for up to 3 feet for 30 minutes; Integrated with Dexcom CGM	www.tandemdiabetes.com/products/t-slim-x2-insulin-pump

Basal insulin is needed to allow cells to take in the glucose for energy, but it also helps regulate gluconeogenesis and suppresses ketone production. Insulin pumps allow for small amounts of insulin to be delivered steadily throughout the day, and basal increments vary among different pumps. Basal rates are preprogrammed into the pump and are measured in units per hour. Most patients have one to four different basal rates, which change with time of day. For example, patients with diabetes who experience the dawn phenomenon, when glucose levels rise in the early morning before waking due to endogenous growth hormone and cortisol surges, may have an increase in the basal rate programmed in the middle of the night when their blood glucose starts to rise. Patients also may have lower basal rates set for the time of day they are most active to decrease the risk hypoglycemia. Some patients may require lower overnight basal rates. Some patients also have different basal profiles for different days (e.g., workdays, exercise days, sickdays). Total basal insulin is usually ~50% of total daily insulin dose.

Bolus Delivery. Bolus insulin accounts for insulin given with meals and snacks, and to correct for elevated glucoses. Insulin pumps allow for preprogrammed ICR and ISF or correction factor. The ICR is the amount of carbohydrate in grams that one unit of insulin covers. For example, an ICR of 1:15 g means that 1 unit of insulin is needed for 15 g of carbohydrate intake. The ISF is used to correct for elevated glucoses. It is an estimate of how much a patients' blood glucose will drop (in mg/dL) with 1 unit of insulin. For example, an ISF of 1:50 mg/dL means that 1 unit of insulin is expected to drop blood glucose by 50 mg/dL. Much like basal rates, ICR and ISF can vary with time of day, and insulin pumps allow for preprogramming of various ICR and ISF over the course of the day. Patients enter the amount of carbohydrates they are eating in grams. Then based on the glucose level (either also entered by the patient or downloaded automatically from connected CMG) the insulin pump would then use the preprogrammed ICR and ISF to calculate a bolus insulin dose. The patient then either agrees to that calculated dose or may manually override to give any dose they choose. Total bolus dose is typically 50% of total daily insulin dose, but for patients who eat large or small amounts of carbohydrates, this can be significantly higher or lower than the basal dose.

Target Blood Glucose Range. The target range is the preset blood glucose range used to calculate a correction dose above and reduction below the target. This target range can be adjusted by time of day. For example, if the daytime target is set at 90–130 mg/dL, then a correction dose will be calculated for any blood glucose level entered into the insulin pump calculator >130 mg/dL.

Square-Wave and Extended Bolus. This insulin pump feature allows a bolus of insulin to be delivered over a specified time, usually 30 min to ≥1 h. This is used in patients with gastroparesis and with high-fat or high-protein meals that result in delayed digestion and elevated glucoses hours after the meal.

Dual-Wave and Combination Bolus. This feature is used to deliver a bolus of insulin immediately followed by the remaining bolus delivered over a specified time period. This type of delivery might be used for meals that are high in both carbohydrates and fat, which may delay digestion.

Active Insulin Time. Active insulin time, also known as insulin on-board, is the insulin pump's way of preventing stacking of insulin doses, which is when an additional correction dose is administered before the previous dose is finished working. When both of these correction doses are working at the same time, or are stacked, it can increase the risk of hypoglycemia. This is a way to keep track of how much insulin is still working and to adjust a bolus dose by taking into account how much insulin is still on-board. The integrated calculator in the insulin pump will automatically subtract the amount of active insulin on-board from a subsequent correction dose to prevent insulin stacking. Active insulin time is usually set for 4 h but often shorter with the new hybrid pumps (see the following).

Infusion Set. An infusion set includes a thin, clear, pliable tubing that attaches the insulin pump to the patient's body. The infusion set is inserted with a needle inside the cannula, which is a plastic catheter that remains in the subcutaneous fat. The needle is necessary to puncture the skin, but it is then withdrawn, leaving only the cannula under the skin. Insertion devices are available to help patients insert the infusion set. Insertion devices are push-button, spring-loaded tools that insert the set. Infusion sets are an important part of insulin pump therapy because if a cannula is kinked in the process of insertion, insulin cannot be successfully delivered, which can lead to hyperglycemia and possibly diabetic ketoacidosis (DKA). Infusion sets need to be changed every 2–3 days to avoid problems with insulin delivery.

Infusion Site. This is the location of infusion set placement. Most patients place infusion sets on the abdomen, but infusion sets also can be placed on the upper arm or thighs. Infusion sets and sites need to be changed every 2–3 days.

Reservoir. Also known as cartridge or syringe, a reservoir is where insulin is stored in the pump. Most reservoirs hold 200–300 units of insulin.

Temporary Basal Rate. This is a basal rate that can be programmed separate from the patient's usual basal rates. This can be set to last for a certain period of time. Temporary basal rates are useful for hospitalized patients who may have increased or decreased insulin requirements while ill or NPO.

Suspend. The suspend feature allows insulin delivery to be stopped. This can be used when changing infusion sets, refilling cartridges, or replacing batteries. It is important to remember to resume insulin delivery when ready.

Patient Selection

Not all patients who are admitted to the hospital on an insulin pump should stay on an insulin pump. Patients need to be evaluated for their physical and mental ability to self-manage their insulin pump each time they are readmitted into the hospital.

Who Can Stay on an Insulin Pump. Patients who will be continuing CSII during their hospitalization need to be able to demonstrate the ability to safely manage their insulin pump. Insulin pump users should be capable of displaying basal rates, ICR, and ISF rates on their pump and to make adjustments to those rates when asked. They also need to be able to bolus for the amount of carbohydrates they consume per meal and to correct for hyperglycemia by using the pump bolus calculator or be able to demonstrate appropriate calculation and administration of a bolus manually. Patients must demonstrate the ability to suspend their insulin pump and set temporary basal rates if needed during their hospitalization. Any patient coming into the hospital needs to have enough pump supplies, including infusion sets and batteries, to last during the duration of their hospital stay as these materials are not kept in or supplied by the hospital. They also need to be able to change their own infusion set and site every 2–3 days and to fill the pump reservoir or syringe with insulin.

Who Should Come off an Insulin Pump. Each time patients are admitted into the hospital, they should be evaluated for the physical and mental ability to

Table 12.2. Contraindications for CSII in Hospitalized Patients

1. Altered mental status or cognitive impairment
2. Metabolic instability (DKA or HHS)
3. Critically ill patients
4. Poor manual dexterity
5. Suicidal ideation
6. Lack of pump supplies at bedside
7. Unwillingness to comply with hospital CSII policy
8. Inability to demonstrate CSII competency
9. Patient preference
10. Caregiver manages CSII and not at bedside 24 h/day
11. Physician judgment

self-manage their insulin pumps. Table 12.2 summarizes a list of recommended con-traindications for CSII self-management in the hospital. CSII should not be used in patients with altered mental status or cognitive impairment. This includes patients who are drowsy while on narcotic medications. Patients who are in DKA or HHS should be transitioned over to hospital protocols for DKA/HHS, usually with initia-tion of IV insulin infusion. Before removal of the insulin pump, however, the infu-sion set and insulin pump need to be evaluated for site infection, kinking of tubing or pump malfunction so that the issue can be remedied. Once the metabolic abnor-malities related to DKA/HHS resolve, then patients can be transitioned back to CSII. In patients with hand injury or trauma, or those who do not have the manual dexterity to adjust insulin pump settings and give insulin boluses, CSII should be discontinued and the patient should be transitioned to subcutaneous or IV insulin. Also any patient who is having suicidal ideation should have CSII discontinued.

All patients need to be willing to comply with hospital policies of CSII self-management. They must also have their own CSII supplies present in the hospital. Given the multitude of different infusion sets and insulin pump supplies available on the market, it is unrealistic for hospital pharmacies to have all of the different pump supplies in stock. Patients must be able to bring in their own supplies to continue using CSII during their hospitalization.

It is extremely important to discuss continuing CSII in house with the patient rather than assume that all patients on CSII want to continue using their insulin pumps. Some patients feel overwhelmed with their current illness and may not want to deal with glycemic control on top of everything else that is going on. It is reasonable to transition patients to subcutaneous basal-bolus insulin therapy dur-ing hospitalization, if patients prefer.

In cases in which a caregiver manages the insulin pump, it is reasonable to leave the insulin pump in place if the caregiver can be at the bedside 24 h/day with the patient and is able to administer all insulin boluses and change the infusion sets accordingly. If the caregiver is unable to reliably perform these tasks, it would be appropriate to transition the patient to basal-bolus insulin therapy so that hospital staff can administer and adjust insulin dosing.

Most important, physician judgment should be used to determine whether or not a patient is clinically able to self-manage CSII. If there is any doubt as to the patient's ability to manage CSII, then the insulin pump should be removed and the patient should be converted to basal-bolus insulin therapy. Removing an insulin pump from an unwilling patient can be extremely challenging. Insulin pump users are used to controlling their own insulin doses and relinquishing that control to others is not easy. In situations in which the patient is unwilling to take off the insulin pump, it is essential to carefully explain why the pump needs to be removed and to provide reassurance that as soon as the patient is stable, willing, and able, insulin pump therapy can be reinitiated. Involving other family members in the discussion is often helpful as well.

Continuing CSII in the Hospital

If a patient is deemed appropriate for CSII use in the hospital, it is important to have institutional protocols to ensure safe use of insulin pumps in the hospital setting. Because most hospital staff, including the nurse and primary medical team, will not be familiar with insulin pumps or management, having the necessary steps clearly outlined and accessible is important.

Hospital Requirements for CSII Use

All institutions should have an inpatient policy for CSII use supported by guidelines, order sets, and patient contracts. Ideally, the cascade of necessary steps would be initiated using a computerized order set, which then would propagate other essential components of the protocol. Necessary components of the order set include the following:

1. Order to use the insulin pump including a medication administration record (MAR) entry for the specific type of insulin to be used for continuous subcutaneous infusion (Figure 12.1).
2. Insulin pump settings, including basal rates, ICRs, ISFs, active insulin times, and target blood glucose range.
3. Consult by pump specialist or outpatient provider.
4. Printed documents, including the following:

   A. Patient contract for patient to sign documenting patient willingness and commitment to—
   - manage the pump in the hospital and adhere to hospital policy
   - provide all insulin pump supplies including infusion sets, reservoirs and batteries
   - supply insulin if required
   - use hospital glucose meter at least 4x/day (ac/hs)
   - use hospital glucose meter only for insulin dosing
   - turn closed-loop pump to manual mode (not use auto mode)
   - document basal rates and all boluses administered on patient flowsheet
   - discuss with medical staff before making any changes to the basal and bolus insulin doses

   B. Patient flowsheet (Figure 12.2)
   C. Nursing tip sheet

Consultation with an endocrinologist, physician with expertise in diabetes, certified diabetes educator, or diabetes resource person trained in insulin pump management should be required to help make appropriate adjustments during hospitalization and troubleshoot any issues that may arise. If someone with insulin pump expertise is not available in-house, then consider consultation with patient's outpatient insulin pump provider either in person or via phone. If the outpatient provider is not available, the patient can be transitioned to subcutaneous basal-bolus insulin during hospitalization. Pump manufacturers also provide 24-h helplines for assistance with device-related questions or problems. The telephone number can usually be found on the back of the pump or controller. However, it should not be expected that hospital personnel will need to seek advice in this

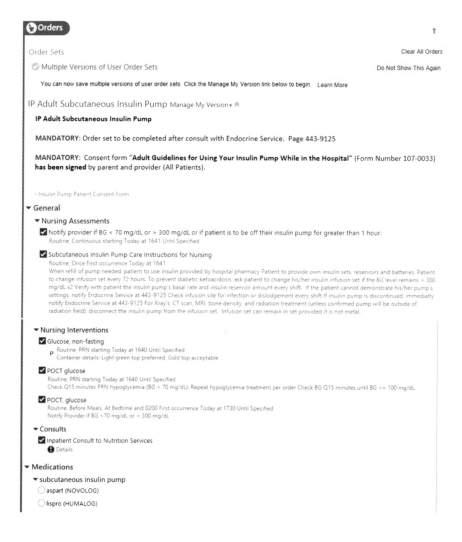

▼ Hypoglycemia Protocol
  ▼ Hypoglycemia protocol
    ☑ dextrose 50% injection syringe 12.5 g
      12.5 g, Intravenous
      Every 15 Min PRN, treat hypoglycemia, starting Today at 1640 Until Discontinued
      Give if BG < 100 mg/dL and patient is incoherent/unconscious or alert but cannot take PO. Repeat check and treatment every 15 minutes until BG >/= 100 mg/dL. If patient is incoherent/unconscious, temporarily disconnect pump tubing from the infusion set or turn off pump.

    ☑ glucose chewable tablet 20 g
      20 g, Oral, Every 15 Min PRN, treat hypoglycemia, starting Today at 1640 Until Discontinued
      Give if BG < 100 mg/dL and patient is alert and can take PO. May substitute 6 oz fruit juice or milk per patient's preference and document in flowsheet. Repeat every 15 minutes until BG >/= 100 mg/dL.

Insulin Pump Instructions:

A. Basal Rate:
Start Time: Midnight to {Time: 0100-2400:14903}.   Infusion Dose: *** units/hr
Start Time: {Time; 0100-2400:14903} to {Time; 0100-2400:14903}. Infusion Dose: *** units/hr
Start Time: {Time; 0100-2400:14903} to {Time; 0100-2400:14903}. Infusion Dose: *** units/hr
Start Time: {Time; 0100-2400:14903} to {Time; 0100-2400:14903}. Infusion Dose: *** units/hr
Start Time: {Time; 0100-2400:14903} to {Time; 0100-2400:14903}. Infusion Dose: *** units/hr
Start Time: {Time; 0100-2400:14903} to {Time; 0100-2400:14903}. Infusion Dose: *** units/hr

B. Carbohydrate Ratio:
Breakfast Dose = 1 unit per {UCSF RXIP CARBOHYDRATE INSULIN DOSE:22484} grams of carbohydrates taken.
Lunch Dose = 1 unit per {UCSF RXIP CARBOHYDRATE INSULIN DOSE:22484} grams of carbohydrates taken.
Dinner Dose = 1 unit per {UCSF RXIP CARBOHYDRATE INSULIN DOSE:22484} grams of carbohydrates taken.
Snack Dose =1 unit per {UCSF RXIP CARBOHYDRATE INSULIN DOSE:22484} grams of carbohydrates taken.

C. High Glucose Correction:
Mealtime: 1 unit per *** mg/dL over target of *** mg/dL.
Bedtime and 2am: 1 unit per *** mg/dL over target of *** mg/dL

D. If patient's BG < 70 mg/dL: check BG every 15 minutes per POCT order and repeat hypoglycemia treatment until BG > = 100 mg/dL. See PRN orders for IV Dextrose and Glucose tabs. Notify provider for BG < 70 mg/dL and > 300 mg/dL.

Figure 12.1. Medication administration record entry.

UC San Diego Health

PATIENT'S OWN INSULIN PUMP – BEDSIDE DOCUMENTATION SHEET
(To be completed by patient)

Patient Identification

Date: _____/_____/_____

Pump model and manufacturer: _____
Type of Insulin (check one): ☐ aspart (Novolog®)   ☐ lispro (Humalog®)   ☐ glulisine (Apidra®)

Time	1a	2a	3a	4a	5a	6a	7a	8a	9a	10a	11a	Noon	1p	2p	3p	4p	5p	6p	7p	8p	9p	10p	11p	MN
Glucose																								
Nutritional bolus																								
Correctional bolus																								
Basal Rate (units/hr)																								

Carbohydrate Ratio
_____ units per _____ grams of carbohydrate (Breakfast)
_____ units per _____ grams of carbohydrate (Lunch)
_____ units per _____ grams of carbohydrate (Dinner)

<u>OR</u>   **Fixed Doses**
_____ units at breakfast
_____ units at lunch
_____ units at dinner
_____ units with snacks

High Glucose Correction
_____ unit for every _____ mg/dL over _____ mg/dL (target glucose) <u>OR</u> *provide copy of written scale*

Completed by: _____   Reviewed by: _____ / _____
           (Patient Name)   *PM Nurse(s)*   *AM Nurse(s)*

D2041 (12-10) ref: MCP 818.4

Figure 12.2. Patient flowsheet.

manner. If there are pump issues, the pump should be discontinued and the patient transitioned to subcutaneous basal-bolus or IV infusion insulin.

The signed patient contract and daily patient flowsheets will become part of the patient medical record. Some institutions require nurses to input each insulin bolus in the MAR so it can be viewed by providers in the electronic medical record (EMR), but others scan the flowsheet into the EMR to be viewed in that manner.

A nursing tip sheet is helpful to quickly familiarize the patient's bedside nurse with the insulin pump and nursing responsibilities, including the following:

- Continually assessing the patient's mental and physical ability to manage the insulin pump
- Assessing the insertion site daily for erythema, swelling, or leakage
- Using a hospital meter to check blood glucose at least 4x/day (ac/hs)
- Documenting location and condition of the infusion site as well as CSII site changes

Initial Assessment

In addition to these minimum requirements, it is also important to assess the patient's insulin pump settings and self-management behaviors to determine whether initial adjustments need to be made. Inpatient glucose targets for non-critically ill patients are <140 mg/dL premeal and <180 mg/dL other times.[7] It is important that patients are aware that inpatient targets are more relaxed than their typical outpatient targets, because of the multiple complicating factors at play in the hospital, including illness, stress, variable renal function, glucocorticoids, and intermittent NPO periods.

The patient should be able to access and show the provider several current settings, including basal rates, ICR, correction factor, active insulin time, and target blood glucose range. Some initial questions to ask the patient include the following:

1. How often do you check your blood glucose at home? Do you have a continuous glucose monitor?
2. What do your blood glucose levels typically run at home?
3. How often do you have low blood glucose level <70mg/dL? If they do occur, do they occur during the day or night?
4. How often do you have high blood glucose level >200 mg/dL?
5. Do you manually calculate your bolus or do you use the bolus calculator/wizard in your pump?
6. How often do you bolus at home?
7. How often do you change your infusion set? When was the last time you changed your infusion set?

If patients are not checking blood glucose levels very often at home, then the A1C and frequency of hyperglycemia or hypoglycemia symptoms will be important to help determine whether the initial settings need to be adjusted. For patients with excellent, tight control in the outpatient setting, basal settings should be decreased by 10–20% or target blood glucose increased to avoid hypoglycemia in the inpatient setting. If patients are experiencing recurrent hypoglycemia at home, daytime lows point to issues with carbohydrate counting, ICR, correction factor, or daytime basal (if lows occur during the day when a meal is skipped). Overnight or early morning hypoglycemia are more concerning for issues with overnight basal rates, unless the patient is bolusing close to bed or overnight.

For patients not using the bolus calculator or wizard, their ICR and correction factor settings do not apply and their ability to accurately calculate meal and correction coverage themselves becomes imperative. Patients should be provided accurate carbohydrate counts for meals in the hospital so appropriate nutritional insulin doses can be calculated. If patients are not bolusing for every meal and snack at home, they may be relying on higher basal rates to cover carbohydrate intake or frequent snacking. This increases the risk of hypoglycemia in the hospital. In this case, total daily doses of insulin may need to be redistributed or basal rates reduced. Typically, insulin requirements are split evenly between basal and bolus insulin, unless carbohydrate intake is very high or low. Infusion sets need to be changed every 48–72 h and patients should be able to do this independently. It is important to note on admission when the infusion set was last changed and ensure that the patient has enough supplies going forward to continue CSII in the hospital.

Daily Assessments

The patient's mental and physical capability to manage CSII should be assessed daily by both the primary provider and nurse. The patient's flowsheet also should be assessed daily to ensure that they are documenting insulin boluses appropriately as well as for the glucose trend over the past 24 h so adjustments can be made accordingly. Subsequent adjustments should be made cautiously, typically in increments of no more than 10–20% of the total daily dose per day. It is usually preferable to avoid making changes to the preprogrammed home settings to account for temporary hospital adjustments as patients likely will need to return to their home settings when their acute illness resolves. Rather, changes can be made by setting an alternate basal pattern, using temporary basal rates that need to be reset at least daily, or adding additional subcutaneous insulin that can be titrated up or down over time.

Troubleshooting

Hyperglycemia. Several factors in the inpatient setting can lead to hyperglycemia including stress, illness, glucocorticoid use, and decreased activity. Table 12.3 addresses common causes of hyperglycemia in the hospital and associated treatment strategies.

Hypoglycemia. Hypoglycemia does not typically warrant pump removal unless it is prolonged or profound. Rather, hypoglycemia warrants immediate treatment per hospital hypoglycemia protocol and investigation into the cause of hypoglycemia. Table 12.4 outlines common causes of hypoglycemia in the hospital setting and associated treatment strategies.

Radiographic Studies. Insulin pumps must be removed or shielded for various radiographic studies. Temporary suspension and disconnection of the pump for short radiographic procedure may be warranted if the device is going to be in the field of ionizing radiation. These studies include magnetic resonance imaging (MRI), X-ray, computed tomagraphy (CT), and fluoroscopy. Infusion sets with a

Table 12.3. Common Causes of Hyperglycemia and Treatment Options

Hyperglycemia	Problem	Treatment
Daytime Hyperglycemia	Poor carbohydrate counting	Provide menus with appropriately labeled carbohydrates
	Stress hyperglycemia	Increase daytime ICR
		Increase daytime basal (set temporary basal rate or an alternate basal pattern)
		Increase ISF
	Once daily morning-dosed glucocorticoid	Increase daytime ICR
		Increase daytime basal (set temporary basal rate or an Alternate basal pattern)
		Increase ISF
Overnight Hyperglycemia	Uncovered snacks	Provide zero-carbohydrate snacks or snacks with appropriately labeled carbohydrates
	Stress hyperglycemia	Increase overnight basal rate (set temporary basal rate or an alternate basal pattern)
		Increase ISF
	Once daily evening-dosed glucocorticoid	Increase overnight basal rate (set temporary basal rate or an alternate basal pattern)
		Increase ISF
Severe Hyperglycemia not responding to boluses	Kinked catheter	Check ketones and basic metabolic panel
		Replace infusion set
	Poor infusion site	Check ketones and chemistry
		Replace infusion set
	Pump removed and not reconnected	Reconnect pump and administer bolus
		Administer bolus using insulin pen, vial/syringe, or IV insulin
	Pump malfunction	Transition to subcutaneous basal-bolus insulin
		Call number on back of pump

ICR, insulin-to-carbohydrate ration; ISF, insulin sensitivity factor; IV, intravenous.

Table 12.4. Common Causes of Hypoglycemia in the Hospital Setting

Hypoglycemia	Problem	Treatment
Fasting Hypoglycemia	Too high basal rates	Decrease overnight basal rate (set temporary basal rate or an alternate basal pattern)
		Change times of different basal rates
	Undocumented bolus	Check pump bolus history to see if bolus administered
Hypoglycemia after meal	Poor carbohydrate counting	Provide menus with appropriately labeled carbohydrates
	Too high ICR	Decrease carbohydrate ratio
	Poor absorption or gastroparesis	Square-wave or dual-wave bolus
	Overcorrection	Decrease ISF
	Undocumented bolus	Check pump bolus history to see if bolus administered, if so evaluate as above
Hypoglycemia between meals	Poor carbohydrate counting	Provide menus with appropriately labeled carbohydrates
	Too high ICR	Decrease carbohydrate ratio
	Too high basal rates	Decrease daytime basal rates (set temporary basal rate or an alternate basal pattern)
	Overcorrection	Decrease ISF
	Undocumented bolus	Check pump bolus history to see if bolus administered

ICR, insulin-to-carbohydrate ration; ISF, insulin sensitivity factor.

stainless steel cannula must also be removed from the patient's body before MRI procedures in particular, but infusion sets with soft synthetic cannula do not require removal. See Table 12.5 for changes required to CSII for various radiographic studies and procedures.

Generally, CSII can be suspended and disconnected for up to an hour without issue. However, when patients will be disconnected for 1–3 h, supplemental insulin should be administered either as a separate injection or as a bolus before pump removal. The bolus dose can be calculated as an hourly basal rate multiplied by the time the pump will be disconnected. If the patient will be disconnected for >3 h, they should be transitioned to IV insulin infusion or subcutaneous basal-bolus therapy to prevent DKA.

CSII in the Emergency Department

The Institute for Safe Medication Practices recommends patients on CSII who present to the hospital (inpatient or the emergency department [ED]), should have CSII use and settings verified within 12 h. Historically, EDs have not had protocols for managing patients on CSII. Without CSII orders or scheduled

Table 12.5. Changes Required to CSII for Radiographic Studies and Procedures

MRI	Pump and metal infusion set should be removed from patient and the MRI room
CT Scan	Pump should be shielded with lead apron or removed
X-Ray	Pump should be shielded with lead apron or removed
Ultrasound	Pump and infusion set can remain on/in
Cardiac Catheterization	Pump should be shielded with lead apron or removed
Pacemaker/AICD	Pump should be shielded with lead apron or removed
EKG	Pump and infusion set can remain on/in
Fluoroscopy	Pump should be shielded with lead apron or removed
Colonoscopy	Pump and infusion set can remain on/in
Laser Surgery	Pump and infusion set can remain on/in
Electrocautery	Pump with metal infusion set should be removed from patient

glucose checks in the ED, adverse glycemic excursions from insulin pump misadventures can occur, increasing risk of DKA or severe hypoglycemia.

To improve safety in the ED, the University of California–San Francisco has implemented the following:

1. Triage (part of the EMR) to identify any patient who comes into the ED with CSII, check point-of-care (POC) glucose, and have patient sign CSII waiver.
2. Include the CSII ED specific order set in the EMR, which note the specific options for adult and pediatric patients and include the following:

   a. Insulin order in MAR without restriction of complete directions (provides the MAR location for nursing to document any patient insulin boluses);
   b. Hypoglycemia medications and protocol in place;
   c. Scheduled POC blood glucose testing q4 hours with "notify provider" orders for glycemic excursions; and
   d. Orders to remove CGM or insulin pump for MRI.

3. Registered nurse (RN) ED protocols (part of order set):

   a. Allows start of POC glucose (reminds patient and RN that CGM blood glucose readings are not allowed for clinical decision making in the ED or hospital; cosignature is required within 24 h);
   b. Allows urinalysis for BG >300 mg/dL to assess for ketones; and
   c. Integrates RN and patient early in the presentation to discuss and sign the CSII/CGM patient waiver to increase compliance.

Transitions

Transition from CSII to IV Insulin Infusion. The insulin pump can be suspended, disconnected, and removed after the initiation of the IV insulin infusion.

Transition from CSII to Subcutaneous Basal-Bolus Therapy. If a patient needs to be transitioned to subcutaneous basal-bolus therapy, doses can be calculated using the pump settings. If they cannot be accessed, then the patient's weight and renal function can be used. If the patient can display the total daily doses for the past few days, then the average total daily dose can be divided by two and administered as glargine or Levemir given once daily or as a divided dose twice daily. Or, if the patient can access the basal settings, the total basal dose can be calculated or displayed and administered as glargine or Levemir once daily or as a divided dose twice daily. Patients typically need ~20% less insulin when delivered via CSII compared to basal-bolus therapy; therefore, it can be reasonable to increase the basal dose by 20% of these calculations if the patient has moderate or poor control. If, however, the patient has frequent hypoglycemia, decreased PO intake, or a basal-heavy insulin regimen (basal dose of >50% total daily dose in setting of normal p.o. intake) a reduction of 10–20% could be warranted. The insulin pump should be discontinued 2 h after the first injection of basal insulin.

For mealtime insulin doses, patients can use the ICR in their CSII for nutritional bolus injections of rapid-acting analog. Alternatively, the basal insulin dose can be divided by three to calculate an appropriate mealtime insulin dose. A correction scale should be ordered based on the ISF set in their insulin pump or based on the total daily dose of insulin.

Transition from IV Insulin Infusion to CSII. When patients are transitioning back to CSII from IV insulin, the overnight IV insulin rates can be observed to estimate the patient's insulin requirements. If IV insulin rates vary greatly from previous pump settings, then preadmission settings and glucose control, weight-based calculations, and assessment of any glucocorticoids or concomitant dextrose-containing IV fluids or medications should be considered before adjusting the insulin pump settings. A temporary basal increase or decrease, or an alternate pattern, can be set to avoid making permanent changes to the outpatient insulin pump settings. IV insulin should be overlapped with initiation of CSII by 1–2 h.

Transition from Subcutaneous Basal-Bolus Therapy to CSII. When transitioning back to CSII from basal-bolus therapy, CSII can be resumed 24 h after the last long-acting basal insulin injection. If CSII is to be resumed <24 h after the last long-acting basal injection, a temporary basal rate should be set reducing the basal to 0–10% and timed to expire 24 h after the last dose of basal insulin. If the basal dose is split into two injections, then the CSII can be resumed 12 h after the last long-acting basal injection and a temporary basal rate set to 50% and timed to expire 12 h after the last dose of basal insulin.

Transition from Hospital to Home. Patients typically can resume their previous home settings unless there has been a significant change in their clinical course or insulin requirements during the hospitalization, such as a change in renal function or an initiation of glucocorticoids. They should have plenty of insulin and pump supplies at home and should be followed by a provider knowledgeable in CSII management and technology. Post-hospitalization follow-up is essential and should be arranged before discharge.

CGM

More outpatients with diabetes are using a variety of CGM devices. The newest CGMs no longer require finger-stick glucoses using POC meters to be done for calibration or to make decisions on therapeutic interventions. Caution has been advised that these CGM devices may not be as reliable as promised, however, and POC glucoses may still be required.[15] Other CGM require calibration at least twice per day and still require utilizing POC glucose measurements for any therapeutic decisions. Depending on the device, oxidants such at uric acid, acetaminophen, and salicylic acid may interfere with the glucose oxidase reaction used in these products, leading to false results. In addition, the CGM results may lag behind POC results by up to 30 min. These sensors are generally changed every 7–12 days and require a 2- to 12-h equilibration time after insertion before becoming active. During these equilibration times, no glucose results are reported.

As of this time, no CGM device has been approved by the U.S. Food and Drug Administration for inpatient use. These devices are not regulated as POC devices and, as such, are not under the purview of hospital POC committees, and there are no standards for any aspect of their use for hospitalized patients. Nevertheless, continuation of outpatient CGM when a patient is hospitalized should be considered as patients feel more comfortable continuing with this device, which may improve patient satisfaction. Continued CGM use in the hospital has the potential to improve outcomes by assisting professionals with identifying hypoglycemic and hyperglycemic events. Patients and medical personnel should understand, however, that no intervention should be made based on the CGM readings in the hospital and that POC measurements using a hospital glucose meter remain mandatory.

Practical Approach to Patients Using CGM Who Come to the Hospital

The following guidelines were developed at a consensus conference on CGM use in the hospital.[16]

1. Develop institutional policies, procedures, and guidelines.
2. Patients should be required to sign patient safety waivers, similar to documentation used with insulin pumps, to illustrate the risks and benefits to the patient with continued use. Waivers should specify that medical providers have the right to remove the CGM from the patient in cases in which they feel the device is not being used properly or the patient is not safe to use the device.
3. The waiver should state and patient should understand that no intervention will be based on the CGM in the hospital, but that a glucose measurement utilizing the hospital POC device will be required.
4. The device will need to be removed for imaging studies such as MRI or CT scans and a new device will be inserted after the procedure.
5. Patients will need to manage these devices themselves as there is no expectation that hospital personnel will be knowledgeable about the increasing number of devices. If this is not possible, the device should be removed.
6. If calibration of the device is required, the hospital POC glucose meter needs to be used.
7. Although CGM data may be particularly useful in patients with altered mental status who cannot report hypoglycemic symptoms, there may be increased liability with continued use of these devices in such patients.

8. There should be an agreement within any institution regarding specific acuities and diagnoses in which CGM use would be contraindicated.
9. Waivers should specify that patients must have their own CGM supplies available to reinsert the device as needed. If the patient lacks appropriate supplies, then the device must be removed.

Future Directions for Inpatient CGM

At this time, large prospective studies are required to examine outcomes and accuracy with these devices in hospitalized patients. Testing will need to be done in patients with vasoconstriction, dehydration, edema, hypoxemia, and medications used on inpatients. Frequent MRI/CT scans requiring the devices to be removed and then replaced may limit usefulness. Studies are needed on cost analysis of CGM to the institution, the effects on nursing workload (decrease or increase), and provider ease of use. In addition, how the CGM data will be entered into the EMR and utilized remains to be established.

Ultimately, CGM may be initiated for some inpatients. The data can be monitored centrally to catch and/or prevent hypo- and hyperglycemia. However, who would be appropriate for this monitoring, what interventions would be made, and whether any outcomes would actually be improved remain to be determined.

Hybrid CSII Inpatient Use

New CSII pumps are becoming more automated. Previously, pumps with a wireless connection to the CGM could be programmed to suspend basal insulin infusions if the glucose reached a specific low glucose or if the glucose level was decreasing too rapidly. As of late 2017, hybrid CSII pumps were introduced. The MiniMed 670G was the first hybrid system on the market and allowed for automated basal rate changes based on continuous glucose data. Once in the "auto mode," there is no set basal rate. Patients still administer bolus insulin according to individualized ICRs.

No studies or databased guidelines have specified the use of the low-glucose suspend pump or the hybrid CSII pump for inpatient use. Thus, all recommendations are based on expert opinions.

There are many potential concerns regarding use of these systems in the hospital, all of which need to be addressed through research studies and experience. Documentation of basal rates is more difficult because there is no set basal rate on these devices when operating in auto mode. Instead, as the basal rate is continually changing based on glucose monitoring data, a common link to the EMR will need to be established on how to document variable basal rates in the medical record. Patients may be switching between "auto" and "manual" modes (either knowingly or not), which further complicates the ability to assess patient competency to use or adjust basal pump settings.

As with any patient with diabetes, acute illness, infections, IV fluids, NPO status, frequent procedures, glucocorticoid therapy and other medications, changes in kidney function, and abrupt dietary changes can all result in variability in glucose levels and insulin sensitivity. The basal rates of the new hybrid CSII systems are totally dependent on the CGM. As discussed for inpatient use of CGM in general, the accuracy of these CGM devices under all of the typical inpatient situations remains unknown. Thus, the basal rates could be directly affected by false CGM values. Also, how the algorithms in these pumps will adjust to these same inpatient situations is not known.

Having the patient move back to manual mode, with their previously programmed basal settings also has potential drawbacks. Just as with CSII in general, for a patient with auto mode, asking them to turn off the auto mode could potentially contribute to decreased patient satisfaction. In addition, it is possible that the basal rate used in the auto mode may be significantly different than the previously programmed basal doses.

Practical Approach to Patients Using Hybrid CSIIs Who Come to the Hospital

The following guidelines were developed as part of a consensus conference on CSII use in the hospital.[17]

1. Contraindications should remain for use of CSII in general.
2. Institution policies and procedures need to be established.
3. Waiver forms for patient to sign are required (as for pumps and CSII in general).
4. Low-glucose suspend should be turned off when patient is hospitalized. CGM has not been accurate enough to avoid false low-glucose readings with insulin infusion being suspended when glucose is not low.
5. The auto mode should be turned off for patient who is hospitalized. There are no data to evaluate how the algorithms will adjust to the changes in glucoses and insulin sensitivity in the inpatient setting.
6. Because hospital glucose meters must be calibrated frequently per regulation, hospital personnel can be assured that these POC values are accurate. Accuracy is absolutely necessary because these values will be used to determine insulin doses when entered into the insulin pump.
7. Patients must agree to use hospital POC values for insulin-dosing decisions and calibration.
8. Until more data are available on how patients are using this newest technology, converting the 670G or any other hybrid CSII pump from auto to manual control would be the best option if used in the hospital. Conversion to manual mode also facilitates entry of discrete basal data into the EMR.
9. Documentation that the patient is able to use this device in the manual mode remains necessary and if the patient is not able to demonstrate this, the pump should be removed.

REFERENCES

1. Umpierrez GE, Klonoff DC. Diabetes Technology Update: Use of Insulin Pumps and Continuous Glucose Monitoring in the Hospital. *Diabetes Care* 2018;41(8):1579–1589

2. Aro S, Kangas T, Reunanen A, Salinto M, Koivisto V. Hospital use among diabetic patients and the general population. *Diabetes Care* 1994;17(11):1320–1329

3. Bo S, Ciccone G, Grassi G, et al. Patients with type 2 diabetes had higher rates of hospitalization than the general population. *J Clin Epidemiol* 2004;57(11): 1196–1201

4. Rosenthal MJ, Fajardo M, Gilmore S, Morley JE, Naliboff BD. Hospitalization and mortality of diabetes in older adults. A 3-year prospective study. *Diabetes Care* 1998;21(2):231–235

5. Donnan PT, Leese GP, Morris AD, Diabetes Audit and Research in Tayside SoMMUC. Hospitalizations for people with type 1 and type 2 diabetes compared with the nondiabetic population of Tayside, Scotland: a retrospective cohort study of resource use. *Diabetes Care* 2000;23(12):1774–1779

6. De Berardis G, D'Ettorre A, Graziano G, et al. The burden of hospitalization related to diabetes mellitus: a population-based study. *Nutr Metab Cardiovasc Dis* 2012;22(7):605–612

7. Umpierrez GE, Hellman R, Korytkowski MT, et al. Management of hyperglycemia in hospitalized patients in non-critical care setting: an endocrine society clinical practice guideline. *J Clin Endocrinol Metab* 2012;97(1):16–38

8. American Diabetes Association. Diabetes care in the hospital. *Diabetes Care* 2018;41(Suppl. 1):S144–S151

9. Cook CB, Boyle ME, Cisar NS, et al. Use of continuous subcutaneous insulin infusion (insulin pump) therapy in the hospital setting: proposed guidelines and outcome measures. *Diabetes Educ* 2005;31(6):849–857

10. Noschese ML, DiNardo MM, Donihi AC, et al. Patient outcomes after implementation of a protocol for inpatient insulin pump therapy. *Endocr Pract* 2009;15(5):415–424

11. Bailon RM, Partlow BJ, Miller-Cage V, et al. Continuous subcutaneous insulin infusion (insulin pump) therapy can be safely used in the hospital in select patients. *Endocr Pract* 2009;15(1):24–29

12. Cook CB, Beer KA, Seifert KM, Boyle ME, Mackey PA, Castro JC. Transitioning insulin pump therapy from the outpatient to the inpatient setting: a review of 6 years' experience with 253 cases. *J Diabetes Sci Technol* 2012;6(5):995–1002

13. Shah AD, Rushakoff RJ. Patient self-management of diabetes care in the inpatient setting: con. *J Diabetes Sci Technol* 2015;9(5):1155–1157

14. Insulin Pumps, 2018. Consumer Guide. Available from http://main.diabetes.org/dforg/pdfs/2018/2018-cg-insulin-pumps.pdf

15. Shapiro AR. FDA approval of nonadjunctive use of continuous glucose monitors for insulin dosing: a potentially risky decision. *JAMA.* 2017;318(16):1541–1542

16. Wallia A, Umpierrez GE, Rushakoff RJ, et al. Consensus statement on inpatient use of continuous glucose monitoring. *J Diabetes Sci Technol* 2017;11(5):1036–1044

17. Thompson B, Korytkowski M, Klonoff DC, Cook CB. Consensus statement on use of continuous subcutaneous insulin infusion therapy in the hospital. *J Diabetes Sci Technol* 2018;12(4):880–889

Chapter 13
Perioperative Continuous Subcutaneous Insulin Infusion Use

Sandra Indacochea Sobel, MD;[1] Mary Korytkowski, MD;[1] and Amy Donihi, PharmD[2]

INTRODUCTION

Individuals with diabetes have an increased risk of requiring surgery in their lifetime compared to individuals without diabetes, regardless of whether they are on noninsulin or insulin therapy.[1,2] Individuals with type 1 diabetes (T1D) and many with type 2 diabetes (T2D) use multiple daily insulin injections (MDI) or insulin pump therapy (also referred to as continuous subcutaneous insulin infusion [CSII]) for their glycemic management. Since the 1970s, patients have used CSII therapy, with recent estimates of more than 1.5 million insulin pump users in the U.S. alone.[3] The sophistication of CSII pump technology appeals to many insulin-treated individuals as a way to provide more control and precision with insulin delivery while trying to achieve desired glycemic targets. Studies have shown that motivated individuals on CSII therapy can improve their glycemic control without increased risk of hypoglycemia.[4]

Given the increased use of CSII therapy in the outpatient setting, it is not surprising that we see an increased number of individuals with diabetes on CSII therapy in the surgical arena admitted for elective surgical procedures. This is true for both hospitals and independent outpatient surgical centers. Many patients prefer to remain on their pump throughout the procedure, if this option is available. When allowed to continue CSII therapy in the inpatient setting, patients report a higher level of satisfaction with care received.[5,6] Historically, evidence-based recommendations were lacking in this area. Over the past several years, a handful of institutions have published their experiences with continuation of CSII during elective surgical procedures and have described the processes used to standardize an approach for CSII use in the perioperative period.[7–10]

The objective of this chapter is to highlight the challenges that exist in the glycemic management of individuals treated with CSII admitted for *elective* surgical procedures. This chapter presents a practical, evidence-based strategy for preparing patients and providers for the care of individuals using CSII during the perioperative period with attention given to minimizing risk. The chapter also includes illustrative patient cases that highlight the application of some of these strategies.

---

[1]Department of Medicine, Department of Endocrinology and Metabolism, University of Pittsburgh Medical Center, Pittsburgh, PA. [2]Department of Pharmacy and Therapeutics, University of Pittsburgh School of Pharmacy, Pittsburgh, PA.

CHALLENGES

As noted, some institutions have policies and protocols in place to guide a patient on CSII therapy safely through elective surgery. These policies were often created by multidisciplinary teams in response to the absence of any prior standardization of care for these patients that resulted in discontinuation of CSII in some patients without administration of subcutaneous (SQ) insulin, or continuation of use without documentation that this was occurring.[11] In situations in which an institution does not have existing policies and procedures, diabetes providers have the opportunity to engage surgical staff and the institution in developing a standardized approach to managing patients on CSII therapy. Regardless of whether the institution has existing policies or protocols, there are many challenges to coordinating the care of patients on CSII therapy in the perioperative setting.

One important challenge is predicting the impact of the planned procedure on glycemic control. Another challenge is an assessment of an individual's ability to self-manage his or her insulin pump immediately following surgery. The type of surgery planned, the type of anesthesia used (local vs. regional vs. general), length of surgery, potential need for hospitalization following the procedure, and need for postoperative pain management can all affect insulin requirements during and after surgery. Patient factors, including how patients use their CSII device, the degree of medical complexity, appetite or ability to eat, and level of consciousness, can affect insulin requirements as well as the ability to self-manage one's own insulin pump.[4,12]

An ongoing challenge is the fast pace of advances in diabetes technology, which has produced a variety of different models and types of CSII devices by different manufacturers.[3,8] Today's devices are smarter, more user-friendly, and designed to improve accuracy, safety, and the overall experience of glycemic management in people living with diabetes. It can be difficult, however, for providers not directly involved with outpatient diabetes management to maintain familiarity with the different pump devices and features that currently are available. Providers who are unfamiliar with how CSII devices work require assurances that they can be safely used in the perioperative period and require education about how to ensure that safety.

Yet another challenge is coordinating communication among all providers involved in the care of patients with diabetes throughout the perioperative experience. Key players include the patient, the outpatient diabetes management team, the hospital's inpatient diabetes management team in places where they exist (which may differ from the outpatient team), preoperative surgery staff, postanesthesia care unit (PACU) staff, and finally the anesthesiologists and surgeons.[8,13] Clear communication and documentation is required to ensure that patient-specific recommendations are followed to achieve successful glycemic control.

This raises a final challenge, which is defining successful perioperative glycemic control. Studies of CSII perioperative therapy are retrospective with few having looked at defined glycemic targets.[10,14,15] Without a standardized definition of acceptable perioperative glycemic control and lack of prospective randomized studies that address this issue, providers and institutions will be left to define their own glycemic goal range, which may result in targets that are either too stringent with a higher risk for hypoglycemia or too lax, which increases risk for hyperglycemia.

PERIOPERATIVE MANAGEMENT

The days leading up to surgery play an important role in preparing an individual for planned elective procedures and contribute in a major way to glycemic control the day of surgery. Boyle et al.[7] defined four different components of the surgical process as the *1)* preadmission phase, *2)* perioperative phase, *3)* intraoperative phase, and *4)* postoperative management phase. Implementation of different strategies during each of these phases minimizes risk and optimizes the care of patients using CSII therapy.

Preadmission

Diabetes History. Outpatient diabetes providers must communicate to the surgical team the important details about the patient's diabetes history. This can include the duration of the diabetes diagnosis, degree of glycemic control as measured by hemoglobin A_{1c}, risk and frequency of hypoglycemia, presence of diabetes-related complications, type of diabetes technology used, and patient's comfort level and familiarity with their CSII device. In addition, the provider should document the type of CSII device, pump settings (basal, bolus, correction insulin doses, glucose targets) (Table 13.1), and type of insulin into the electronic medical record so that it is available to everyone providing care for the patient. The patient should be encouraged to bring a copy of this information to the surgical suite the day of the procedure along with any recommendations provided by their diabetes care provider for perioperative insulin management. This preemptive documentation is particularly useful in the event that the patient requires a hospital stay and may not be able to provide this important information during the postoperative period. Should the patient require an inpatient stay, documentation of this information will also provide the inpatient teams with the tools needed to allow a smooth transition of glycemic management following surgery. This is particularly important in institutions without a dedicated institutional diabetes management team.

Hemoglobin A_{1c}. Measuring a hemoglobin A_{1c} (A1C) before surgery provides some information related to an individual's glycemic control and can help inform medical teams as to whether the timing of the surgery is appropriate. Studies have shown that individuals with A1C levels >8% who undergo elective surgeries have a greater risk of postoperative complications. This suggests that individuals with A1C levels >8% postpone the elective procedure until glycemic control improves, to minimize postoperative complications.[16]

Patient Preference. It is important to determine and document the willingness of a patient to continue CSII therapy during the planned elective procedure. Understanding the patient's preference is instrumental in providing meaningful recommendations related to his or her perioperative glycemic management.

If the patient elects not to continue CSII therapy for the elective procedure, the patient's outpatient diabetes provider should provide recommendations for converting the patient from CSII to MDI basal-bolus therapy with MDI, preferably several days in advance of the procedure.

One example of how to transition from CSII to basal-bolus MDI therapy is first to determine the amount of basal insulin the patient needs. If the patient does not have a history of frequent hypoglycemia, then the total basal dose of insulin can be summed and rounded down to the nearest whole number; this would be

Table 13.1. Definition of Common CSII Terms

CSII Term	Unit	Definition
Basal Rate(s)	units/hour	Indicates the amount of insulin given per hour during the day. Differing rates can be entered to account for periods of the day when less (i.e., consistent afternoon increased activity) or more (i.e., significant dawn phenomenon) basal insulin may be needed. The 24-h total basal insulin dose can usually be found on the basal rate homescreen.
Temporary (Temp) Basal	%	A percentage of the basal rate that can be set to increase or decrease, respectively, basal rates that are higher or lower than the programmed basal rate. In addition to the percent increase or decrease, the duration of the temporary basal rate needs to be determined and entered into the pump (can be up to 24 h).
Insulin-to-Carbohydrate Ratio (ICR)	grams (g)	ICR indicates how many grams of carbohydrates 1 unit of insulin covers. This ratio determines the amount of insulin delivered as a bolus to cover nutritional intake. A higher ratio indicates a person who is more insulin sensitive, whereas a lower ratio indicates more insulin resistance.
Sensitivity/Correction Factor	mg/dL	This refers to the anticipated decrease in serum glucose for each administered 1 unit of insulin. A higher sensitivity/correction is seen in more insulin sensitive individuals. The correction corrects blood glucose to the target range (see below).
Target	mg/dL	The glucose range or number to which the pump will aim to correct glucose levels outside of the target range. Targets can vary at different times of day.
Duration of Insulin action	hours (h)	Amount of time the insulin bolus lasts to lower glucose after a bolus is administered.

the amount of basal insulin the individual would use the day before the procedure. For example, if the individual's total basal dose of insulin is 22.6 units/day, then the individual would inject 22 units of a basal insulin (i.e., glargine or degludec insulin). If the patient experiences frequent hypoglycemia or is on a basal heavy regimen (i.e., the basal insulin dose represents >50% of the daily insulin requirement), then one should consider dropping the total basal dose of insulin by 20% to 50% (17 or 11 units, respectively, in this example). The individual should be instructed to inject the calculated basal dose at dinnertime and remain on the pump until 2 h after the injection of the SQ basal dose. The pump still can be used for dinnertime bolus insulin. Once 2 h has lapsed since the basal SQ injection, the patient should disconnect the pump. The pump and supplies will stay at home during the surgical procedure and any inpatient stay that may be necessary.

The morning of the procedure, the majority of patients will be fasting in accordance with their preoperative instructions, which means that there is no need to administer prandial insulin that day. If, however, the fasting capillary blood glucose (CBG) is >180 mg/dL, the patient can administer a SQ correction dose of rapid-acting insulin according to the previously established insulin sensitivity factor, which should be recorded from the pump settings. Again, the patient should bring a copy of their pump settings on an information sheet to the surgical suite because this can guide the perioperative team into knowing how much correctional insulin to give for glucose levels outside of the designated perioperative target range. The patient should provide information to the postanesthesia care unit regarding the type, time, and dose of the last basal insulin given, as well as type, time, and dose of the last rapid-acting insulin given. In the event that a patient does not provide this information, correction insulin doses (often referred to as correction or sliding scale insulin) based on current institutional algorithms can be used.[1,17]

If the patient's preference is to continue CSII therapy during the elective surgery, then it is important to know whether the institution has preexisting protocols related to perioperative CSII glycemic management as well as whether the surgical team has experience and comfort with perioperative CSII use.

CSII Settings. Outpatient diabetes providers should guide changes in CSII settings to achieve desired glucose targets in the days leading up to surgery. This provides the opportunity for a reevaluation of basal settings, as patients who remain on their pump intraoperatively will have basal rates running continuously throughout the procedure. If the patient reports drops in glucose levels during periods of fasting, it would be important to lower basal settings, for example, by 10–20% during the observed times of drop in glucose. Conversely, if glucose levels rise during periods of fasting >180–200 mg/dL and are unrelated to the infusion set or site issues, consider increasing basal settings by 10–20% during the observed time periods reported. Some authors have advocated for basal rate testing and have outlined their approach to doing so in the preadmission phase,[13] whereas others advocate for a standard 20% basal rate reduction the day before surgery.[13,18]

Another important pump setting to evaluate is the programmed sensitivity or correction value. The sensitivity or correction factor refers to the serum glucose drop elicited by 1 unit of insulin (Table 13.1). If the individual is hyperglycemic (CBG >180–200 mg/dL) the day of surgery, he or she will require a correction bolus before or after the procedure to achieve glucose levels back into target range, that is, 100–200 mg/dL.[10,17] Inaccurately conservative or overly aggressive sensitivity or correction values place the individual at risk for persistent hyperglycemia or hypoglycemia, respectively. Extreme glucose levels in the perioperative surgery area can cause delays in operative start time or even risk cancelation of the procedure. Reviewing CSII pump downloads before the procedure and potentially using information extracted from personal or professional continuous glucose monitor (CGM) devices allow for the determination of glycemic trends several days before surgery and also may help provide a more informed recommendation for any CSII pump-setting change. Providing the patient with a copy of the pump settings is helpful if hospital admission is required postoperatively and the hospital team needs access to the information.

CSII Supplies. Patients should bring all of their insulin pump supplies with them to the surgical suite on the day of the procedure. Even if the elective procedure is a planned outpatient procedure, unforeseen complications may arise that could require the availability of the pump supplies. In addition to the pump, these supplies include infusion sets, batteries, connecting cable (if the pump requires charging), and potentially even insulin and syringes for refilling the reservoirs (Figure 13.1). Properly labeling all supplies with the patient name can ensure that they remain with the rest of the patient's belongings and do not get misplaced, or worse, discarded. The outpatient diabetes providers can set glycemic management expectations for the patient for the day of surgery.

Patients may express a wish to bring their own glucose meters to the hospital. Although this may be permissible, it is also an opportunity for the providers to explain how management decisions for correcting glucose levels outside of the target

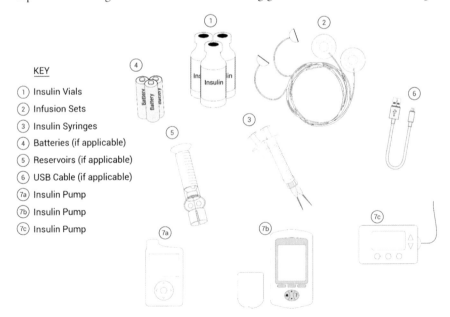

Figure 13.1. Examples of CSII models and CSII supplies to take to the hospital in preparation for elective surgery.

range should be made using the hospital's point-of-care (POC) meters, which automatically upload into the electronic system's records and allow care providers to identify why certain insulin treatment decisions were taken.[19] In addition, explaining how glycemic targets in the perioperative phase may differ from the preprogrammed pump settings is helpful in setting glycemic management expectations.

CSII Placement. Knowing the part of the body involved in the planned elective surgical procedure allows providers to guide patients where to place the CSII pump before surgery. It is recommended that the infusion site be placed outside of the surgical field.[7-10,13] For example, if a laparoscopic cholecystectomy surgery is planned, recommending placement of the pump on the left arm or left upper-outer thigh ensures that the CSII site is out of the surgical field and also renders the pump easily accessible by the anesthesiologist, should she or he need access to the pump during the surgery (Figure 13.2).

Another important recommendation is to have the patient insert a new CSII site at least the evening before surgery, with consideration being ~12 h before the surgical admission.[7,17] Some authors recommend changing the site the morning before surgery as long as there is the opportunity to obtain at least two self-monitored

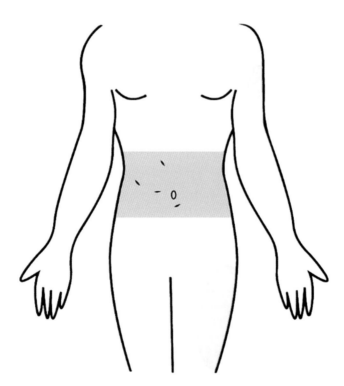

Figure 13.2. Shaded area indicates planned surgical field and CSII should not be placed in this area. Highlighted areas on arm and leg indicate appropriate placement sites for CSII infusion site.

Table 13.2. Preadmission Procedures for CSII Users before Elective Surgery

Suggested Preadmission Procedures before Elective Surgery for Patients Receiving CSII Therapy	
Preadmission Nurse	Notifies the primary diabetes care provider when a patient using an insulin pump is scheduled for planned or elective surgery
Primary Diabetes Provider	Prior to surgery date contacts patient to do the following: • Verify basal rate settings and insulin to carbohydrate ratio, correction factor, and type of insulin used in pump • Obtain recent blood glucose levels/trends and information about episodes of hypoglycemia • Recommends insulin pump settings to the patient before surgery • Remind patient to bring additional insulin and pump supplies to hospital (see Figure 13.1) • Remind patient to place a new pump infusion site away from the surgical site within 24 h before surgery (for an abdominal procedure, the infusion set should be inserted in arm or leg, see Figure 13.2) • Review institutional requirements for continued use of insulin pump in the event of admission • Advise patient to identify self as an insulin pump user at admission for surgery

Source: Adapted from Boyle et al.[7]

glucose measures before leaving home. Patients need to ensure that the new site is working properly and that any type of glycemic excursion with the new site is identified and acted on in advance of arrival at the institution.[13] Both hypo- and hyperglycemia can lead to delays or cancelation of a planned procedure, so one should strive for goal glucose levels on the morning of surgery.

For an overview of preadmission procedures for CSII users, see Table 13.2.

Preoperative Period

Identification and Documentation. Upon presentation to the presurgical admission area, patients should identify themselves as using CSII therapy. Presurgical staff should document the location of pump and the date of the last site change.[7,8] This last detail is especially pertinent in the event that the individual requires postoperative hospital admission, in which case the inpatient team will need to know when the next site change should take place. If CSII therapy is continued during the preoperative period, an order that includes the basal rate of insulin should be placed in the medical record. The preoperative nurse should chart any bolus doses that the patient self-administers in the medication administration record so that all providers are aware.

CBG Monitoring. The appropriate presurgical staff member should measure the patient's POC capillary blood glucose upon arrival to the presurgical area. Any BG level outside of the goal target range (100–200 mg/dL) should result in corrective measures either via hypoglycemia management protocols or by asking the patient to administer a bolus corrective dose of insulin.[10,17] Nursing should clearly document any corrective insulin doses in the medication administration section of the medical record and clearly communicate this to the anesthesia and surgical teams to keep them informed of patient status.

Intraoperative Glycemic Management Plan. The final decision as to whether the patient will remain on CSII therapy during the surgery rests with the anesthesiologist. The decision to have the patient disconnect from CSII therapy can be due to the following factors: persistent CBGs outside of target range, planned use of electromagnetic imaging during the procedure, expected long surgical time, anesthesiologist's comfort level with CSII technology, lack of an institutional CSII perioperative glycemic management protocol, or factors that could later impact oral intake.[13] In these cases, patients need to be transitioned to IV or SQ insulin therapy. In our institution, we continue CSII therapy if the plan is to discharge a patient home following surgery or if the planned procedure will be ≤2 h. If the estimated surgical time is >2 h, the patient is transitioned from CSII to IV insulin infusion therapy.[10]

Separate IV access for IV insulin infusion is needed for patients disconnected from the insulin pump. The initial insulin infusion rate can be based on the programmed basal settings in the insulin pump (Table 13.3). For example, if the pump setting has a programmed basal rate of 1.2 units/h, then insulin infusion rate should start at 1 unit/h). The CSII device can be removed 30 min after the initiation of IV insulin infusion.[10] CBG monitoring and insulin infusion titration would then proceed as per institutional protocol.

For hypoglycemia, defined as a CBG <70mg/dL, it is recommended that the IV insulin infusion be stopped for 1 h. It is also recommended that 25 mg D50 (1/2 amp) be administered with a repeat CBG in another 15 min. In 1 h, if CBG is >100 mg/dL, the insulin infusion can be resumed at 1 unit/h and adjusted hourly.[17]

Some authors have reported discontinuation of CSII therapy without transition to alternative insulin therapy for procedures planned to last 1–3 h long.[18] We do not support these recommendations and caution that this practice can increase the risk for severe hyperglycemia and diabetic ketoacidosis.

If the plan is to proceed with use of CSII intraoperatively, then presurgical staff should ensure that the pump is on and delivering insulin. Patient consent for continued use should be documented and an order placed into the electronic medical record that the pump will be continued during the procedure,[7,9,18]

Intraoperative Period

Identification and Documentation. Confirmation and EMR documentation of CSII pump location and proper functioning should occur when the patient

Table 13.3. Starting Rate for IV Insulin Infusion for Patients Taken Off of CSII Therapy before Surgery

Current Hourly Basal Rate (using insulin pump)	Starting Rate for IV Insulin (units/h)
≤0.5	0.5
0.5–1.5	1
1.5–2.5	2
>2.5	2.5

arrives in the operating room (OR). This confirms the plan of relying on the CSII pump as the primary source of basal insulin delivery to achieve and maintain glycemic control during the operation.

CBG Monitoring and Therapy. CBG monitoring should occur at least every hour.[7,14] If a CBG measurement is significantly discordant from prior CBG measurements, confirmation of this level is prudent with either another CBG measurement or using an alternate method, such as from an arterial blood sample or laboratory testing.[9,18] There should be no delay in treatment if the CBG is <70 mg/dL while awaiting confirmation of the result. Intraoperative glycemic targets should be well defined and are often institution specific, ranging from 100–200 mg/dL in many published reports.[10,13,14] We recommend a target of 100–180 mg/dL that reduces risk for hypoglycemia and hyperglycemia. For levels exceeding the predefined target, the anesthesiologist will typically administer SQ corrective insulin doses as per the institutions protocol.[9,10] That is, the CSII device is not used for bolus dosing during surgery. For hypoglycemia, defined as any CBG <70 mg/dL, the CSII device can be disconnected with conversion to IV insulin therapy after following the interventions described previously for correction of hypoglycemia while on IV insulin infusion. In cases in which it may not be feasible for surgical personnel to remove the device or adjust current basal rates, the patient can be treated with dextrose infusions and frequent glucose monitoring.

Protocol Example. Figure 13.3 is an example of our institution's CSII perioperative glycemic management protocol (PGMP).[10] We have reported on its safety and efficacy, which was defined as a first postoperative CBG <200 mg/dL. The demonstrated efficacy of this CSII PGMP was independent of surgical time in surgeries <120 min in length. The protocol initially guides management of CSII according to whether or not the patient is expected to require hospital admission. If it is a planned outpatient procedure, regardless of estimated surgical length, CSII is continued and the patient continues the usual basal settings unless otherwise instructed for concerns regarding hyper- or hypoglycemia (see prior discussion). If hospital admission is planned after the procedure, then the next tier in the management algorithm is estimated surgical length. If estimated surgical length is <120 min, the protocol recommends continuation of CSII, where the recommendation for procedures >120 min is conversion from CSII to IV insulin infusion.[10]

Troubleshooting. In the event of intraoperative pump malfunction or dislodgement, prompt recognition of the problem helps avoid severe hyperglycemia and development of DKA. Some CSII pumps come equipped with alarms that can indicate infusion errors; however, with the other sounds present in the operating room, it may be difficult to hear the pump alarm. Hourly CBG monitoring allows for early identification of any significant changes in glucose levels, which can prompt a therapeutic intervention. In the situation of pump malfunction or other complication, the patient can be disconnected from the pump and converted to IV insulin therapy, especially if a longer surgical time is anticipated. Another option would be to administer frequent SQ insulin boluses until the patient is back in the PACU, but caution is advised in this scenario to avoid insulin stacking and a potential reversal in CBG trend to hypoglycemia. In some cases, ongoing IV or SQ insulin may be required, whereas in other cases, the patient may be able to resume CSII therapy once they are awake enough to do so.[9,10,18]

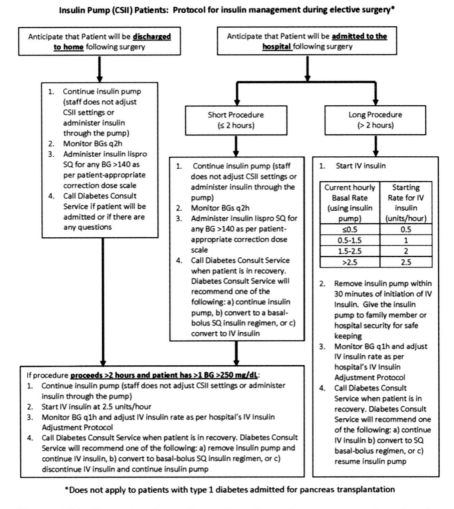

Insulin Pump (CSII) Patients: Protocol for insulin management during elective surgery*

Figure 13.3. Example of a perioperative glycemic management protocol.

Postoperative Period

Identification and Documentation. Confirmation, followed by verification, of CSII pump location and proper functioning should be documented upon arrival to the PACU.

CBG Monitoring and Therapy. A CBG on arrival, followed by hourly monitoring, helps ensure that glycemic targets are being met. Until the patient is awake and alert, PACU staff may need to provide SQ insulin correction doses for any hyperglycemic excursions. Continued assessment of patient's alertness and ability to self-manage the pump should also occur so that the patient may resume self-management of CSII when it is safe to do so.[14,18]

If the patient was converted to IV insulin therapy, the surgical team will determine whether this modality should be continued or consult the endocrine or diabetes service for guidance for transition off the IV insulin infusion.[7,10]

MISCELLANEOUS

Continuous Glucose Monitors

Given the rapidity with which diabetes technology continues to develop, it is important to comment on the increasing use of CGM devices. In the U.S., there are presently three primary stand-alone CGMs on the market (DexCom, Abbott, and Medtronic). They each estimate capillary glucose levels via interstitial glucose. The accuracy of each of these CGMs differs and for some models can be altered by changes in fluid status, ambient temperature, and some medications (e.g., acetaminophen). Although CGM use in the outpatient setting has been shown in several well-designed trials to improve glycemic control and reduce hypoglycemia, only a few studies have examined the inpatient setting and perioperative period.[19–21] For this reason, in addition to the perioperative factors aforementioned that can affect the accuracy readings, use of the patient's CGM technology to guide hospital insulin dosing is not recommended.[19] This is especially important for patients using the hybrid closed-loop CSII therapy. In the automatic mode, the pump uses the sensor readings to adjust the basal settings for a target of 120 mg/dL.[22] It is also necessary, however, for the patient to perform several calibrations with their meter throughout the day to ensure accuracy of the sensor. During anesthesia, these calibrations cannot occur. For this reason, the pump should be placed on manual mode (in which it is not dependent on the sensor readings) and pump adjustments can be made manually based on the hospital's POC meter.

PATIENT CASES

Case Study 1

A 23-year-old woman with a history of T1D for 18 years on CSII therapy, preoperative A1C of 6.5%, was scheduled for a right carpal tunnel release. Planned duration of surgery was 15 min with anticipated disposition to home. Her insulin pump settings were as follows:

Basal
12 A.M.: 1.0 units/h
8 A.M.: 0.85 units/h

Carbohydrate Ratio
1:9

Sensitivity Factor
1:30

Target
90–120 mg/dL

Five days before her planned procedure, she contacted her endocrinologist for instructions. She reported having tight glycemic control in the morning over the previous weeks and was instructed to program a 10% basal rate reduction starting at 4 A.M. the day of her surgery for 24 h. She was continued on CSII therapy during surgery and in the postoperative period as well.

Her blood glucose trend was as follows:

	Presurgical	First OR	Last OR	Postanesthesia Unit
Glucose mg/dL	106	95		105

Case Study 2

A 46-year-old woman with a history of T1D for 20 years on CSII therapy, preoperative A1C of 7.1%, was scheduled for a total thyroidectomy with planned surgical length of 90 min and planned transfer to the floor thereafter. Her insulin pump settings were as follows:

Basal
12 A.M.: 0.95 units/h
6 A.M.: 1.45 units/h
12 P.M.: 1.55 units/h
10 P.M.: 1.25 units/h

Carbohydrate Ratio
1:8

Sensitivity Factor
1:50

Given that her procedure was estimated to last <120 min, she was continued on CSII therapy. Pump status was documented during surgery and continued in the postoperative period as well.

Her blood glucose trend was as follows:

	Presurgical	First OR	Last OR	Postanesthesia Unit
Glucose mg/dL	290	148	123	92

Case Study 3

A 43-year-old woman with a history of obesity, T2D for 8 years on CSII therapy, preoperative A1C of 8.1%, was scheduled for a robotic distal pancreatectomy and splenectomy with planned surgical length of 360 min (6 h) and planned transfer to the floor thereafter. Her insulin pump settings were as follows:

Basal
12 A.M.: 3.2 units/h
5:30 A.M.: 3.4 units/h

Carbohydrate Ratio
1:5

Sensitivity Factor
1:20

Given that her procedure was estimated to last >120 min, she was transitioned from CSII therapy to IV insulin infusion. She was started at a rate of 4 units/h and total duration of surgery was 6 h 46 min, as surgery required conversion to open procedure. Her insulin infusion rate at the end of the surgery was 2 units/h. Her blood glucose trend was as follows:

	Presurgical	First OR	Last OR	Postanesthesia Unit
Glucose mg/dL	155	136	179	187

She was transferred to the ICU after surgery and the inpatient endocrine consult service was called for glycemic control recommendations. Given the patient's NPO and postoperative mental status, she was kept on the IV insulin infusion overnight at a rate of 3 units/h.

CONCLUSION

Diabetes care providers must consider the patient's preference regarding whether he or she would like to remain on CSII therapy during an elective surgical procedure. If so, it is important to have a systematic approach in place that explains how to prepare these patients for elective surgery. This plan includes a review of what the planned surgical procedure and anticipated surgical length is, an explanation of whether or not an inpatient stay postprocedure is planned, and then a focus on CSII settings and adjusting the settings as necessary in advance of the procedure with proper documentation communicated to and accessible by the surgical team. Ultimately, the decision to continue CSII therapy perioperatively will fall on the surgical team, so it is also important to familiarize oneself with the hospital's policies on CSII use during elective surgeries.

REFERENCES

1. Umpierrez GE, Smiley D, Jacobs S, Peng L, Temponi A, Mulligan P, Umpierrez D, Newton C, Olson D, Rizzo M. Randomized Study of Basal-Bolus Insulin Therapy in the Inpatient Management of Patients With Type 2 Diabetes Undergoing General Surgery (RABBIT 2 Surgery). *Diabetes Care* 2011; 34:256–261

2. Clement S, Braithwaite SS, Magee MF, Ahmann A, Smith EP, Schafer RG, Hirsch IB. Management of diabetes and hyperglycemia in hospitals. *Diabetes Care* 2004;27:553–591

3. Thompson B, Korytkowski M, Klonoff DC, Cook CB. Consensus statement on use of continuous subcutaneous insulin infusion therapy in the hospital. *J Diabetes Sci Technol* 2018;12(4):880–889

4. Edem D, McCarthy P, Ng J, Stefanovic-Racic M, Korytkowski MT. Insulin pump therapy: patient practices and glycemic outcomes. *J Diabetes Sci Technol* 2018;12(6):1250–1251

5. Noschese ML, DiNardo MM, Donihi AC, Gibson JM, Koerbel GL, Saul M, Stefanovic-Racic M, Korytkowski MT. Patient outcomes after implementation of a protocol for inpatient insulin pump therapy. *Endocr Pract* 2009;15: 415–424

6. Grunberger G, Abelseth JM, Bailey TS, Bode BW, Handelsman Y, Hellman R, Jovanovic L, Lane WS, Raskin P, Tamborlane WV, Rothermel C, Force AIPMT. Consensus statement by the American Association of Clinical Endocrinologists/American College of Endocrinology insulin pump management task force. *Endocr Pract* 2014;20:463–489

7. Boyle ME, Seifert KM, Beer KA, Apsey HA, Nassar AA, Littman SD, Magallanez JM, Schlinkert RT, Stearns JD, Hovan MJ, Cook CB. Guidelines for application of continuous subcutaneous insulin infusion (insulin pump) therapy in the perioperative period. *J Diabetes Sci Technol* 2012;6:184–190

8. Boyle ME, Seifert KM, Beer KA, Mackey P, Schlinkert RT, Stearns JD, Cook CB. Insulin pump therapy in the perioperative period: a review of care after implementation of institutional guidelines. *J Diabetes Sci Technol* 2012;6:1016–1021

9. Mackey PA, Thompson BM, Boyle ME, Apsey HA, Seifert KM, Schlinkert RT, Stearns JD, Cook CB. Update on a quality initiative to standardize perioperative care for continuous subcutaneous insulin infusion therapy. *J Diabetes Sci Technol* 2015;9(6):1299–1306

10. Sobel SI, Augustine MA, Donihi A, Reider J, Forte P, Korytkowski M. Safety and efficacy of a peri-operative protocol for patients with diabetes treated with continuous subcutaneous insulin infusion who are admitted for same-day surgery. *Endocr Pract* 2015;21(11):1269–1276

11. Nassar AA, Boyle ME, Seifert KM, Beer KA, Apsey HA, Schlinkert RT, Stearns JD, Cook CB. Insulin pump therapy in patients with diabetes undergoing surgery. *Endocr Pract* 2012;18:49–55

12. Heinemann L, Fleming GA, Petrie JR, Holl RW, Bergenstal RM, Peters AL. Insulin pump risks and benefits: a clinical appraisal of pump safety standards, adverse event reporting, and research needs: a joint statement of the European Association for the Study of Diabetes and the American Diabetes Association Diabetes Technology Working Group. *Diabetes Care* 2015;38(4): 716–722

13. Partridge H, Perkins B, Mathieu S, Nicholls A, Adeniji K. Clinical recommendations in the management of the patient with type 1 diabetes on insulin pump therapy in the perioperative period: a primer for the anaesthetist. *Br J Anaesth* 2016;116(1):18–26

14. Corney SM, Dukatz T, Rosenblatt S, Harrison B, Murray R, Sakharova A, Balasubramaniam M. Comparison of insulin pump therapy (continuous subcutaneous insulin infusion) to alternative methods for perioperative glycemic management in patients with planned postoperative admissions. *J Diabetes Sci Technol* 2012;6:1003–1015

15. Ma D, Chen C, Lu Y, Ma J, Yin P, Xie J, Yang Y, Shao S, Liu Z, Zhou X, Yuan G, Yu X. Short-term effects of continuous subcutaneous insulin infusion therapy in perioperative patients with diabetes mellitus. *Diabetes Technol Therapeut* 2013;15(12):1010–1018

16. Underwood P, Askari R, Hurwitz S, Chamarthi B, Garg R. Preoperative A1C and clinical outcomes in patients with diabetes undergoing major noncardiac surgical procedures. *Diabetes Care* 2014;37:611–616

17. DiNardo M, Donihi AC, Forte P, Gieraltowski L, Korytkowski M. Standardized glycemic management and perioperative glycemic outcomes in patients with diabetes mellitus who undergo same-day surgery. *Endocr Pract* 2011;17:404–411

18. Abdelmalak B, Ibrahim M, Yared JP, Modic MB, Nasr C. Perioperative glycemic management in insulin pump patients undergoing noncardiac surgery. *Curr Pharmaceut Design* 2012;18:6204–6214

19. Peters AL, Ahmann AJ, Battelino T, Evert A, Hirsch IB, Murad MH, Winter WE, Wolpert H. Diabetes technology—continuous subcutaneous insulin infusion therapy and continuous glucose monitoring in adults: and endocrine society clinical practice guideline. *J Clin Endocrinol Metab* 2016;101(11): 3922-3937

20. Song IK, Lee JH, Kang JE, Park YH, Kim HS, Kim JT. Continuous glucose monitoring systems in the operating room and intensive care unit: any difference according to measurement sites? *J Clin Monit Comput* 2017;31(1):187–194

21. Grunberger G, Handelsman Y, Bloomgarden ZT, Fonseca VA, Garber AJ, Haas RA, Roberts VL, Umpierrez GE. American Association of Clinical Endocrinologists and American College of Endocrinology 2018 position statement on integration of insulin pumps and continuous glucose monitoring in patients with diabetes mellitus. *Endocr Pract* 2018;24(3):302–308

22. MiniMed 670G Insulin Pump System. Available from www.medtronicdiabetes.com/products/minimed-670g-insulin-pump-system. Accessed May 2018

Chapter 1

Benefits of Continuous Glucose Monitoring: A Case of Burnout

Adriana Valencia, RD, CDE[1]

CASE PRESENTATION

P.G. is a 41-year-old Asian woman with type 2 diabetes. She has been coming to the endocrinology clinic since November 2010. She was diagnosed with diabetes at the age of 21 years. Her initial treatment consisted of oral medication only: metformin and sulfonylurea. When she became pregnant in 2008, she started on basal-bolus insulin and states she had excellent control. P.G. also has a history of issues with her kidneys. She started seeing nephrology around 2009. When she transferred to the University of California, San Diego (UCSD) for her care in 2011 she was considered to have chronic kidney disease (CKD) stage 3, which is believed to be related to her poor blood glucose control before pregnancy.

P.G. and I initially met at the end of December 2016. At this time, her A1C was 7.1% in the setting of CKD. She did not bring her meter to this visit, but she did state that she checked her blood glucose ~5–7 days a week. At her NP visit about a week prior, her meter was downloaded. Between 13 November 2016 and 12 December 2016, she had four blood glucose readings with an average of 116 mg/dL (Figure 1.1). P.G.'s main concern at her RD visit was working toward weight loss and increasing her level of physical activity. We reviewed her carb goal of 45 g/meal and low-carbohydrate snacks between meals. Her BMI at the time was ~29 kg/m². We also discussed the importance of checking her blood glucose levels, which she seems to have struggled with for a long period of time.

At a follow-up visit with her MD in May 2017 between 20 April 2017 and 19 May 2017, she had taken 13 blood glucose readings with an average of 214 mg/dL (Figure 1.2). P.G. was feeling burned out at this time and was not checking her blood glucose levels frequently. Her MD suggested she consider a continuous glucose monitor (CGM). P.G.'s A1C at this time was taken and was still 7.1%.

P.G. met with her RD about 5 months later. She had many questions about CGM that were answered. She decided to move forward with the process, and we faxed over a form for her insurance company to get the approval process started. Her main motivation at the time was feeling that actually seeing her blood glucose values numbers would motivate her to give her insulin. Her hope was also that having a CGM would reduce her fear of her blood glucose levels dropping when she exercised. She came to the clinic in January to receive assistance with her Dexcom placement with our nurse practitioner. P.G. came back

---

[1]University of California–San Diego Medical Center, University of California, La Jolla, CA.

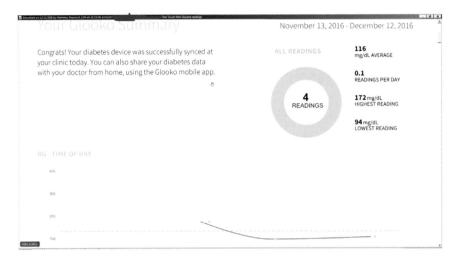

Figure 1.1. Glooko summary: November 13–December 12, 2016.

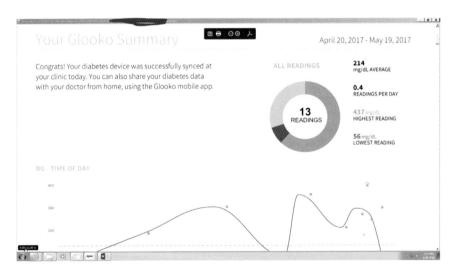

Figure 1.2. Glooko summary: April 20–May 19, 2017.

to the clinic to see her MD and RD for follow-up with her Dexcom 11 days after her CGM placement on 17 January. This was her first visit since her placement. At this time, she reported loving her CGM. The MD's notes from this visit briefly describe her feelings toward her CGM and give her average blood glucose levels, which have improved (Figure 1.3). The RD's notes describe the changes P.G. made to her diet after having the information from her Dexcom (Figure 1.4).

Currently, P.G. is taking insulin detemir 45 units twice a day, insulin aspart, and liraglutide for her diabetes management. Her regimen is as follows: breakfast 45 units, lunch 45 units, and dinner 20–45 units depending on meal size. Since having her CGM, P.G. has reported feeling more in control of her diabetes. She also felt more comfortable participating in physical activity. P.G. continues to struggle with stress eating, which we discuss at almost every visit.

P.G.'s most recent CGM trend in January 2018 shows much improvement compared to her previous blood glucose readings. Her average blood glucose is 165 mg/dL with a standard deviation of 48 (Figure 1.5). Having her CGM has helped P.G. feel more empowered and has allowed her MD and NP to make appropriate changes in her insulin regimen.

dexcom
Mean 165 SD 48
Much better
Calibrating wrongly
Loves it

Figure 1.3. MD note from visit in January 2018.

Discussion:
RD meet with patient for follow up. She also meet with MD today, patient discussed. Is really liking her CGM. She had questions regarding placing it that were answered today. Has found her dexcom very helpful and it has made her realize how much eating rice really affects her blood sugars. Has been trying to work on reducing her rice intake. Feels that has been the most difficult thing to change in her diet. We dicussed the idea of trying cauilflower rice. We talked about different recipes she could try. Suggested at least mixing it with 1/2 rice and 1/2 cauliflower rice. RD present during MD visit as well today. Reminded her of goal of non starchy vegetables with her meals. Would like to continue to work on weight loss. Overall blood sugars are looking much better.

Figure 1.4. RD note from visit in January 2018.

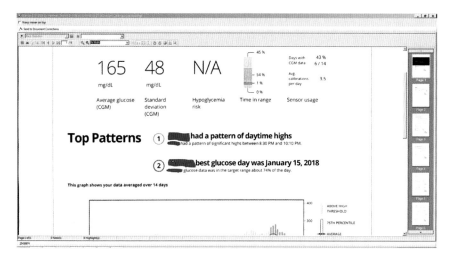

Figure 1.5. P.G.'s CGM data from January 2018.

Chapter 2
Technology-Facilitated Diabetes and Pregnancy Management

Donna Jornsay, MS, BSN, CPNP, BC-ADM, CDE, CDTC,[1] and
Lara DeLeuw, BSN, RN, CDE[1]

The prevalence of both type 1 diabetes (T1D) and type 2 diabetes (T2D) has been increasing in the U.S., as has the prevalence of diabetes complicating pregnancy. Both preexisting T1D and T2D in pregnancy cause significantly greater maternal and fetal risks, including spontaneous abortions, preeclampsia, fetal anomalies (most notably cardiac and spinal cord abnormalities), and other complications such as macrosomia, neonatal hypoglycemia and hyperbilirubinemia, and fetal demise, than does gestational diabetes (GDM). The specific risk of fetal malformations is directly proportional to the degree of maternal hyperglycemia, as evidenced by the a HbA_{1c} value, in the first 9–10 weeks of gestation.[1] Preconception counseling and management should be directed at the importance of establishing glycemic control as close to normal as possible. Ideally, a HbA_{1c} value < 6.5% should be obtained before discontinuing contraception.

The risk of hypoglycemia in early pregnancy is particularly increased for women with T1D, and the altered counterregulatory hormone responses seen in pregnant women may decrease hypoglycemia awareness. Management of insulin-requiring diabetes, whether T1D or T2D, and coexisting nausea and vomiting can make hypoglycemia management even more challenging. This makes insulin pump therapy and continuous glucose monitoring particularly advantageous for women with preexisting diabetes.[2] Ideally, insulin pump therapy, with or without continuous glucose monitoring, should be initiated before conception. This provides the woman with the opportunity to become thoroughly comfortable with the technology and to collaboratively work with her diabetes team to maximize her glycemic control and to minimize both her glucose variability and hypoglycemia.

CASE PRESENTATION

C.C. is a 28-year-old woman who has had T1D for 23 years. She uses insulin lispro (Humalog) via a tethered insulin pump. Her endocrinologist, who is adept with diabetes technology, but not comfortable with pregnancy management, referred her to the Diabetes and Pregnancy Program for preconception education and management. C.C. started the preconception program in October 2017 with

---

[1]Diabetes and Pregnancy Program, Mills-Peninsula Medical Center, Burlingame, CA.

a HbA_{1c} of 6.6%, which was decreased from the 7.0%–7.2% range in spring 2017. At this time, her endocrinologist put her on the Abbott Libre PRO glucose sensor to detect any hidden hypoglycemia and to determine her willingness to wear a continuous glucose monitor (CGM) during pregnancy. Despite a HbA_{1c} value of 7.0% in April 2017, the sensor uncovered significant hypoglycemia, postmeal hyperglycemia, and glucose variability as shown in Figure 2.1.

C.C. had a baseline preconception assessment to evaluate diabetes complications. This assessment included a 24-h urine test for protein/creatinine, thyroid function test, a HbA_{1c}, an electrocardiogram (ECG), and dilated ophthalmologic exam, all of which were within normal limits. Although it is common for patients to have had an annual dilated eye exam, frequently the 24-h urine and ECG have not been performed. It is important to assess the woman's understanding of all aspects of diabetes self-management and to provide her with the necessary education on the changes intrinsic to pregnancy. This assessment and education is a top priority to identify any unmet needs or barriers she may present to achieving excellent glycemic control. Often our focus on diabetes technology is to the exclusion of the holistic approach to the person living with diabetes.

Based on her Libre sensor download, both basal and bolus adjustments were necessary to eliminate her hypoglycemia and postmeal hyperglycemia. The experience of wearing the Libre sensor and seeing the glucose data convinced C.C. that she wanted to wear a full-time CGM during her pregnancy.

CGM devices measure interstitial fluid glucose, which correlates typically within 9–13% of capillary blood glucose values, although often with a 5- to 15-minute lag behind capillary glucose in women who are not pregnant. The U.S. Food and Drug Administration (FDA) has not currently approved any of the three glucose-monitoring systems commercially available in the U.S. for use during pregnancy. Despite this lack of approval, research has demonstrated similar margins of error in pregnant women.[3] The CGM Group within the Working Group Diabetes Technology of the German Diabetes Association has

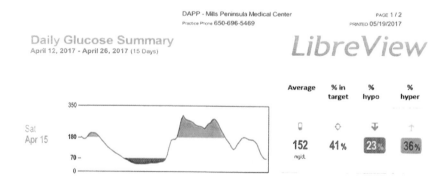

Figure 2.1. Daily glucose summary: Saturday, April 15.

defined evidence-based indications for the practical use of CGM and two of these indications are "pregnancy associated with inadequate blood glucose results" and the "need for more than 10 blood glucose measurements per day."[4] Clearly, both of these indications apply to pregnancy complicated by preexisting T1D.

C.C. received education on her pregnancy meal plan, including small, frequent meals to avoid postmeal glucose spikes and snacking to avoid premeal hypoglycemia. The importance of meal consistency with lean protein and balanced carbohydrate portion sizes was stressed. In addition, the frequency of blood glucose monitoring and the importance of morning ketone testing was reviewed. Of particular importance was teaching C.C.'s husband the use of the glucagon emergency kit secondary to the increased risk of hypoglycemia in the first half of pregnancy.

During this preconception period, C.C. was discovered to have some degree of lipohypertrophy, which was contributing to her glucose variability.[5] The download of her pump revealed that she typically changed pump sites every 3–4 days, rather than the recommended 2–3 days. She had been using a traditional tethered insulin pump for several years, which limited her infusion site rotation to her abdominal areas. Her thighs are too muscular to accommodate an infusion site and she had difficulty reaching her upper outer hip area. After exploring different anatomical infusion sites, she chose to use an untethered Insulet insulin pump, which, because of its ability to self insert, allowed her greater flexibility in the placement of the Pod in previously unused tissue. This change resulted in improved insulin absorption. At this point, C.C. also chose to go on a Dexcom CGM because the Libre sensor she tried prior to pregnancy did not have alarms to detect hypoglycemia or hyperglycemia. Her HbA_{1c} in early January 2018, following these changes, reduced to 6.4%.

The Glooko download (Figure 2.2) of her Insulet pump from early February 2018 showed many postmeal and overnight high glucose values (Figure 2.3). Her overnight basal rates at this time were increased to 1.20 units/h and 1.35 units/h. Her insulin-to-carbohydrate ratio (ICR) at this time was 1 unit/6 g of carbohydrate at breakfast, 1 unit/8 g of carbohydrate at lunch, and 1 unit/7 g of carbohydrate at dinnertime.

With the continuous glucose sensor data, and some diet and exercise changes, her HbA_{1c} was further reduced to 6.1% in early March 2018. Shortly afterward, she had a positive pregnancy test.

Now that C.C. is pregnant, the importance of changing infusion sites every 48 h to avoid both site infections and infusion site failure was emphasized. At 12 weeks' gestation, C.C.'s Dexcom download showed both overnight and postmeal hypoglycemia (Figure 2.4). This is not unusual at this time in pregnancy and frequently persists until ~20 weeks' gestation secondary to decreasing levels of maternal alanine and fetal energy demands. Her basal rates needed to be lowered to first 1.00 units/h overnight and then 0.80 units/h overnight. The patient commented that she had never been on basal rates this low.

Glucagon teaching and hypoglycemia prevention and treatment were again reviewed with C.C. and her partner. Also stressed with C.C. were the tighter pregnancy blood glucose targets, with fasting blood glucose values ideally in the 70–80 mg/dL range, and no higher than 90 mg/dL, and 1-h postmeal values no

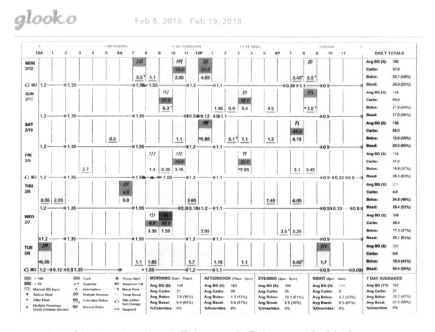

Figure 2.2. Glooko download: February 5–February 19, 2018.

higher than 140 mg/dL. Women are often surprised to hear that pregnant women without diabetes have fasting glucose values of 55–65 mg/dL. HbA$_{1c}$ values during pregnancy should be maintained at <6% provided that the woman is not experiencing clinically significant hypoglycemia.

Now at 15 weeks' gestation, C.C. has almost no premeal hypoglycemia, and her postmeal blood glucose values are becoming elevated (Figures 2.5 and 2.6). C.C. required a decrease in her ICR to prevent this premeal hyperglycemia. It was also important to discuss the need for a 15-min lag between the premeal insulin bolus and the meal, even with the rapid-acting insulin analogs.

For pregnant women with T1D, the first trimester glycemic management can be the most problematic. Increasing pregnancy hormones can cause postmeal highs, but without vigilance as to snack times, frequent hypoglycemia occurs 2.5 h following the premeal rapid-acting insulin administration. The first trimester is even more difficult if the woman experiences frequent nausea and vomiting or hyperemesis. As she progresses through the second trimester, we can expect to see greater consistency with blood glucose trends and increasing basal and prandial insulin requirements as human placental lactogen (HPL) levels increase.

The preconception percentage distribution of basal-bolus insulin (typically 50%/50% in nonpregnant people) also changes as the pregnancy progresses. It is not unusual for women to need only 30–40% of their total daily insulin dose as basal and 60–70% as bolus because of the impact of HPL on postmeals blood glucose values in particular.

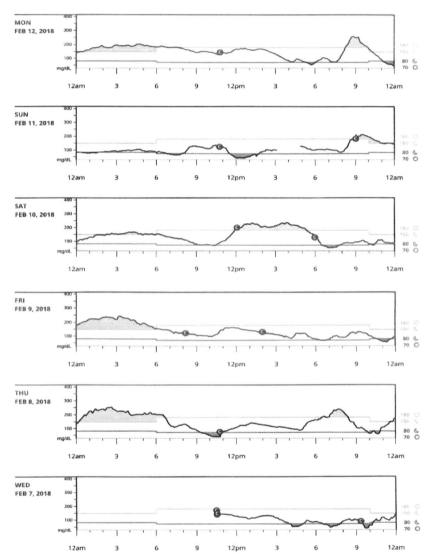

Figure 2.3. Dexcom download: February 7–February 12, 2018.

Technology offers significant assistance with clinical decision making in the management of diabetes during pregnancy. CGM alarms alert the woman to hypoglycemia, especially overnight at which time it otherwise would go unrecognized.

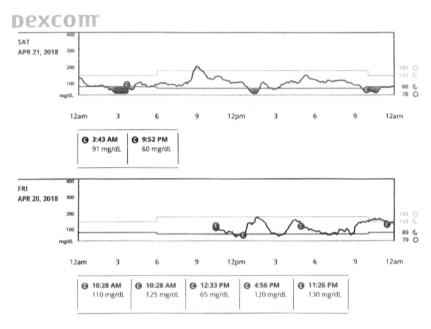

Figure 2.4. Dexcom download: April 20–April 21, 2018.

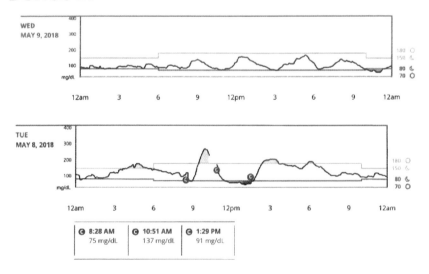

Figure 2.5. Dexcom download: May 8–May 9, 2018.

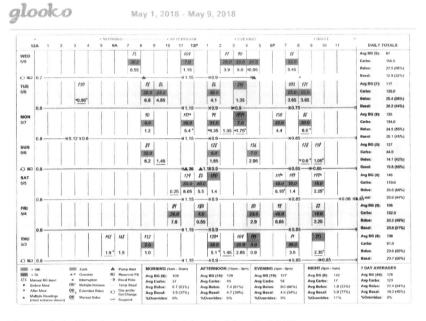

Figure 2.6. Glooko download: May 1–May 9, 2018.

This allows the woman and her partner to feel that she is safe while sleeping or napping. Insulin pump therapy provides the multiple overnight basal insulin rates needed to prevent hypoglycemia and to overcome the predictable dawn phenomenon seen more frequently with pregnancy. As the use of diabetes technology increases, providers will want to expand their knowledge and experience to promote maternal normoglycemia and prevent the maternal and fetal consequences of malglycemia.

　　Addendum: C.C. had a spontaneous vaginal delivery of a healthy baby boy at 38 weeks and 5 days whose Apgar scores were 9 at 1 min and 9 at 5 min. His birth weight was 3245 g, putting him at an appropriate weight for his gestational age.

REFERENCES

1. Jensen DM, Korsholm L, Ovesen P, Beck-Nielsen H, Moelsted-Pedersen L, Westergaard JG, Damm P. Peri-conceptional A1C and risk of serious adverse pregnancy outcome in 933 women with type 1 diabetes. *Diabetes Care* 2009;32(6):1046–1048

2. Murphy HR, Elleri D, Allen JM, Harris J, Simmons D, Rayman G, Wilinska ME. Closed-loop insulin delivery during pregnancy complicated by type 1 diabetes. *Diabetes Care* 2011;34(2):406–411

3. Kovatchev B, Anderson S, Heinemann L, Clarke W. Comparison of the numerical and clinical accuracy of four continuous glucose monitors. *Diabetes Care* 2008;31(6):1160–1164

4. Liebl A, Henrichs HR, Heinemann L, Freckmann G, Biermann E, Thomas A, Continuous Glucose Monitoring Working Group of the Working Group Diabetes Technology of the German Diabetes Association. Continuous glucose monitoring: evidence and consensus statement for clinical use. *J Diabetes Sci Technol* 2013;7(2):500–519

5. Blanco M, Hernandez MT, Strauss KW, Amaya M. Prevalence and risk factors in insulin-injecting patients with diabetes. *Diabetes Metab* 2013; 39(5):445–453

Chapter 3

Effective Utilization of Continuous Glucose Monitoring in a Patient with Type 2 Diabetes and an A1C of 9.3%

Jane Jeffrie Seley, DNP, MPH, BC-ADM, CDE, CDTC,[1]
and Naina Sinha Gregory, MD[2]

Although clinicians often think about continuous glucose monitoring (CGM) systems as a tool to identify patterns of hypo- and hyperglycemia and to select and titrate diabetes medications, sensor glucose (SG) information offers additional support for those who wish to modify lifestyle behaviors, such as meals, physical activity, and stress management.[1] Until recently, CGM was a consideration for patients with type 1 diabetes (T1D) but was rarely offered to patients with type 2 diabetes (T2D). In truth, because patients with T2D become increasingly insulin deficient over time, the availability of numerous pre- and post-meal SG determinations instead of, or in addition to, self-monitoring of blood glucose (SMBG) would be useful in guiding therapy and achieving glycemic targets.

CGM studies in the population with T2D has been limited. Vigersky et al.[2] conducted a randomized controlled trial (RCT) with 100 patients with T2D on any diabetes regimen (orals, injectables, or lifestyle changes) with the exception of prandial insulin. The intervention group (intermittent CGM 2 weeks on/1 week off for 12 weeks) was compared to usual care (self-monitoring of blood glucose 4 times/day) and both groups were followed for an additional 40 weeks. At the end of the intervention (12 weeks), the mean A1C was lowered by 1.0% in the CGM group and 0.5% in the SMBG group. Fonda[3] and others have shown that CGM use in patients with T2D can promote positive lifestyle changes and A1C reductions independent of insulin use.

The 2016 AACE/ACE Consensus Statement on Continuous Glucose Monitoring[4] strongly recommends CGM for patients with T1D of all ages, and states that CGM may be of value in patients with T2D. In light of the improved accuracy, no calibration, and ease of use of newer CGM systems, adoption by patients with T2D should grow. The International Consensus on Use of Continuous Glucose Monitoring cites several T2D CGM studies that show benefits for patients, including motivating patients to make behavioral changes when A1C levels are above target.[5]

[1]New York–Presbyterian, Weill Cornell Medical Center, New York, NY. [2]Weill Cornell Medicine, New York, NY.

CASE PRESENTATION

A.G. is a 69-year-old South Asian male physician who has had T2D for >20 years. On initial consultation in July 2017, his A1C was suboptimal at 9.3%. His current diabetes regimen consisted of metformin 1,000 mg twice daily (b.i.d.), glimepiride 2 mg b.i.d., and glargine 26 units at 10 P.M.

Our goal was to introduce strategies to decrease glucose variability and increase time in range in a patient with long-standing T2D and an A1C well above target.

Previous Diabetes History

A.G. has been on a variety of diabetes medications in the past but had to discontinue several of them because of side effects. While on SGLT2 inhibitor therapy, he had two urinary tract infections, with a DPP-4 inhibitor he developed a skin rash, and with a thiazolidinedione (TZD) he had significant fluid retention. He also had been on a once-daily GLP-1 RA injection over a year ago, which was stopped because of significant nausea and abdominal discomfort.

A.G. had never seen a diabetes educator or nutritionist and had decided to become vegetarian two years ago. He was not physically active despite having a treadmill, stationary bike, and free weights at home, which his wife uses regularly.

He works very long hours and has a stressful job that requires a high level of cognitive functioning. He is concerned about maintaining his mental clarity at the workplace.

After his diabetes was initially diagnosed, he was able to maintain an A1C between 6.5% and 7.2% for the first 10 years. During the next 10 years, his A1C gradually increased from 7.3% to 8.4%. During this time period, he was on a combination of oral agents, including metformin, sulfonylureas, TZDs, and DPP-4 inhibitors. He has a history of HTN and hyperlipidemia that are both under optimal control with rosuvastatin 10 mg daily and telmisartan 40 mg daily. He has no known micro- or macrovascular complications.

At the time of his initial visit, he was complaining of increasing fatigue and was experiencing intermittent polyuria and polydipsia. He was not performing SMBG because when he checked his blood glucose it was always >250 mg/dL. He expressed frustration about not being able to manage his diabetes and was feeling depressed about the situation. His wife implored him to seek an endocrine consultation, and he was at the visit primarily at her urging.

At this visit, we were concerned about adequate dietary protein intake and he was referred the same day to a dietitian in our practice (a certified diabetes educator) who saw the patient for diabetes self-management education support and medical nutrition therapy.

The following information was gathered at the time of the initial nutrition visit:

Breakfast

7 A.M.　　smoothie made with almond milk, kale, and blueberries

Lunch	(Brought from home)
1 P.M.	2 pieces of whole-wheat roti flatbread (2 oz by weight at visit)
	1 hardboiled egg every other day
	sautéed vegetables in olive oil (e.g., lima beans, peas)

Snacks	
3:30 P.M.	handful of peanuts
5:30 P.M.	medium apple

Dinner	
8 P.M.	2 pieces of whole-wheat roti flatbread sautéed vegetables in olive oil
	(similar to lunch)
Weight:	207 pounds
BMI:	27.19 kg/m^2

The importance of adequate dietary protein with a low glycemic diet and its impact on postmeal BG excursions was discussed at length with the patient. Two suggestions to increase his daily protein intake were to add whey protein powder to his breakfast smoothie and add low-fat plain Greek yogurt to his lunch or dinner.

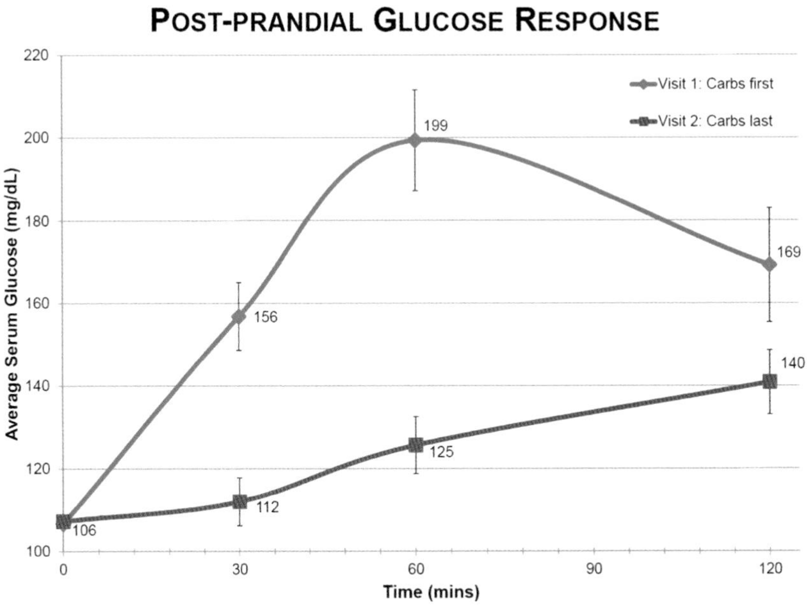

Figure 3.1. Carbohydrate-last meal pattern lowers postprandial glucose excursions in T2D.

We reviewed the results of a recent study from our institution showing the impact of food order on postprandial rises in BG with A.G.[6] The study showed that a carbohydrate-last meal pattern can be an effective behavioral strategy to blunt postprandial glycemic rises. The graph depicting this impact (Figure 3.1) was shared with him at the visit. He was amazed to learn this information and was empowered to try this in his own meal planning.

The plan at the end of the initial visit was to continue his current regimen of metformin 1,000 mg b.i.d., glimepiride 2 mg b.i.d., and glargine 26 units at 10 P.M. He agreed to focus on a low glycemic meal plan with adequate dietary protein intake and to start a regular exercise regimen of 150 min/week including a combination of cardiovascular and resistance training.

We discussed a Dexcom G5 CGM trial with A.G., and he agreed with the plan to use it as a temporary tool to provide real-time feedback to see the impact of lifestyle and dietary modification on his glycemic pattern.

A.G. returned to the office 2 weeks after the Dexcom had been placed to review the download and see the effect of his lifestyle efforts. The pattern of post-lunch and nocturnal hyperglycemia was reviewed. He found the information from the Dexcom very useful and did see the benefit of real-time feedback on reducing postprandial hyperglycemia.

The average blood glucose level on the Dexcom download was 170 mg/dL (Figure 3.2), which was incongruent with his recent A1C of 9.3%. This data showed that the recent glucose pattern was a marked improvement from his previous glycemic control.

The plan after this visit was to continue use of the Dexcom at least intermittently and work on improving postprandial BG control. A weight loss goal of 5 lb was discussed to address his BMI of 27 kg/m².

After 2 weeks, A.G. called to review his postdinner blood glucose values, which were still averaging 220 mg/dL. He still had not been able to lose any weight. It was decided to proceed with a gastric-emptying study to determine whether he

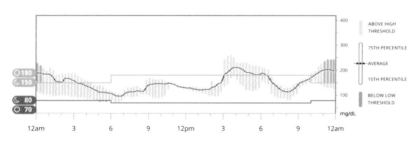

Figure 3.2. DEXCOM Saturday, 15 July, to Friday, 21 July 2017.

had any gastroparesis given the abdominal symptoms he experienced with GLP-1 therapy. A nuclear medicine gastric-emptying study was performed in August 2017 revealing normal gastric emptying of solids (97% emptying at 4 h).

It was decided to stop the sulfonylurea because it was not enabling A.G. to achieve the target postdinner blood glucose and may have been contributing to difficulty losing weight. Given the normal gastric-emptying study, we discussed a trial of a lower dose of GLP-1 RA treatment. This lower dose was decided upon given the history that the patient had significant nausea and abdominal pain with his last trial of a GLP-1 RA agent.

A.G. returned to the office in September 2017 and his A1C had decreased from 9.3% to 7.7% in 9 weeks. He was tolerating liraglutide 1.2 mg daily and his postdinner blood glucose values were averaging <180 mg/dL. He was feeling more energetic and had lost 8 lb. He was proud of his new diabetes control and was hopeful it would continue to improve.

He started to send in his Dexcom downloads for review every 2 weeks for the next 2 months and then every 4 weeks as his time in range increased. Reports were reviewed within a few days by either the endocrinologist or the diabetes educator, and feedback was given when needed. The review of the data and timely feedback was a key factor in motivating the patient to make positive lifestyle changes. A.G. was seen in the office every 3 months for a physical exam, bloodwork, and a consultation with both the endocrinologist and the diabetes educator.

A.G.'s A1C continued to improve. A March 2018 Dexcom download revealed a continued improvement in reaching postmeal BG targets and overall glycemic control (Figure 3.3).

A.G.'s most recent A1C in May 2018 was 6.9%, with no hypoglycemia indicated on his Dexcom downloads. He has lost a total of 14 lb and continues to choose his meals wisely and exercise regularly. We initially thought the Dexcom would be a temporary or perhaps intermittent tool, but he is keen to keep it on for continued real-time feedback and improved quality of life. To keep

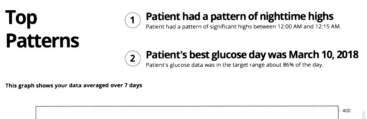

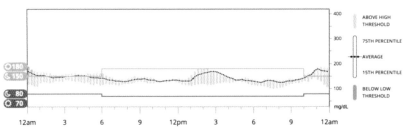

Figure 3.3. DEXCOM Download 7–13 March 2018.

A.G. motivated to wear the CGM, we upgraded him to the Dexcom G6 so that he could benefit from features such as no finger-stick calibration, a smaller transmitter, and extended wear time.

REFERENCES

1. Carlson AL, Mullen DM, Bergenstal RM. Clinical use of continuous glucose monitoring in adults with type 2 diabetes. *Diabetes Technol Therap* 2017;19(S2):S4–S11

2. Vigersky R, Shrivastav M. Role of continuous glucose monitoring for type 2 in diabetes management and research. *J Diabetes Complic* 2017;31(1):280–287

3. Fonda SJ, Graham C, Munakata J, Powers JM, Price D, Vigersky RA. The cost-effectiveness of real-time continuous glucose monitoring (RT-CGM) in type 2 diabetes. *J Diabetes Sci Technol* 2016;10(4):898–904

4. Fonseca VA, Grunberger G, Anhalt A, Bailey TS, Blevins T, Garg SK, Tamborlane W. Continuous glucose monitoring: a consensus conference of the American Association of Clinical Endocrinologists and American College of Endocrinology. *Endocr Pract* 2016;22(8):1008–1021

5. Danne T, Nimri R, Battelino T, Bergenstal RM, Close KL, DeVries JH, Beck R. International consensus on use of continuous glucose monitoring. *Diabetes Care* 2017;40(12):1631–1640

6. Shukla AP, Andono J, Touhamy SH, Casper A, Iliescu RG, Mauer E, Aronne LJ. Carbohydrate-last meal pattern lowers postprandial glucose and insulin excursions in type 2 diabetes. *BMJ Open Diabetes Res Care* 2017;5(1):e000440

Chapter 4

Coaching Insulin Pump Uploads When an Individual Inputs "Phantom Carbohydrates"

Margaret Pellizzari, MBA, MS, RN, CDE, CDTC[1]

CASE STUDY 1

A.S. is a 17-year-old man with type 1 diabetes (T1D) for 2.5 years. He has been wearing a Dexcom G5 continuous glucose monitoring (CGM) for the past 1.5 years. He has been using an Omnipod insulin pump for the past 1 year. He was in the office for his 3-month follow-up visit. His A1C was 6.3%. His A1C is usually <7% (target range for A1C pediatrics according to the American Diabetes Association's clinical recommendation is <7.5%). He was commended on his efforts; certainly living with T1D as a teenager has its challenges. His BMI is at the 81st percentile. His insulin pump was uploaded to Diasend for review.

Figure 4.1 shows one blood glucose check for the day. According to Dexcom G5, calibrations should be taken every 12 h. He is taking multiple boluses of carbohydrates throughout the day.

Figure 4.2 shows no glucose values in that 24-h period of time and, once again, multiple boluses of carbohydrates. A.S.'s body weight is not an issue as evidenced by his BMI of 81%. He reports consuming 418 g carbohydrates for this day. Upon further conversation, A.S. reports that he notices his Dexcom arrows going up and to minimize elevated glucoses, he boluses for "phantom carbohydrates," that is, carbohydrates that he does not consume but adds to the calculations to avoid hyperglycemia.

Figures 4.3–4.5 show a comparable value of blood glucose to CGM values. For this 2-week period of data, however, only four blood glucose values were taken. In December 2016, the Dexcom G5 was approved by the U.S. Food and Drug Administration (FDA) for making treatment decisions without the need for a confirmatory blood glucose finger-stick test; however, 12-h calibrations were recommended. Newer CGM models (Abbott Libre and Dexcom G6) are FDA approved to replace finger-stick blood glucose monitoring. For the 2017 Endocrine Society meeting, a pediatric worksheet tool was developed to utilize Dexcom G5 trend arrows to adjust insulin doses (https://s3-us-west-2.amazonaws.com/dexcompdf/HCP_Website/Pediatric_Worksheet_CGM_G5_V4.pdf).

Figure 4.6 shows the distribution of basal and bolus insulins. Because of A.S.'s many boluses of fictitious carbohydrates to avoid hyperglycemia, his basal delivery is 27%. A.S. has his original basal rates from 1 year ago. He has grown 2 inches in height and gained 8 lb over the past year.

[1]Program Coordinator, Pediatric Endocrinology, Cohen Children's Medical Center, Northwell Health, Lake Success, NY.

	00:00	01:00	02:00	03:00	04:00	05:00	06:00	07:00	08:00	09:00	10:00	11:00	12:00	13:00	14:00	15:00	16:00	17:00	18:00	19:00	20:00	21:00	22:00	23:00	Daily totals
Fr 3/2																									Average (1): 73mg/dl Carbs: 567g Insulin: 52.7U Bolus: 77%

Figure 4.1. Dexcom download for Friday, March 2.

Tu 3/6					Average (0): -- Carbs: 418g Insulin: 36.7U Bolus: 71%

Figure 4.2. Dexcom download for Tuesday, March 6.

Compilation

Glucose	CGM	Insulin	Carbs	Activity	
Average	**Average**	**Average daily dose**	**Average carbs / day**	**Avg steps / day**	**Avg kcal / day**
126 mg/dl	**127** mg/dl	**39.8 U**	**443 g**	**0** steps	**0** kcal
SD = 72 # = 3	SD = 44 # = 3641	SD = 15 # days = 14	SD = 192 # = 250	0% of 10000 (target)	0% of 2500 (target)
Avg # / day = 0.2	Avg # / day = 260.1	Avg # bolus doses/day = 17.9	Avg # / day = 17.9		

Figure 4.3. Averages for glucose, CGM, insulin, carbs, and activity.

Glucose (mg/dl)

Glucose values summary		Interval	Avg BG	# BG	SD
Average (mg/dl)	126	00:00-06:00	0	0	0
Median (mg/dl)	78	06:00-08:00	0	0	0
Highest value (mg/dl)	228	08:00-10:00	0	0	0
Lowest value (mg/dl)	73	10:00-12:00	0	0	0
Standard deviation (SD)	72	12:00-14:00	0	0	0
Values per day	0.2	14:00-16:00	0	0	0
Number of values	3	16:00-18:00	0	0	0
Values above goal (180 mg/dl)	1	18:00-20:00	228	1	0
Values within goal (70-180 mg/dl)	2	20:00-22:00	73	1	0
Values below goal (70 mg/dl)	0	22:00-24:00	78	1	0

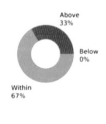

Above 33%

Below 0%

Within 67%

Figure 4.4. Glucose values summary.

CGM (mg/dl)

CGM readings summary	
Average (mg/dl)	127
Median (mg/dl)	118
AUC high > 180 mg/dl	4
AUC low < 70 mg/dl	1
Highest value (mg/dl)	318
Lowest value (mg/dl)	39
Standard deviation (SD)	44
Values per day	260.1
Number of values	3641
Values above goal (180 mg/dl)	406
Values within goal (70-180 mg/dl)	3029
Values below goal (70 mg/dl)	206
Average daily CGM sensor duration	21:40 (90%)
Total CGM sensor duration	12 days 15:25

Interval	Avg	#	SD
00:00-06:00	122	979	47
06:00-08:00	128	277	46
08:00-10:00	123	290	36
10:00-12:00	113	310	26
12:00-14:00	127	310	52
14:00-16:00	137	307	46
16:00-18:00	143	296	46
18:00-20:00	132	265	31
20:00-22:00	133	306	47
22:00-24:00	117	306	38

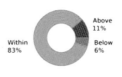

Figure 4.5. CGM readings summary.

Insulin

Insulin doses summary	
Average daily insulin (U)	39.8
Standard deviation (SD)	14.6
Average daily basal (U)	10.6
Average daily bolus (U)	29.2
Average bolus doses/day	17.9
Average days between cannula fills	2.4
Average days between primes	2.4

Carb summary	
Avg # carbs/day	443 g
Standard deviation (SD)	192

Bolus calculation summary	
Avg # Normal Boluses/day	17.9 (100%)
Bolus overrides/total boluses	1%
Avg # bolus overrides/day	0.2

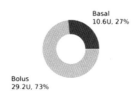

Figure 4.6. Insulin doses summary.

Concerns

We raised the following concerns:

- Multiple bolus of carbohydrates
- Minimal blood glucose checks
- Minimal calibrations for Dexcom G5 device
- Basal insulin = 27%

Coaching Points

A.S. is doing an amazing job with his blood glucose management and he should be commended for his efforts. Additionally, we should inform him that his insulin pump is not working hard enough for him; he is exerting a lot of effort and thought process to ensure good glycemic control.

He is working extra hard to "guesstimate" carbohydrate amounts (phantom carbohydrates) to ensure extra insulin delivery to minimize elevated glucoses. The plan was to

- discuss the idea of basal-bolus distribution of 50%/50% or similar values to increase basal insulin delivery;

- inform A.S. that as he comes out of the honeymoon phase and is in puberty, his insulin requirements will increase;

- discuss basal rate checks without having food or factious carbohydrate input so that basal delivery may be set to target range; and

- discuss importance of basal insulin delivery and dosing in the event he may need/want to go on injections.

CASE STUDY 2

A.C. is a 10-year-old girl who has been living with T1D for 1 year. She has been on an Omnipod insulin pump for 2 years. Her A1C is 6.8% and the family was commended for their efforts at their visit. She does not wear a CGM; she reports that she does not want to wear two pieces of equipment on her body. Her insulin pump was uploaded. Figure 4.7 shows her upload.

AC's mother is getting up in the middle of the night to check her daughter's blood glucose. Mom reports that she is concerned that if she doesn't give A.C. insulin as a bolus at that time, her daughter's glucose will be elevated. Mom reports that she inputs a random amount of factious carbohydrates into the pump so that it calculates insulin and she boluses that amount of insulin. A.C. wakes up in target range. At school, the nurse inputs the actual amount of carbohydrates into the pump. When A.C. is home, mom continues to input erroneous amounts of

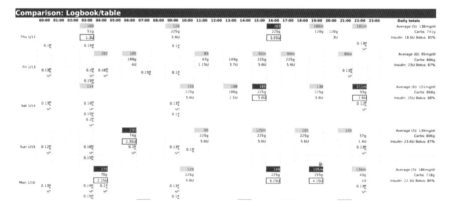

Figure 4.7. Insulin pump upload: January 12–January 16.

carbohydrates so that A.C. gets enough insulin to avoid hyperglycemia. Figure 4.8 depicts an inappropriate amount of daily carbohydrates for this child (824 g/day). On average, this child should consume 30–60 g carbohydrates per meal and 15–30 g carbohydrates for snacks (after school and bedtime). On average, A.C.'s basal constitutes 12% of her daily needs according to her pump upload. In reality, A.C.'s mom is using bolus feature to compensate for the inaccurate basal settings.

Her insulin dosing was recalculated based on weight as well as total daily dose using the 1,800 and 500 rule. A decision was made to choose best dosing based on glucose values when the child was not given "phantom carbohydrate intake." The family should be commended on their efforts. In addition, we—

- asked the family to upload pump to Diasend weekly for review;

- asked the family to do some basal rate testing overnight as well as early morning (the child was not willing to skip lunch or dinner);

- discussed with her mom the need to gain trust in the pump and the need for more accurate dosing in the pump settings;

- discussed with the family the use of CGM to assist with glucose management; and

- offered positive support to the family.

A.C.'s mom is doing a lot of work to control glucoses and the outcomes were great as evidenced by A1C of 6.8%. Table 4.1 shows simplification strategies for working with children with diabetes who are using insulin pumps.

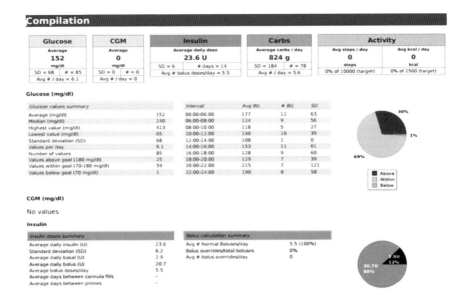

Figure 4.8. Averages for glucose, CGM, insulin, carbs, and activity; demonstrating inappropriate amount of daily carbohydrate for A.C.

Table 4.1. Strategies for Children with Diabetes

Concerns	Actions to Take
Insulin requirements change over time especially during growth spurts and during puberty	Basal rate testing will help identify insulin requirements. Adjustments should be made within 1–2 h before the trend occurs.
Trust in the insulin pump basal delivery	Utilization of CGM to assess glucose patterns. Education regarding dose adjustments based on CGM trend arrows.
Accuracy of carbohydrate counting especially during transition periods	Yearly nutrition visit to assess carbohydrate counting as well as healthy growth and development with proper nourishment.
Diabetes burnout	Positive coaching to support families.

REFERENCES

1. American Diabetes Association. Standards of medical care in diabetes, 2018. *Diabetes Care* 2018;41:S126–S133

2. Laffel LM, Aleppo G, Buckingham BA, Forlenza GP, Rasbach LE, Tsalikan E, Weinzimer SA, Harris DR. A practical approach to using trend arrows on the Dexcom G5 CGM system to manage children and adolescents with diabetes. *J Endocr Soc* 2017;1:1461–1476

3. Scheiner G. *Practical CGM: A Guide to Improving Outcomes through Continuous Glucose Monitoring.* Arlington, VA, American Diabetes Association, 2015

4. Walsh J, Roberts R. *Pumping Insulin: Everything for Success on an Insulin Pump and CGM.* San Diego, CA, Torrey Pines Press, 2016

Chapter 5

A Teenager with Chronic Hyperglycemia

Neesha Ramchandani, PNP, CDE[1]

CASE STUDY

Anna is a 15-year-old girl who was diagnosed with type 1 diabetes (T1D) when she was 8 years old. She is a sophomore in high school and is doing well academically. She has been on the honor roll every quarter. She also participates in a variety of extracurricular activities, including sports. She is co-captain of the junior varsity girls' soccer team this year. Overall, she is a highly motivated individual. She lives with her mother and father in New York City. The family is financially stable.

Now that Anna is a teenager, she is in charge of her own diabetes self-management (DSM). Her mother used to check her blood glucose (BG) levels and give all of her insulin. Over the past few years, as Anna has gotten older and desired more independence, responsibility for the various DSM tasks has shifted from parent to child.

Anna has been using an insulin pump for the past 3 years. She changes her pump site by herself every 2–3 days. She checks her BG as requested by her diabetes clinicians, ≥4 times/day. Her mother checks her BG levels overnight when necessary. Anna is also able to count carbohydrates with ease. However, she is not bolusing (taking insulin through her pump) for most of her food intake. Her biggest problem areas are during and immediately after school. When asked why, she just shrugs her shoulders and looks sheepish.

INTERVENTIONS

The initial interventions that we tried included discussions about the relationship of hyperglycemia to microvascular complications of diabetes using graphs from the Diabetes Control and Complications Trial studies.[1] We explained that getting her BG levels closer to the target range of 70–150 mg/dL would help Anna play soccer better and focus better in school (practical, real-life information), encouraging her to set bolus reminder alarms on her pump, and scheduling monthly clinic visits to impress upon her the severity of the situation. However, none of these interventions had any impact on her glycemic control. Her HbA$_{1c}$ remained in the 11–12% range and her average BG over the 2 weeks preceding each clinic

[1]New York University, Rory Meyers College of Nursing, New York, NY.

visit was in the 300 mg/dL range. Additionally, she continued to not give herself boluses during and after school.

After a discussion between the pediatric diabetes team and Anna and her mother, it was decided that Anna should start using a continuous glucose monitor (CGM). The team believed that if Anna could see her glucose values in real time, she might actually do something to bring down her glucose levels. We ordered a CGM for Anna. When it arrived, Anna and her mother were instructed on its use by Anna's diabetes educator. During the CGM training, Anna was advised that it would be best if she wore the CGM all the time and that it should be worn for a minimum of 1 week every month. Anna's mother said that Anna would wear it all the time. Anna was agreeable to this. Initial high- and low-glucose alerts were set to 350 mg/dL and 80 mg/dL, respectively, so as not to create alarm fatigue. No other alerts or alarms were set. The plan was to decrease the value of the high-glucose alert to something closer to the recommended target range for adolescents with diabetes as Anna's glycemic control improved.

Anna returned for a follow-up visit 2 weeks after starting CGM (January 2008). Her initial 7-day sensor glucose tracing and glucose distribution appear in Figures 5.1*A* and 5.1*B*. Although much of what is depicted in these figures was already known to both the diabetes team and the family, Anna and her mother were shocked when they saw this download. It had a greater impact on both of them than months of looking at elevated BG values on the meter and in the logbook. The baseline CGM data highlighted the extent of the problem to Anna and her mother by putting it right in front of their faces. Anna had significantly elevated glucose values throughout the day and night on a continuous basis (Figure 5.1*B*). More than 90% of her glucose values were >220 mg/dL (12.2 mmol/L), and nearly two-thirds of her glucose values were >300 mg/dL (16.7 mmol/L). Her median sensor glucose was 331 mg/dL (18.4 mmol/L) (Figure 5.1*A*). Additionally, as was known from self blood glucose monitoring prior to CGM initiation, Anna's biggest problem areas were during and immediately after school, and into the evening (Figure 5.1*A*). This was when she was the least likely to give herself a bolus.

Anna wore her CGM religiously, usually 6–7 days per week. She did not mind it. She and her mother continued to come in every 1–2 months for follow-up visits. During the visits, Anna's CGM was downloaded and the results were reviewed and compared to those from the previous visit. Every success was praised, no matter how small, and every area that did not improve or worsened was investigated in a nonaccusatory manner. In between visits, neither Anna nor her mother downloaded her CGM at home. Anna also did not pay too much attention to her CGM in between visits, although she found it helpful that she could look at it at any time and get a glucose reading in real time. She also appreciated the high- and low-glucose alerts.

This progress required taking baby steps, as an adolescent's first priority is usually not optimal glycemic control.[2] However, over the next 16 months Anna's glucose values and HbA$_{1c}$ slowly decreased. Her high sensor-glucose limit was slowly lowered as well. No other CGM alerts were ever added. Anna continued to miss boluses, especially during and immediately after school, but she became increasingly likely to bolus for her food intake the longer she used her CGM. Her CGM download from May 2009 appears in Figures 5.2*A* and 5.2*B*. Although she

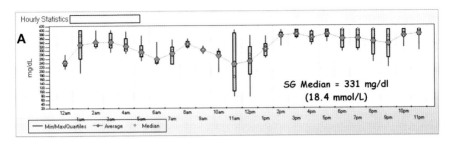

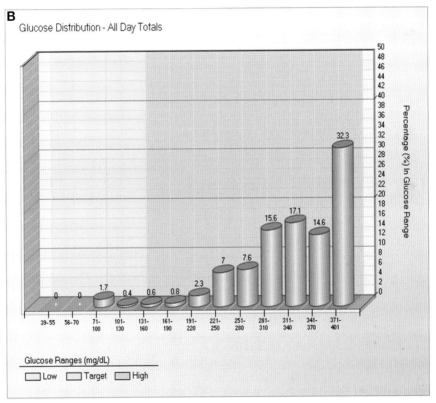

Figure 5.1. A: Baseline CGM Hourly Statistics. **B:** Baseline CGM Glucose Distribution.

continued to have hyperglycemia reaching into 300mg/dL (16–17 mmol/L) range after school and in the early evening, Anna's median sensor glucose had decreased to 195 mg/dL (10.8 mmol/L) (Figure 5.2*A*) and her glucose distribution had significantly improved (Figure 5.2*B*). After months of CGM use and frequent follow-up visits, 63.5% of Anna's sensor glucose values were <220 mg/dL (12.2 mmol/L),

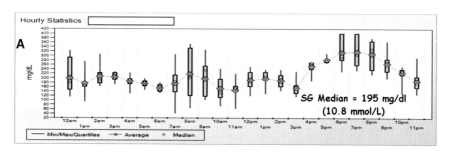

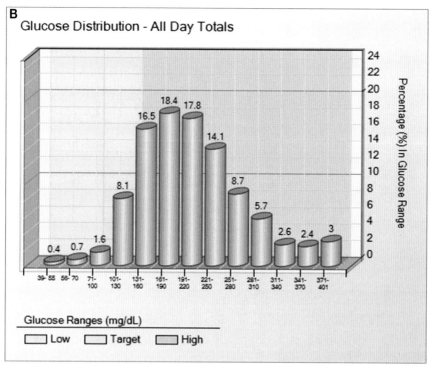

Figure 5.2. A: CGM Hourly Statistics, 16 Months Post-CGM Start. **B:** CGM Glucose Distribution, 16 Months Post-CGM Start.

and <10% were >300 mg/dL (16.7 mmol/L). All of this was achieved without a notable increase in hypoglycemia. Her HbA$_{1c}$ had also decreased to the 8–9% range. Anna and her mother were thrilled.

DISCUSSION

Two important issues need to be considered in Anna's case. First, she was diagnosed when she was young, and although she was receiving a developmentally appropriate transition in the transfer of DSM tasks from parent to child, she had not necessarily been equipped with the knowledge needed for optimal DSM. This is an issue that has recently started to receive recognition in the literature.[3] But diabetes education alone is not the key. Research has shown that adolescents with T1D can tell you everything they are supposed to be doing to manage their diabetes, but still not be doing it.[4] This brings us to the second issue: Anna is an adolescent.

During the adolescent years, there is often an internal tug-of-war between normal adolescent behaviors and optimal glycemic control.[2] Normal adolescent behavior often wins. For many adolescents with T1D, no amount of abstract reasoning or lecturing about diabetes complications will have any impact on their glycemic control. Putting the effects of hyperglycemia in the context of the adolescent's life (making it real) may or may not inspire them to improve their glycemic control, depending on their current performance in these other areas. The majority of adolescents are more concerned about how they appear to others than about taking care of their diabetes, especially when they run the risk of making a fool of themselves in front of their friends if they have a hypoglycemic event, but the negative sequelae of hyperglycemia do not appear for years.[2] Many adolescents also do not want to do anything that makes them look different in front of their peers, such as taking an insulin bolus or insulin injection or checking their BG levels.[2] It is not clear which of these issues was affecting Anna's glycemic control in particular, but all of them may have played a part.

Optimal glycemic control in adolescents, however, is not an insurmountable task. Given the right tools, adolescents can do well, or at least much better, with their DSM. A recent large study of adolescents with T1D and their mothers (total $n = 1,040$ subjects) found CGM use to be associated with both lower HbA_{1c} levels and less adolescent distress when compared to no technology use and insulin pump use without CGM.[5] Using a CGM empowers adolescents (and their parents as well) by equipping them with previously unavailable information that can be easily accessed without calling undue attention to oneself.[6] With the push of a button, the adolescent can see both their sensor glucose and a directional arrow indicating the rate of change. High- and low-glucose alerts, rate-of-change alerts, and predictive alerts can be set on the CGM so that the adolescent can be alerted to problematic glucose levels without needing to look at the receiver frequently. Alerts should be set judiciously to avoid alarm fatigue from the device alerting too frequently. The alerts do not need to ring; they also can be set to vibrate. Parents, too, can monitor their adolescent's sensor glucose values from afar using apps and web portals, giving them peace of mind about their adolescent's glycemic well-being,[5] without the perceived constant parental nagging about "Did you check your sugar?" or "What's your number?"

CONCLUSION

Anna continued to use her CGM and continued to do well with it. Her glucose levels did not decrease much more over the next 2 years from where they had reached in May 2009, but they did not increase to pre-CGM levels either. Her HbA_{1c} remained in the 8% range throughout the remainder of her high school years.

CGM technology has enabled Anna and many like her to do much better with their glycemic control and DSM than they did with insulin pump therapy and BG monitoring alone. CGM is an important tool that should be considered for all adolescents with insulin-requiring diabetes.

REFERENCES

1. Skyler JS. Diabetic complications. The importance of glucose control. *Endocrinol Metab Clin North Am* 1996;25(2):243–254

2. Kupper F, Peters LWH, Stuijfzand SM, den Besten HAA, van Kesteren NMC. Usefulness of image theater workshops for exploring dilemmas in diabetes self-management among adolescents. *Glob Qual Nurs Res* 2018;5: 2333393618755007. doi: 10.1177/2333393618755007

3. Sullivan-Bolyai S, Crawford S, Johnson K, Ramchandani N, Quinn D, D'Alesandro B, Streisand R. PREP-T1 (Preteen Re-Education With Parents-Type 1 Diabetes) feasibility intervention results. *J Fam Nurs* 2016;22(4):579–605. doi: 10.1177/1074840716676589

4. Wysocki T, Hough BS, Ward KM, Green LB. Diabetes mellitus in the transition to adulthood: adjustment, self-care, and health status. *J Dev Behav Pediatr* 1992;13(3):194–201

5. Vesco AT, Jedraszko AM, Garza KP, Weissberg-Benchell J. Continuous glucose monitoring associated with less diabetes-specific emotional distress and lower A1C among adolescents with type 1 diabetes. *J Diabetes Sci Technol* 2016;1932296818766381. doi: 10.1177/1932296818766381

6. Lawton J, Blackburn M, Allen J, Campbell F, Elleri D, Leelarathna L, Hovorka R. Patients' and caregivers' experiences of using continuous glucose monitoring to support diabetes self-management: qualitative study. *BMC Endocr Disord* 2018;18(1):12. doi: 10.1186/s12902-018-0239-1

Chapter 6

Adjustments in Insulin Pump Settings Can Improve Glycemic Control

Laura Barba, NP, MS, CDE[1]

FIRST VISIT: 24 MARCH 2018

S.B. is a 28-year-old woman with type 1 diabetes (T1D), a history of hypothyroidism and lupus, and chronic kidney disease stage 3 due to lupus nephritis. During my first visit with this patient, I made the following assessment:

- Diagnosis: 2006 she went into diabetic ketoacidosis.

- Profound hypoglycemia requiring admission ~3 years ago. Had a seizure resulting from hypoglycemia. No recent hypoglycemia.

- Past regimens: On multiple daily insulin injections until 2017 when she started using an insulin pump (Medtronic). Lost her continuous glucose monitoring (CGM) sensor (MiniMed with Enlite) and stopped using it.

The focus of the visit was on diabetes self-management and developing a better understanding of insulin pump therapy. S.B. is not using the pump in a conventional way. She rarely enters carbohydrates for bolus and she suspends the pump for hours each day. Most nights, the pump is suspended all night long. She has concerns about hypoglycemia; however, every morning, her blood glucose numbers are >200–300 mg/dL. She also complains of nausea, so I suspect she may have positive ketones, but she does not check for ketones.

Looking at her pump settings and based on her total daily dose (TDD) of insulin, her settings are heavy basal and heavy for carbohydrate coverage as well as for blood glucose correction. This matches her clinical situation, because she has hypoglycemia if she uses the suggestions for bolus made by her pump and does not suspend the pump basal.

We made adjustments in her pump settings (see Table 6.1). S.B. is planning on moving to the new Medtronic 670G in 1–2 months.

S.B. also states that she has not been feeling well lately and feels that she may be having a recurrence of her lupus. She was referred to her rheumatologist. I also noted from her labs that her current glomerular filtration rate (GFR) is 29. She was referred to her nephrologist for evaluation as well.

---

[1]Division of Endocrinology, Diabetes and Metabolism, University of California–San Diego Health System, San Diego, CA.

Table 6.1. Current Regime, First Visit

Basal Rates	Bolus Ratios	Correction Factors/Targets
12 A.M. = 0.725 units/h	12 A.M. = 1 unit for 12 g carbohydrate	Correction factors: 12 A.M. = 46 mg/dL
7 A.M. = 0.775 units/h		Target blood glucose levels:
10 P.M. = 0.725 units/h		12 A.M. = 110–120 mg/dL
		Duration of insulin action: 4 h

Current Diabetes Regimen

Her current regime is as follows:

- Insulin aspart (Novolog)
- Medtronic pump
- MiniMed 630G

Her TDD of insulin is 22 units basal 56%. She rarely enters carbohydrates into the bolus wizard. She suspends the pump for up to 16 h/day. On most days, she is suspending the pump for at least 3–8 h with subsequently high blood glucose post suspend (see Figure 6.1).

S.B. states that she is suspending basal because if she does not, she will have low blood glucose levels (Table 6.2). She suspends the pump almost every night. Current basal each day was 12.18 units daily (56% of TDD); however, basal insulin, if she did not suspend, would be 18.15 units daily (which is way too much basal). See Table 6.3 for her other medications.

Complications and Pertinent Medical History

S.B. is experiencing several complications:

- Hypertension: Yes, on meds. Goal: <140/80: 126/90 (at goal today).
- Hyperlipidemia: No.
- Retinopathy: No. Last eye exam: Within the last 8 months.
- Nephropathy: Yes. Has lupus nephritis. Is followed by nephrology.
- Neuropathy: Yes. Occasional numbness and tingling in the feet.
- Coronary artery disease/cardiovascular disease/peripheral vascular disease: No.
- Other: Lupus. States that she is "having the start of a recurrence" of her lupus and is referred to rheumatology.
- Hypothyroidism: Takes LT4 175 mcg daily (recent thyrotropin 0.02). Dose recently reduced.

(continued)

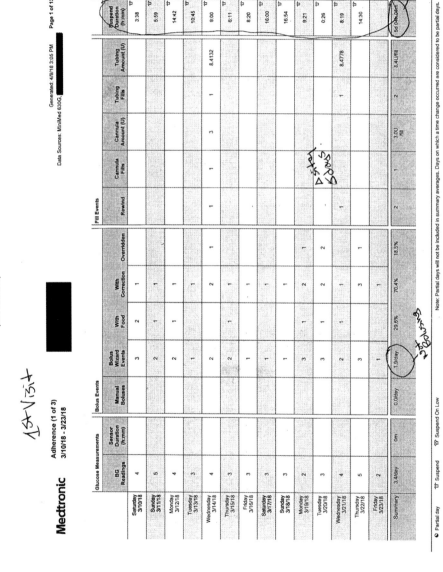

Figure 6.1. Medtronic 630G report on first visit: March 10–March 23, 2018.

Medtronic

Adherence (2 of 3)
3/24/18 - 4/6/18

Data Sources: MiniMed 630G,

Generated: 4/9/18 3:05 PM

Date	Glucose Measurements		Bolus Events					Fill Events					Suspend Duration (h:mm)
	BG Readings	Sensor Duration (h:mm)	Manual Boluses	Bolus Wizard Events	With Food	With Correction	Overridden	Rewind	Cannula Fills	Cannula Amount (U)	Tubing Fills	Tubing Amount (U)	
Saturday 3/24/18	4			4	2	2	1						6:54
Sunday 3/25/18	4			3	1	2							8:06
Monday 3/26/18	2			1	1			1			1	8.238	0:05
Tuesday 3/27/18	2			1	1								4:11
Wednesday 3/28/18	4												1:05
Thursday 3/29/18	4			3	1	2							17:18
Friday 3/30/18	4			3	1	2	2						13:58
Saturday 3/31/18	5			2		2	2						14:33
Sunday 4/1/18	5			3	1	2	1						10:40
Monday 4/2/18	3			3	2	1	1						9:16
Tuesday 4/3/18	22			21		21	16	5			4	25.3504	8:16
Wednesday 4/4/18	6			4	1	4	1						14:19
Thursday 4/5/18	3			3	1	2	1						3:04
Friday 4/6/18	5			6	2	4	2	1			1	9.1328	0:04
Summary	5.2/day	0m	0.0/day	4.1/day	22.8%	77.2%	47.4%	7	0	–	6	7.1U/fill	4d 15h 49m

⬤ Partial day   ⊍ Suspend   ⊍ Suspend On Low

Note: Partial days will not be included in summary averages. Days on which a time change occurred are considered to be partial days.

Figure 6.1. *(continued)*

Medtronic

Adherence (3 of 3)
4/7/18 - 4/9/18

Generated: 4/9/18 3:05 PM
Data Sources: MiniMed 630G,
Page 3 of 12

| | Glucose Measurements | | Bolus Events | | | | | Fill Events | | | | | |
	BG Readings	Sensor Duration (h:mm)	Manual Boluses	Bolus Wizard Events	With Food	With Correction	Overridden	Rewind	Cannula Fills	Cannula Amount (U)	Tubing Fills	Tubing Amount (U)	Suspend Duration (h:mm)
Saturday 4/7/18	4			3		3	1						
Sunday 4/8/18	3			4	1	3							1:48
Monday 4/9/18	2			2	1	1							0:04
Summary	3.5/day	0m	0.0/day	3.5/day	22.2%	77.8%	11.1%	0	0	—	0	—	1h 52m

⊙ Partial day   ⇪ Suspend   ⇪ Suspend On Low   Note: Partial days will not be included in summary averages. Days on which a time change occurred are considered to be partial days.

Figure 6.1. *(continued)*

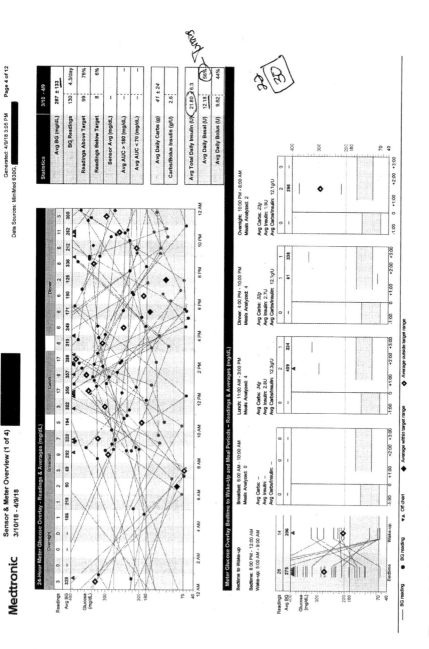

Figure 6.1. *(continued)*

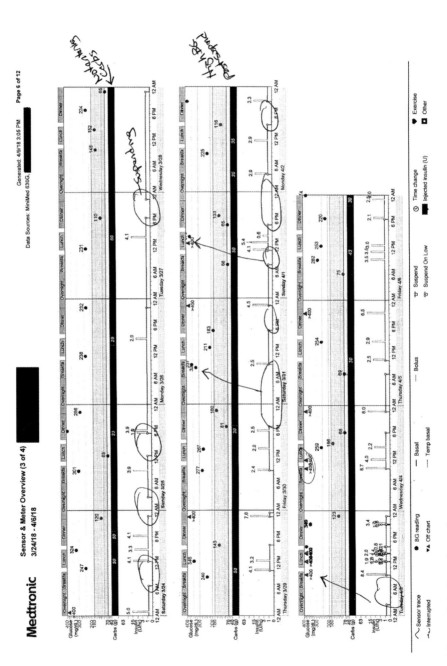

Figure 6.1. (continued)

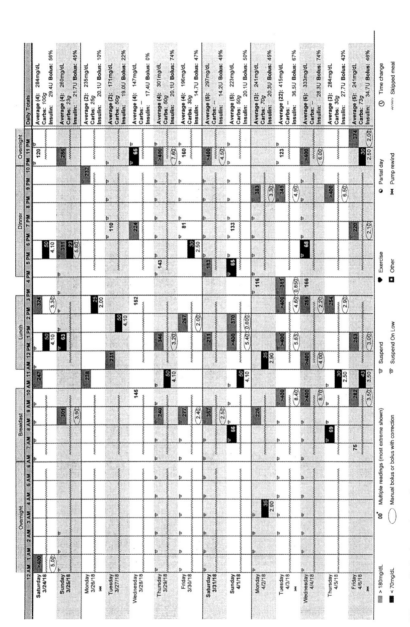

Figure 6.1. *(continued)*

Figure 6.1. *(continued)*

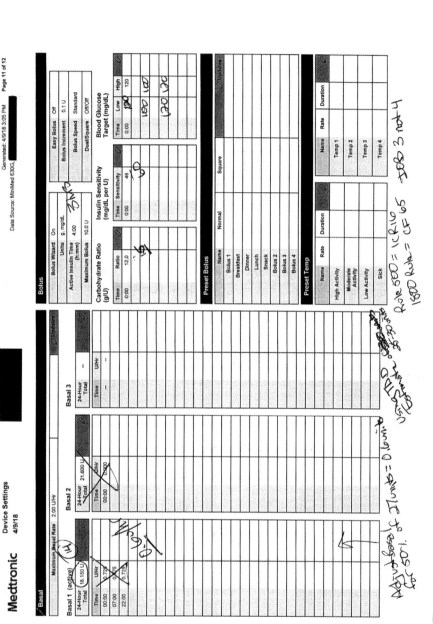

Figure 6.1. *(continued)*

Table 6.2. A1C History

Lab Results		
Component	Value	Date
A1C	9.6	04/02/2018
Lab Results		
Component	Value	Date
MICALB	430.9	04/02/2018
MACRR	1381	04/02/2018
Lab Results		
Component	Value	Date
GLU	121	04/02/2018
CREAT	2.08	04/02/2018

Notably, the patient denies any symptoms of hypothyroidism, including fatigue, weight gain, or cold intolerance. She exhibits no symptoms of hyperthyroidism, including palpitation, heat intolerance, or weight loss. She gets her periods every 4–6 weeks.

Blood Glucose Monitoring

Following is a review of S.B.'s blood glucose testing and results:

- Testing frequency: 4.3 times/day
- 14-day average: 287 mg/dL; SD 133 mg/dL
- Blood glucose (BG) range: 45–505 mg/dL
- Fasting blood glucose (FBG): 275 mg/dL
- ACL: 225 mg/dL
- ACD: 227 mg/dL
- HS: 155 mg/dL
- Frequency of lows: 8 events <70 mg/dL in the past month
- Normal BG: 80–130 mg/dL

CGM Interpretation

S.B. will start Medtronic's Guardian CGM soon.

Nutrition Management and Current Meal Plan

S.B. met briefly with the registered dietician and certified diabetes educator. She does not enter carbohydrates very often. Currently, she is entering only carbohydrates for food 0–2 times/day (41 g of carbohydrates daily per download). She recognizes this as a problem but also has concerns that when she enters all her carbohydrates, she has hypoglycemia.

State-of-Care Medical History

S.B. lives with her husband and works as a child daycare provider 5 days a week.

Allergies

Sulfa drugs

Labs from December 2017

Creatinine: 1.6

BUN: 28

Ca: 9.6

GFR: 44

LDL: 107

HDL: 45

TG: 94

A1C: 9.1%

ROS: Gen: no recent weight gain/weight loss, + fatigue. **Eyes:** no visual disturbance. **CV:** no chest pain, no palpitations. **Resp:** no shortness of breath, + LE edema. **GI:** occasional nausea, no vomiting, no abdominal pain, no diarrhea. **GU:** No hematuria, no dysuria. **Skin:** no bruising, no rashes, no hyperpigmentation. **Neuro:** no paresthesias, no tremor. **Endo:** no polyuria, no polydipsia.

Physical Examination

- BP: 126/90 (BP Location: Left arm, BP Patient Position: Sitting, BP cuff size: Large)
- Pulse: 94
- Temperature: 98.6°F (37°C) (Oral)
- Respiratory: 12
- Weight: 88.5 kg (195 lb)
- BMI: 33.47 kg/m^2
- General: Well-developed, well-nourished; in no acute distress.
- Hent: Within normal limits.
- Eyes: No lid lag or proptosis. No icterus, no scleral injection, no periorbital edema.
- Respiratory: Easy WOB in no distress.

Table 6.3. Medications

Current Outpatient Prescriptions	
Medication	**Sig**
• amLODIPINE (Norvasc) 10 mg tablet	Take 10 mg by mouth daily.
• glucagon (Glucagon) 1 mg injection	1 mg by intramuscular route as needed for low blood glucose.
• hydroxychloroquine (Plaquenil) 200 mg tablet	Take 200 mg by mouth 2 times daily.
• mycoPHENOLate mofetil (Cellcept) 500 mg tablet	Take 500 mg by mouth 2 times daily.
• Novolog 100 unit/mL injection	Up to 40 units of insulin aspart (Novolog)/day via pump
• traZODone (Desyrel) 100 MG tablet	Take 100 mg by mouth daily.

- CV: Pink well perfused, mild LE edema.
- GI: Soft, non tender.
- MSK: MAE, normal gate.
- Neurologic: Alert and oriented x3. No tremor.
- Psychiatric: Pleasant, normal affect, normal judgment.
- Skin: Warm to touch.

ASSESSMENT AND PLAN

Patient Education

Self-Monitoring of Blood Glucose.

- Reviewed timing and frequency of testing and premeal BG goals.
- Suggested testing a minimum of 4 times/day before meals and bedtime; start CGM soon.
- Discussed testing before bedtime goal for BG. If BG <100–120 mg/dL at bedtime, have a small snack (15 g).
- Discussed benefits of using CGM; will be starting a Guardian sensor with the 670G Medtronic pump.
- Discussed using results for decision making; contact clinic if BGs are consistently <70 mg/dL or >200 mg/dL.

Healthy Eating.

- Discussed making healthy food choices, reading nutrition labels, under-standing portion sizes, carbohydrate counting, and entering carbohydrates into the pump for bolus wizard suggestions.

- Discussed the importance of covering all carbohydrates with an insulin-to-carbohydrate ratio (ICR) to avoid a spike or drop in BG levels.

- Currently, S.B. only rarely is entering carbohydrates into the pump for dos-ing. Reduced ICR so she is not as afraid to bolus because of concerns for hypoglycemia.

Medication and Insulin. TDD 22 with basal-bolus is not balanced. She would have heavy basal if she did not suspend so often. We suspect she needs at least 25–30 units of insulin to get her BG to goal due to the fact that with 22 units, her average BG is 287 mg/dL and her A1C is 9.6%.

- Reduced basal so she does not have to suspend pump all night long.

- Reduced carbohydrate coverage so she feels more comfortable putting car-bohydrates into pump for dosing.

- Discussed importance of taking insulin at least 15–20 min prior to eating.

- Reduced correction as well. Encouraged frequent testing overnight with these changes. Encouraged her to contact us between visits if she needs further adjustments. Goal is for her to bolus for carbohydrates or correc-tion and not to have to suspend the pump to avoid hypoglycemia.

Reducing Risks.

- Reviewed diagnostic labs and discussed prevention and detection of acute or chronic complications.

- Discussed treatment of hypoglycemia and the need to always carry fast-acting carbohydrates to treat lows (4 oz juice, 3–4 glucose tabs, 15 Skittles, 4 Starburst candies).

- Reviewed the "rule of 15"—that is, treating with 15 g of fast carbohydrates when feeling low or if BG is <70 mg/dL; then recheck in 15 min or retreat with 15 g if <70 mg/dL.

- Reminded to check BG before driving and to treat if <100 mg/dL before driving.

- Discussed glucagon/has glucagon.

- Discussed risk of hyperglycemia in T1D and need for ketone testing.

Overall Assessment

S.B. is a 28-year-old woman with poorly controlled diabetes. Her last A1C was 9.6%. She uses a Medtronic pump and is planning on transferring to the 670G very soon. Currently, she is using the pump in an inefficient manner. She rarely enters carbohydrates and she has been suspending the pump for 3–16 h/day. She suspends her pump almost every night with hyperglycemia in the morning. We made adjustments to her pump settings, and she will try a using them (Table 6.4). We will follow her closely.

Patient Goals

- Check BG at bedtime and every 3–4 h overnight for next 3 nights with pump changes.
- Send MyChart in 2–3 days if experiencing BG <70 mg/dL or >200 mg/dL.
- Do not suspend pump at all and keep it on and connected to your body.

Things to remember:

- Check BG before meals and before bedtime (4 times daily).
- If BG at bedtime is <100–120 mg/dL, have a small snack: 15–20 g of carbohydrate; no insulin.
- Cover carbohydrates with insulin aspart (Novolog) bolus.
- Try to take meal insulin coverage at least 15–20 min before eating a meal; If not sure about how many carbs you will eat, cover at least half of the expected carbohydrate intake and then cover the rest when you are done.
- Be prepared to treat lows at all times. Carry fast-acting carbohydrates, such as juice, glucose tablets (3–4 tabs), or candy that is easy to chew and swallow (e.g., Skittles 15 candies, Starburst 4 candies). Let us know if you need a prescription for an emergency glucagon kit.
- If having symptoms of low BG: Check BG on meter: treat with 15 g of fast-acting carbohydrate and retest in 15 min; if BG <70 mg/dL, then treat again and repeat.

Table 6.4. New Settings

Basal Rates	Bolus Ratios	Correction Factors/ Targets
12 A.M. = 0.6 units/h	12 A.M. = 1 unit for 20 g carbohydrate	Correction factors: 12 A.M. = 60 mg/dL
	5 A.M. = 1 unit for 15 g carbohydrate	Target blood glucose levels: 12 A.M. = 120 mg/dL
	8 P.M. = 1 unit for 20 g carbohydrate	5 A.M. = 100 mg/dL
		8 P.M. = 120 mg/dL
		Duration of insulin action: 3 h

- Check BG prior to vigorous physical activity: If <150 mg/dL, eat a 15-g carbohydrate snack to avoid low BG during activity.
- For T1D, check urine ketones if BG >300 mg/dL and when ill or experiencing any nausea and vomiting. If positive, rest, hydrate, and take insulin; continue to test urine ketones until clear. If large and vomiting, go to the emergency department. Pick up strips.
- Call nephrology and be seen soon; also call rheumatology and get in to be seen.
- Use MyChart for communication or call the clinic office to communicate between visits.
- Check BG prior to driving and have a snack if <100 mg/dL.
- Contact us if BG levels are <70 mg/dL or >200 mg/dL consistently so we can adjust your diabetes medications and plan.
- Bring glucose meter or logbook to each appointment.

Visit Diagnoses

- Uncontrolled insulin dependent T1D (CMS-HCC) E10.65
- Hypothyroidism due to Hashimoto's thyroiditis E03.8, E06.3
- Insulin pump in place Z96.41
- Insulin pump titration Z46.81
- Counseling for insulin pump Z46.81

FOLLOW-UP CALL: 11 APRIL 2018

Called and talked to S.B. She has been leaving the pump unsuspended, as instructed. Her BG levels are remaining high regardless (200–300 mg/dL). Over the phone, she was instructed to increase her basal to 0.65 units/h from 0.6 units/h for 24 h. We also increased her coverage for carbohydrates and changed her from 1:15 during the day to 1:10 for better carbohydrate coverage and after dinner 1:15 from 1:20.

If she continues to have higher BG numbers in the morning (>150–180 mg/dL), she was instructed to increase basal to 0.7 units/h.

She was encouraged to call if she has any questions or concerns and if she starts having any low BG levels <70 mg/dL or consistently >200 mg/dL. She was reminded to sign up for MyChart so she can communicate through her electronic medical record or call the office with any questions or concerns.

FOLLOW-UP VISIT: 7 MAY 2018

At her last visit, S.B. stated that she had not been feeling well and might be having a recurrence of her lupus. She was seen by her rheumatologist, who is following her closely and starting her on steroids. She is starting 10 mg of prednisone daily for her rheumatoid arthritis (RA). She has also seen nephrology since the last visit to follow up on her nephritis and GFR 29.

Her A1C dropped from 9.6% to 8.7% since last visit; her 14-day average BG dropped from 287 mg/dL with an SD of 133 to an average BG of 196 mg/dL with an SD of 95 (see Figure 6.2). She feels she is having less variability and feels like the pump is working better. She is now able to enter carbohydrates more regularly (total carbohydrates entered last visit 41 g/day now 88 g/day).

At this visit, she is doing a good job not suspending the pump but admits she takes the pump off now for 1–3 h during the day if she is experiencing lower BGs and is concerned about lows. When she takes the pump off, rather than suspending, it becomes more difficult to track "insulin on board" on the download.

I explained to her that when she is on 670G, the pump will theoretically back off as needed, so disconnecting it will not be necessary to avoid lows. She tends not to enter carbohydrates very often and only corrects BG when it is high. This also leads to higher BG levels. When using the 670G, it will be important to enter all carbohydrates consumed and her BG levels for correction throughout the day to avoid hyperglycemia and prevent getting kicked out of auto mode.

The focus was on diabetes self-management and insulin pump therapy. We discussed issues related to starting steroids and using a temp basal starting at 30% and increasing up to 60% or more for 8 h during the day and correcting BG with the pump every 3–4 h during the day and covering all carbohydrates. S.B. started on 670G with the Guardian sensor (6 May 2018) and will not be in auto mode for at least 1–2 weeks after starting.

Reports having accuracy issues with the sensor. We explained that in the first 12 h, it may not be as accurate as it will be after that. We suggested that she contact MiniMed to be sure nothing is wrong with the sensor. She reports calibrating the device as instructed. Because she just started on 670G, she is not yet in auto mode and reports having been suspended before low was activated; because she is having sensor issues, she is not able to use that feature. She is speaking with a MiniMed representative daily as she gets started using this device.

Current Diabetes Regimen

Her TDD is 24 units (basal 61%). She enters carbohydrates into the bolus wizard more often now than she was at her last visit (0–3 times daily). She has stopped suspending the pump for up to 16 h a day and now will disconnect for 1–3 h if going low (a couple times a week, mostly in the afternoon). She does a good job of entering her BG for correction 1–3 times daily. For more information on her current regimen see Table 6.5. She states she is still disconnecting. She is concerned that if she does not, she will have low BG levels.

Her current regime is as follows:

- Insulin aspart (Novolog)
- Medtronic pump
- MiniMed 630G (she just started the 670G yesterday and is not yet on auto mode)

Blood Glucose Monitoring

Testing Frequency: 4.2 times/day
30-day average: 195 mg/dL down from 227 mg/dL

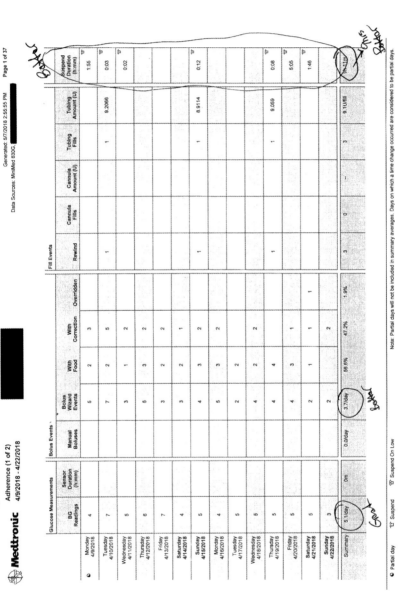

Figure 6.2. Medtronic 630G report on follow-up visit: April 9–April 22, 2018.

Medtronic Adherence (2 of 2)
4/23/2018 - 5/6/2018

	Glucose Measurements		Bolus Events					Fill Events					Suspend Duration (h:mm)
	BG Readings	Sensor Duration (h:mm)	Manual Boluses	Bolus Wizard Events	With Food	With Correction	Overridden	Rewind	Cannula Fills	Cannula Amount (U)	Tubing Fills	Tubing Amount (U)	
Monday 4/23/2018	4			3	2	1							⅏
Tuesday 4/24/2018	3			2	2			1			1	8.8929	0:13
Wednesday 4/25/2018	3												
Thursday 4/26/2018	4			2	2								
Friday 4/27/2018	5			4	1	3	2						
Saturday 4/28/2018	4			1		1							
Sunday 4/29/2018	3			1		1							⅏
Monday 4/30/2018	4			2	1	1							
Tuesday 5/1/2018	3			2	1	2	1	2			1	9.9169	0:10
Wednesday 5/2/2018	2			2	2								
Thursday 5/3/2018	4			4	3	1	1						
Friday 5/4/2018	3			2		2	1						
Saturday 5/5/2018	4			3		3	1						⅏ 0:03
Sunday 5/6/2018	2			3	1	2							⅏ 13:17
Summary	3.4/day	0m	0.0/day	2.2/day	48.4%	54.8%	19.4%	3	0	--	2	9.4U/fill	13h 43m

● Partial day   ⅏ Suspend   ⅏ Suspend On Low

Note: Partial days will not be included in summary averages. Days on which a time change occurred are considered to be partial days.

Figure 6.2. *(continued)*

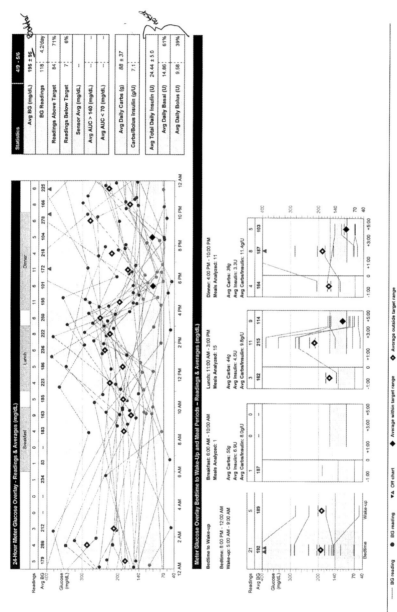

Figure 6.2. *(continued)*

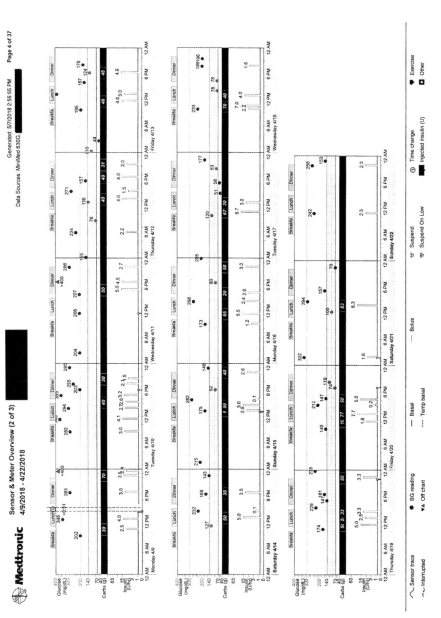

Figure 6.2. *(continued)*

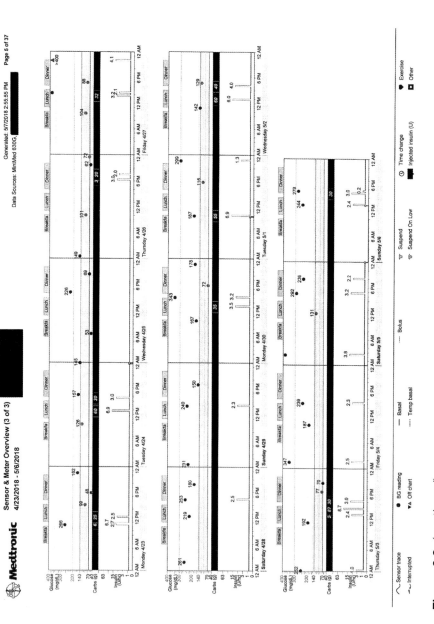

Figure 6.2. *(continued)*

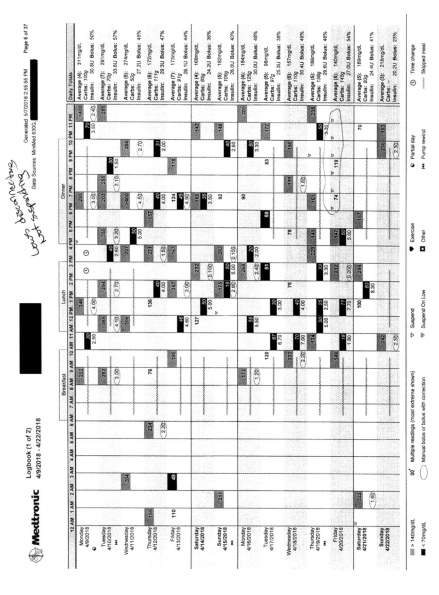

Figure 6.2. *(continued)*

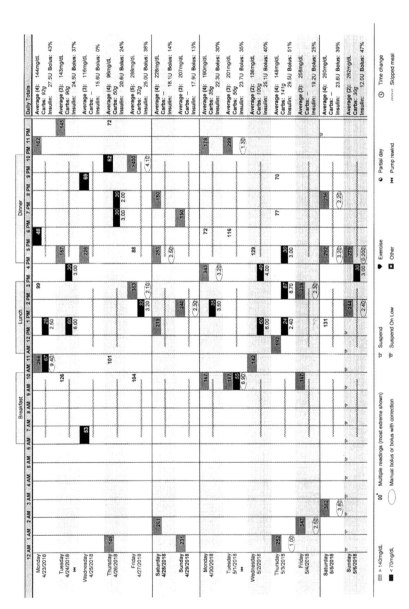

Figure 6.2. *(continued)*

Medtronic

Device Settings Snapshot
Monday 5/7/2018 2:56 PM

Basal

Maximum Basal Rate   2.00 U/Hr

Basal 1 (active)   14.400 U

	Day Off		Workday	
24-Hour Total	—		24-Hour Total	—

Time	U/Hr	Time	U/Hr	Time	U/Hr
0:00	0.600	—	—	—	—

Bolus

Bolus Wizard	On	Easy Bolus	Off
Units	g, mg/dL	Bolus Increment	0.1 U
Active Insulin Time (h:mm)	3:00	Bolus Speed	Standard
Maximum Bolus	10.0 U	Dual/Square	Off/Off

Carbohydrate Ratio (g/U)

Time	Ratio
0:00	15.0
5:00	10.0
20:00	15.0

Insulin Sensitivity (mg/dL per U)

Time	Sensitivity
0:00	60

Blood Glucose Target (mg/dL)

Time	Low	High
0:00	120	120
5:00	100	100
20:00	120	120

Preset Bolus

Name	Normal	Square
Bolus 1		
Breakfast		
Dinner		
Lunch		
Snack		
Bolus 2		
Bolus 3		
Bolus 4		

Preset Temp

Name	Rate	Duration
High Activity		
Moderate Activity		
Low Activity		
Sick		

Name	Rate	Duration
Temp 1		
Temp 2		
Temp 3		
Temp 4		

Sensor

Sensor   Off

High Alerts

On (Snooze 2:00)

Start Time	High (mg/dL)	Alert On High	Alert Before High	Rise Alert Limit (mg/dL)
0:00	300	x		

Low Alerts

On (Snooze 0:20)

Start Time	Low (mg/dL)	Suspend	Alert On Low	Alert Before Low
0:00	70	On Low	x	x

Calibration Reminder   On
Calibration Reminder Time   1:00

Notes

Figure 6.2. *(continued)*

BG range: 45 to >400 mg/dL
FBG: 187 mg/dL
ACL: 162 mg/dL
ACD: 164 mg/dL
HS: 192 mg/dL
Frequency of lows: 7 events <70 mg/dL in the past month
Considers a normal BG: 80–130 mg/dL

CGM Interpretation

S.B. has started Guardian CGM (no data yet).

Labs from 5 February 2018

A1C: 8.7%
UMABCR: Within normal limits
PTH: 42 (15–65 normal)
HCT: 32
Hgb: 10.6
Creatinine: 1.9
GFR: 42
TC: 184
TG: 396
LDL: 71
HDL: 34
Vitamin D: 14

Physical Examination

- BP: 128/89 (BP Location: Left arm, BP Patient Position: Sitting, BP cuff size: Regular)

Table 6.5. Current Regimen, Follow-Up Visit

Basal Rates	Bolus Ratios	Correction Factors/Targets
12 A.M. = 0.65 units/h	12 A.M. = 1 unit for 15 g carbohydrate	Correction factors: 12 A.M. = 60 mg/dL
	5 A.M. = 1 unit for 10 g carbohydrate	Target blood glucose levels:
		12 A.M. = 120 mg/dL
	8 P.M. = 1 unit for 15 g carbohydrate	5 A.M. = 100 mg/dL
		8 P.M. = 120 mg/dL
		Duration of insulin action: 3 h

Table 6.6. A1C History, 5 February 2018

A1C: 8.7%		
Lab Results		
Component	Value	Date
A1C	9.6 (H)	04/02/2018

- Pulse: 92
- Temperature: 99.2°F (37.3°C) (Oral)
- Respiratory: 17
- Height: 5' 4" (1.626 m)
- Weight: 87.5 kg (193 lb)
- BMI: 33.13 kg/m²
- General: Well-developed, well-nourished; in no acute distress.
- Hent: Within normal limits.
- Eyes: No lid lag or proptosis. No icterus, no scleral injection, no periorbital edema.
- Respiratory: Easy WOB in no distress.
- CV: Pink well perfused, mild LE edema.
- GI: Soft, nontender.
- MSK: MAE, normal gate.
- Neurologic: Alert and oriented x3. No tremor.
- Psychiatric: Pleasant, normal affect, normal judgment.
- Skin: Warm to touch.

ASSESSMENT AND PLAN

Patient Education
Self-Monitoring of Blood Glucose.
- Reviewed timing and frequency of testing and premeal BG goals.
- Suggested testing a minimum of 4 times daily prior to meals and bedtime. Calibrate Guardian as needed.

- Discussed testing prior to bedtime goal for BG. If BG <100–120 mg/dL at bedtime, have a small snack (15 g).
- Discussed benefits of using CGM 670G Medtronic pump. Will call MiniMed because of issues with accuracy.
- Discussed using results for decision making; contact clinic if BGs are consistently <70 mg/dL or >200 mg/dL.

Healthy Eating. Discussed importance of covering all carbohydrates with ICR to avoid a spike or drop in BG levels.

Medication and Insulin. Her TDD 24 with basal-bolus is heavy basal. No changes in pump settings.

- Encouraged her to continue working on entering any carbohydrates consumed and BG levels for correction 3–4 times daily. We also suggested getting on auto mode as soon as possible to decrease her fears of low BG levels.
- Keep pump connected; do not disconnect when on auto mode.
- Encouraged her to contact us if she needs further adjustments.
- The goal is for her to bolus for carbohydrates and not to have to suspend or disconnect the pump to avoid hypoglycemia.
- Discussed the importance of taking insulin at least 15–20 min before eating.
- Because her February 2018 labs showed low vitamin D levels, she started 2,000 IU of Vitamin D3 daily.

Overall Assessment

S.B.'s last A1C was 8.7% down from 9.6% (Table 6.6). She uses a Medtronic pump and just started on 670G; she is not yet in auto mode. She started taking steroids for RA and has a plan in place to increase basal during the day. No other pump setting changes today (Table 6.7). We encouraged her to continue working on entering any carbohydrate consumed and her BG levels for correction 3–4 times daily. She should get on auto mode as soon as possible to decrease her fear of low BG levels. We suggested she keep the pump connected; she should not disconnect when on auto mode. We will follow her closely.

- No pump setting change; talk to Medtronic as you get started on 670G.
- If not in auto mode, use temp basal and start at a 30–50% increase for 8 h for a steroid taper. Check BG levels often.
- Send MyChart on Wednesdays if having BG levels <70 mg/dL or >200 mg/dL.
- Do not suspend the pump at all and keep it connected to your body.

Table 6.7. Current Regime, Moving Forward

Basal Rates	Bolus Ratios	Correction Factors/Targets
12 am = 0.6 units/h	12 A.M. = 1 unit for 15 g carbohydrate 5 A.M. = 1 unit for 10 g carbohydrate 8 P.M. = 1 unit for 15 g carbohydrate	Correction factors: 12 A.M. = 60 mg/dL Target blood glucose levels: 12 A.M. = 120 mg/dL 5 A.M. = 100 mg/dL 8 P.M. = 120 mg/dL Duration of insulin action: 3 h

CONCLUSION

S.B. came to the clinic frustrated because she felt her pump was not working. To prevent hypoglycemia she had to suspend her basal for hours on end. She was fearful of entering carbohydrates and BG levels into the pump because when she did, she was having lows. Her pump settings were totally wrong for her insulin needs. After talking to her and discovering how she was using the pump, we were able to gain insight and to make changes in her settings (reducing basal as well as bolus settings) that allowed her to use her pump in a more effective way and improve glycemic control.

With the changes made, S.B. saw improvements in average BG and standard deviation of BG as well as an improvement in A1C. Before our meetings, she was working very hard—suspending the pump and trying to figure out what carbohydrate count she could enter to avoid having a low BG level throughout the day. She came in to her first visit thinking that pumping was not going to work for her and left her second visit with a better understanding of how often we need to adjust pump settings to meet individual needs. She is excited to move forward with the Medtronic 670G and the Guardian sensor. Her next visit will provide even more insight as to how to further refine her pump settings using the Hybrid-AP technology as a guide.

Chapter 7
Continuous Glucose Monitoring: Understanding Strategies to Simplify the Insulin Regimen in Older Patients with Hypoglycemia

Michelle Magee, MD, MBBCh, BAO, LRCPSI;[1,2,3] Claudia Morrison, RD, CDE;[4] and Gretchen Youssef, MS, RD, CDE[1]

CASE PRESENTATION

An otherwise-healthy 78-year-old Caucasian male who is a judge has had type 2 diabetes (T2D) for 30 years. He has successfully kept his A1C in the 6.5–7% range and has no micro- or macrovascular complications. Recently, the court clerks have been giving him candy or juice when he seems to be "thinking less clearly," which was happening several times daily. Our endocrine team was consulted to perform a review of his diabetes relative to his ability to continue serving on the court.

He took glargine 40 units at bedtime with a sliding-scale regimen of insulin aspart with each meal until 2 months ago when his endocrinologist reduced the insulin glargine dose to 20 units for an A1C of 6.2%. He does not write down his meal insulin doses and cannot tell you the sliding scale, but he reports that he may take up to 15 units of insulin aspart with a meal.

He is alert and oriented and knows all of the details of his past medical history. His A1C is now 7.3%, fructosamine is 330 (0–285), and C-peptide is <0.1 mg/mL (1.1–4.4). A cortrosyn stimulation test reveals cortisol at baseline of 18.0 mcg/dL and at 30 min of 22.8 mcg/dL. The results of the cortrosyn stimulation test rules out adrenal gland insufficiency.

The team's registered dietitian (RD) and certified diabetes educator saw the patient for diabetes self-management education support (DSMES), medical nutrition therapy, and continuous glucose monitoring (CGM) system initiation.

HIGHLIGHTS OF DSMES ASSESSMENT

His typical food intake follows:

Breakfast
7 A.M.   1 cup of steel cut oatmeal with 2 T of raisins and 2% milk
                ~60 g carbohydrate or 4 carbohydrate choices

[1]MedStar Diabetes Institute, Washington, D.C. [2]MedStar Health Research Institute, Hyattsville, MD. [3]Georgetown University School of Medicine, Washington, D.C. [4]MedStar Washington Hospital Center, Washington, D.C.

Lunch   (Often lunch is much later.)
~1 P.M.   sandwich, fruit, and yogurt or 2 cups of chili and crackers
           ~60 g carbohydrate or 4 carbohydrate choices
Dinner
7 P.M.   fish, vegetables 1–2 cups and 1 medium-large potato baked/
           boiled, fruit ~60 g carbohydrate or 4 carbohydrate choices
Snack   chocolate if available

Self-monitoring of blood glucose: Checks before breakfast (80–120 mg/dL), dinner (80–90 mg/dL), or bedtime (usually > 100 mg/dL). Does not check blood glucose at work.

Weight: 76 kg
BMI: 25 kg/m^2

Hypoglycemia: Knows signs, symptoms, and treatment of hypoglycemia but has hypoglycemia unawareness.
Assessment of insulin administration:

- Demonstrates proper insulin pen administration technique.

- Storage of insulin is appropriate.

- Rotates injection sites in abdomen.

- Has fair understanding of actions of mealtime and basal insulin.

Physical activity: Walks his dog 20 min each night after dinner.

Sleep: 8 h/day

Table 7.1 shows simplification strategies for older patients with diabetes.

Table 7.1. Simplification Strategies for Older Patients with Diabetes

Barrier to Diabetes Self-Care	Solutions for Consideration
Forgets to take meal insulin	Stop meal insulin if <10 units/meal and start once-daily noninsulin agent that acts to control postmeal blood glucose excursion
Forgets to take basal insulin	Change time of day taken to a time the patient thinks will be easier to remember to take (e.g., with breakfast or supper instead of bedtime, if patient falls asleep after dinner and then forgets to take it).
Cannot follow insulin scale	Stop meal insulin scale and start fixed insulin dose (*strategy used in this case*) or simplified insulin scale with meals
Cannot self-administer insulin	Engage family member or caregiver and minimize number of insulin shots daily by use of noninsulin once-daily alternate antihyperglycemic agents
Forgets to take other diabetes medications	Maximize use of once-daily or once-weekly antihyperglycemic agents

Source: Adapted from Munshi et al.[1]

We discussed with this patient several strategies that may be considered when working with older adults. One useful strategy in older adults with adequate β-cell reserve who forget to take their meal insulin doses, particularly when they are on low doses (i.e., <10 units of insulin/meal) is to replace mealtime insulin with a once-daily noninsulin agent. This patient's C-peptide is low, so replacing his mealtime insulin with a noninsulin agent to simplify his regimen is not an option, as he will need mealtime insulin on-board to control postmeal glucose levels.

The patient was taking insulin glargine at bedtime. Although he does not miss this dose of insulin, he felt that it would be much easier to take the insulin glargine before dinner. Bedtime insulin may be missed because patients often fall asleep and do not take it; therefore, taking it at breakfast or dinner may be preferred.

On the basis of the diabetes team's evaluation, the patient was felt to be over-insulinized. It is unclear what doses of insulin he is taking with each sliding scale at mealtime. Sliding-scale insulin was replaced with a fixed and reduced dose of 10 units of insulin aspart with each meal. Simplification of a patient's insulin plan, by avoiding insulin sliding scales and replacing them with fixed insulin doses before meals, may reduce insulin dosing errors, especially in older adults, such as this patient.

The RD assessed the patient's intake of carbohydrate to be ~60 g at breakfast, lunch, and dinner. The RD reviewed with the patient carbohydrate sources in his diet and the affect of carbohydrate on blood glucose. The importance of eating lunch on time was emphasized. Because the patient is now on a fixed dose of insulin with meals, the need to consume a consistent intake of 4 carbohydrate choices with each meal was stressed. The patient was not interested in learning carbohydrate counting, and thus consistency of carbohydrate intake was emphasized. The mealtime insulin dose would need to be decreased with the consumption of fewer carbohydrates.

The team reinforced a glycemic goal of an A1C <8% based and blood glucose values in the range of 110–180 mg/dL throughout the day to prevent hypoglycemia. A less-stringent A1C goal was targeted because of the patient's past episodes of hypoglycemia and age as recommended in the American Diabetes Association's *Diabetes in Older Adults*[2] guidelines and the Association's *Standards of Medical Care in Diabetes, 2019.*[3]

A professional CGM was initiated on the patient to determine daily glucose trends. The CGM was set at alerts outside of the range of 100–200 mg/dL. CGM technology has been used as a tool to document the incidence and magnitude of both hypoglycemia and hyperglycemia in adults with diabetes. In adults with T2D, even when it is apparently well controlled, CGM has shown that hypoglycemia and excessive postprandial glycemic excursions are common. In older patients, CGM has shown hypoglycemia to be extremely common and often asymptomatic, and even when A1C is ≥8%, CGM has shown hypoglycemia rates to be as high as 65%. Fully 93% of these lows were not detected by traditional finger-stick blood glucose testing, nor by symptoms, which increases risk of harm to the patient.[4] In another study, 25 older patients (mean age of 73.9+/–4.4 years) with an A1C <7.5% were placed on CGM for 144 h and 1 month later another 144 h. Eighty percent of the patients had 103 hypoglycemic events of which 14 of the patients had a blood glucose value of <40 mg/dL.

A download of the patient's first CGM report is shown in Figure 7.1. The data revealed blood glucose patterns of multiple sustained episodes of hypoglycemia noted from 9 A.M. to 6 P.M.[5]

The patient was advised to reduce his meal insulin dose to 7 units at each meal and to continue the 20 units of glargine that he takes at dinner.

We reviewed the treatment and prevention of hypoglycemia with the patient. He stated that he now carries glucose tablets with him to treat hypoglycemia and that he would overtreat hypoglycemia events, resulting in high blood glucose.

The patient requested to use the CGM one more time. A download of the second CGM readings revealed improved blood glucose control but with the patient still experiencing some sustained hypoglycemia episode in the late afternoon (Figure 7.2). The patient stated that he now is taking 7 units of insulin aspart with meals but often is not consuming the 4 carbohydrate choices at lunchtime or is often late for lunch. The patient was advised to decrease lunchtime insulin to 5 units and to continue to take 7 units of insulin aspart with breakfast and dinner.

This patient found the CGM data to be so useful in helping to avert hypoglycemic episodes that he obtained a personal CGM (see the data in Figure 7.3). Note that the hypoglycemic events have decreased with no blood glucose levels <80 mg/dL. At this follow-up visit, the patient and his wife both observed that he was feeling a lot better, was less tired, and was much sharper of mind. It was deemed appropriate from the perspective of his diabetes for him to return to the court bench.

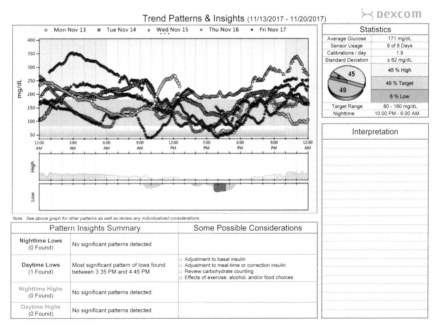

Figure 7.1. Download of the patient's first CGM report.

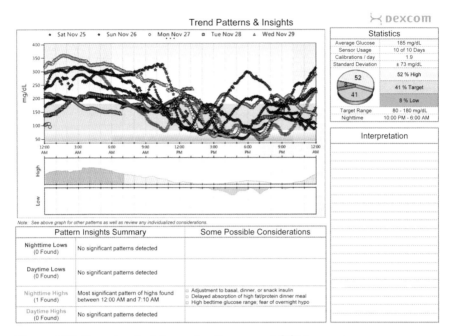

Figure 7.2. Download of the patient's second CGM report.

The patient continues to work with the endocrinologist and diabetes educator to further fine-tune his insulin and lifestyle plan. This case highlights the benefits simplifying strategies for older patient with diabetes. The use of CGM in older adults is a powerful tool and, as such, it provides patients with valuable information that enables them and their healthcare providers to make more informed decisions that have a significant impact on quality of life.

REFERENCES

1. Munshi M. Cognitive dysfunction in older adults with diabetes: what a clinician needs to know. *Diabetes Care* 2017;40:461–467

2. Kirkman MS, Briscoe VJ, Clark N, et al. Diabetes in older adults. *Diabetes Care* 2012;35:2650–2664

3. American Diabetes Association. Standards of medical care in diabetes, 2019. *Diabetes Care* 2019;42(Suppl. 1):S139–S145

4. Munshi, M, Slyne C, Segal AR, et al. Simplification on insulin regiment in older adults and risk of hypoglycemia. *JAMA Intern Med* 2016;176:1023–1025

5. Hay LC, Wilmshurst EG, Fulcher G. Unrecognized hypo- and hyperglycemia in well-controlled patients with type 2 diabetes mellitus: the results of continuous glucose monitoring. *Diabetes Technol Ther* 2003;5(1):19–26

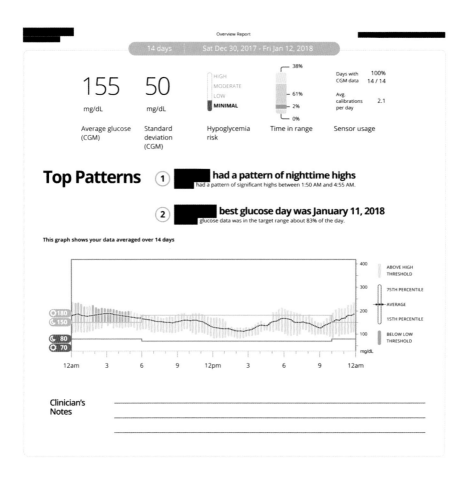

Figure 7.3. Download from patient's personal CGM.

Devices

Dexcom Receiver

CGM ID		**Current Alert Settings for Device**		
Serial Number		Low Alert	On	100 mg/dL
Uploaded On	**January 12, 2018**	High Alert	On	200 mg/dL
		Fall Rate Alert	On	3 mg/dL/min
		Rise Rate Alert	Off	3 mg/dL/min
		Out of Range Alert	On	20 min

Figure 7.3. *(continued)*

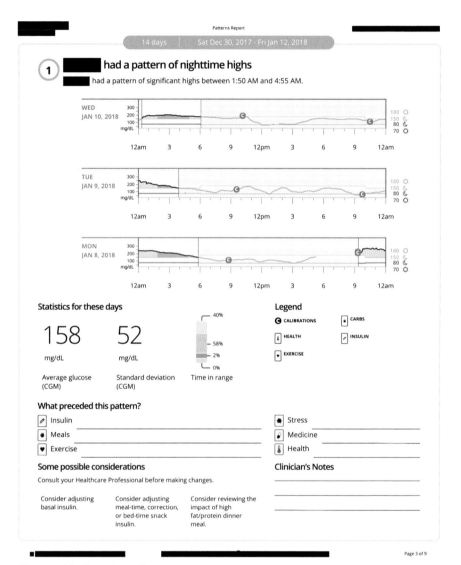

Figure 7.3. *(continued)*

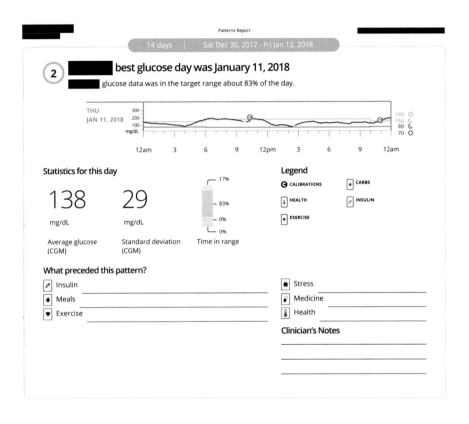

Figure 7.3. *(continued)*

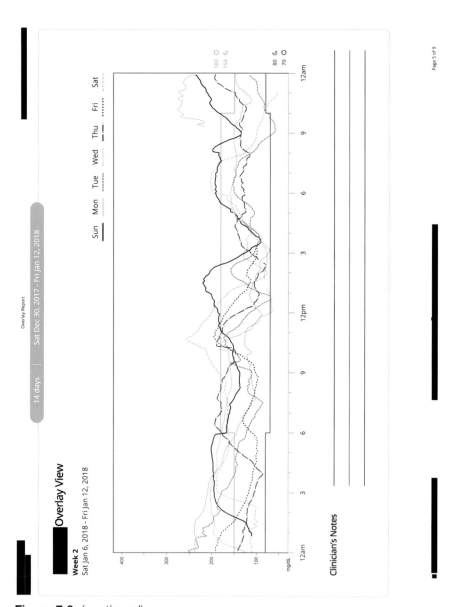

Figure 7.3. *(continued)*

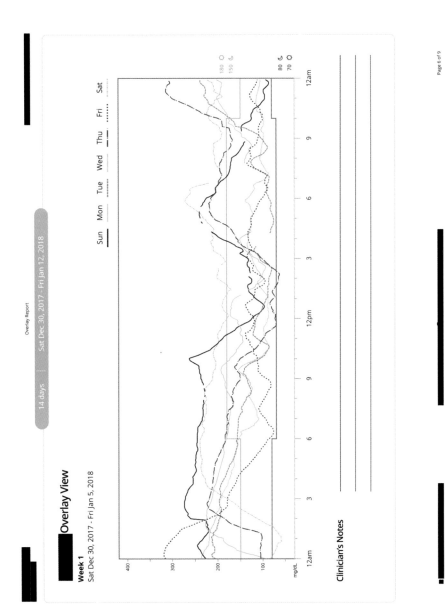

Figure 7.3. *(continued)*

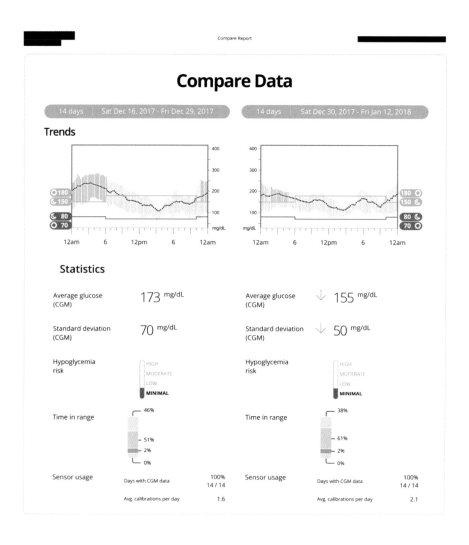

Figure 7.3. *(continued)*

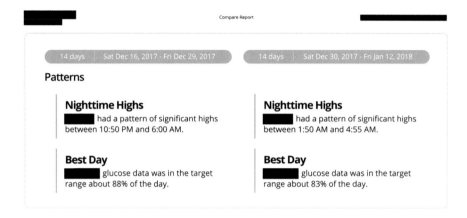

Figure 7.3. *(continued)*

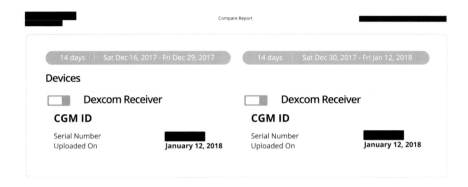

Figure 7.3. *(continued)*

Chapter 8

Helping Patients Understand Predictive Technology with the Use of Professional Continuous Glucose Monitoring

Lucille Hughes, DNP, MSN/Ed, CDE, BC-ADM, FAADE,[1] and Sara Madtes, RD, CDE[2]

For patients with diabetes, professional continuous glucose monitoring (CGM) provides an opportunity to see the future of blood glucose levels.[1] Professional CGM is often the first introduction a patient will have to the world of CGM and often serves as a gateway to personal CGM. With the assistance of the provider, CGM allows an individual to review the past, see the present, and predict the future of their blood glucose control. Better yet, the ongoing heightened awareness resulting from this technology has helped patients lower their A1C.[1–3]

PATIENT CASE REPORT

M.H. is a 68-year-old Caucasian woman; she is married with one son. She is presently retired and her previous profession is unknown. M.H. was diagnosed with type 1 diabetes 35 years ago and was seen in the Diabetes Education Center with a patient-centered goal to reduce A1C to a target range of ≤7%. M.H. has a past medical history significant for hyperlipidemia and essential hypertension. She admitted to having frequent hypoglycemia, with levels ranging as low as 40–70 mg/dL, and infrequent hyperglycemia, which she detected through finger-stick blood glucose monitoring, which she was performing ~5–6 times daily. At this time, M.H. had an A1C of 7.9%.

Upon initial assessment, M.H. reported an insulin regimen consisting of insulin glargine 30–34 units each night, which she adjusted based on bedtime blood glucose level. In addition, she reported taking a fixed premeal dose of 5 units of insulin aspart, and a correction dose based on her blood glucose level (3 units for a blood glucose of 101–150 mg/dL, 4 units for a blood glucose of 151–200 mg/dL, and so on). M.H. was not carbohydrate counting at this time; however, she consumed very few carbohydrates for both her meals and snacks. She understood how to appropriately read the nutrition facts label on packaged foods, but she was not familiar with the various carbohydrate-serving sizes for fruits and vegetables, which were her more frequent carbohydrate choices. At this visit, M.H. agreed to participate in a 2-week professional Libre CGM study to aide in identifying blood glucose patterns. Unfortunately, the sensor came off after 1 week, and she returned

[1]South Nassau Community Hospital, Oceanside, NY. [2]South Nassau Diabetes Education Center, South Nassau Community Hospital, Oceanside, NY.

to the office for initial download. Upon download of the CGM data, we were able to detect multiple hypoglycemic events (N = 13). M.H. was experiencing these events in the afternoon, evening hours, and overnight as well.

M.H. was surprised at the frequency of her hypoglycemia because she had been asymptomatic. At that point, we discussed hypoglycemia unawareness and prevention strategies. Further review of the download revealed glucose variability as seen by wide swings in blood glucose ranging from 40 mg/dL to 300 mg/dL. On the basis of the data review from Libre Pro, we discussed the benefits of intensive insulin management and of using an insulin-to-carbohydrate ratio (ICR) of 1:20 and insulin sensitivity factor of 1:70. Her insulin glargine was reduced to 22 units to address the pattern of overnight blood glucose decline resulting in fasting hypoglycemia (see Figure 8.1).

M.H. returned to the Diabetes Education Center 3 months later to participate in a repeat Libre Pro study. Upon review of the download, it became apparent that the adjustments made in response to the initial CGM study reduced the mean = [standard deviation] by more than 50% (79 mg/dL to 37.8 mg/dL), and time in range increased by more than 50% (43% to 79%; see Figure 8.2). Hyperglycemia decreased from 39% to 1%; however, nocturnal hypoglycemia persisted, which appeared to be an ongoing basal issue (see Figures 8.2 and 8.3).

To correct this pattern of nocturnal hypoglycemia, M.H. transitioned from insulin glargine to insulin degludec, 14 units each night, which has greatly reduced nocturnal hypoglycemia.

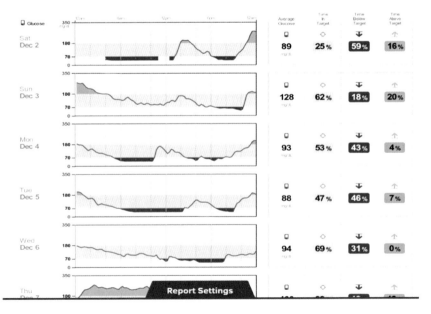

Figure 8.1. Download of patient data.

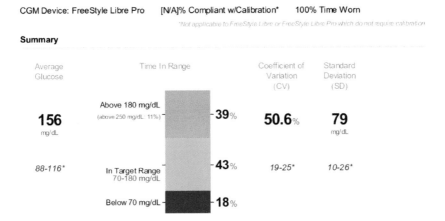

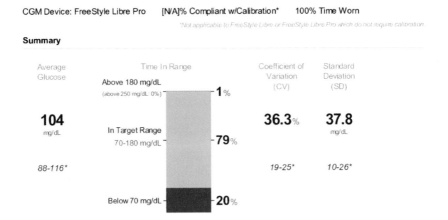

Figure 8.2. Comparison of patient data, 15 December 2017 versus 25 March 2018.

This experience led M.H. to purchase a personal CGM system. Because of her hypoglycemia unawareness, the Dexcom G5 was recommended for the predictive low alarm this system offers. Through this persistent detection and analysis of blood glucose trends and patterns that both professional and personal CGM offers, M.H. has been able to adjust her basal and mealtime insulin doses

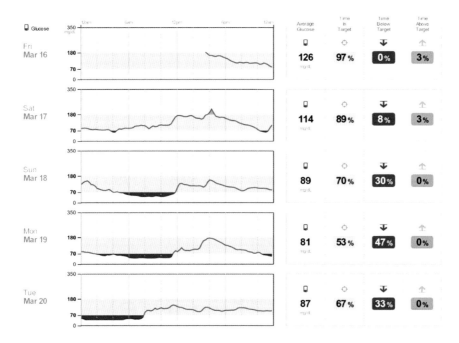

Figure 8.3. Download of patient data 3 months later.

accordingly to reduce her risk for low blood glucose levels as well as to decrease the glucose variability she was experiencing so often. M.H. is now on a suitable dose of insulin degludec, resulting in steady glycemic control overnight and zero occurrences of hypoglycemia. On the basis of M.H.'s most recent personal CGM download, her time in range is 66%, time above range is 32%, and time below range decreased to 1% (see Figure 8.4). Her latest A1C from July, 2018 was 6.2%.

For many patients, professional CGM provides an opportunity for providers to detect the root cause of glycemic variability quicker than relying on self-monitoring of blood glucose results. Furthermore, professional CGM is often the gateway to personal CGM utilization, allowing the patient the opportunity to participate in proactive glycemic self-management aimed at preventing hypo/hyperglycemia, lowering A1C, and ultimately preventing the chronic complications associated with diabetes.

Top Patterns ① Marian's best glucose day was August 20, 2018

Marian's glucose data was in the target range about 100% of the day.

This graph shows your data averaged over 90 days

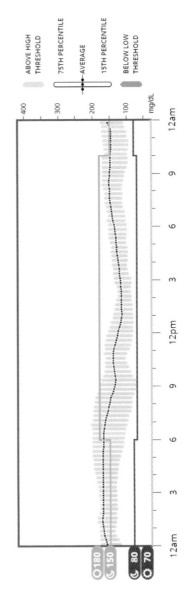

Figure 8.4. Download of patient data, August 2018.

REFERENCES

1. Jensen MH, Christensen TF, Tarnow L, Mahmoudi Z, Johansen MD, Hejlesen OK. Professional continuous glucose monitoring in subjects with type 1 diabetes: Retrospective hypoglycemia detection. *J Diabetes Sci Technol* 2013;7(1):135–143

2. Yeoh E, Choudhary P. Technology to reduce hypoglycemia. *J Diabetes Sci Technol* 2015;9(4):911–916

3. Gehlaut RR, Dogbey GY, Schwartz FL, Marling CR, Shubrook JH. Hypoglycemia in type 2 diabetes- more common than you think: A continuous glucose monitoring study. *J Diabetes Sci Technol* 2015;9(5):999–1005

Chapter 9
The Power of a Sample

Jean Unger, BSN, RN, CDE,[1] and Shannon Christen, RD, CDE[1]

This case study illustrates how flash glucose monitoring (FGM) (FreeStyle Libre; Abbott Diabetes Care, Witney, U.K.) dramatically improved glycemic control versus self-monitoring of blood glucose (SMBG) in a Medicare patient. Before March 2017, Centers for Medicare and Medicaid Services (CMS) coverage for a personal continuous glucose monitoring (CGM) system was limited. Patients on multiple daily insulin injections are encouraged to SMBG at least four times daily, and when patients fail to perform SMBG as prescribed, data to make treatment decisions are limited and hemoglobin A_{1c} is often above target. Access to real-time sensor glucose data and trend graphs can help patients optimally self-manage their chronic disease. For several other patients, including those who are newly diagnosed and are managing their diabetes over a long period of time, this self-testing process is often the cause of added distress, which leads to a decrease in quality of life.[1]

CASE PRESENTATION

The patient is a 68-year-old man who works as a biologist in an academic research laboratory. He was diagnosed with type 2 diabetes at the age of 55 years and developed mild retinopathy and chronic kidney disease stage 3. He was initially treated with metformin for 2 years and started insulin therapy in 2007. Since 2016, the patient was followed by his primary care physician with hemoglobin A_{1c} in the 12–13% range; he was referred to an endocrinologist in 2016.

In 2016, the endocrinologist advised the patient to titrate up insulin glargine by 2–3 units every 5–7 days to achieve a fasting average of 120 mg/dL and to start rapid-acting insulin aspart with a 4-unit fixed dose at each meal. He was instructed to check blood glucose every morning and 1–2 h after meals. From 2017 to 2018, however, the patient's hemoglobin A_{1c} ranged from 11% to 12%. He continued to check blood glucose once daily. The patient reported he had been too busy to take care of his diabetes. He was feeling burdened to take the time to leave the laboratory to check his blood glucose.

In February 2018, the patient was seen by the endocrinologist and hemoglobin A_{1c} was 12.3%. He reported work-related stress and continued to express that he was feeling burdened to check glucose during the workday. The patient was

---

[1]Division of Endocrinology, Diabetes and Metabolism, Department of Medicine, University of Colorado Anschutz Medical Campus, Lone Tree Medical Center, Lone Tree, CO.

taking insulin glargine 54 units before bed, 20 units in the morning, and insulin aspart 8–12 units with meals (taking about half a dose before a meal and half after a meal per his request). Therapy options were reviewed: SGLT2 inhibitors, metformin, and GLP-1 agonist therapy was contraindicated based on his renal status. He admitted that he is "not too careful" with his carbohydrate intake. His fasting blood glucose average was 220 mg/dL. Patient failed to bring his Free-Style Lite meter to his visits, but instead would keep a typed-up blood glucose log for review to include details to explain why his blood glucoses are out of target range (Table 9.1). CGM options were reviewed with the patient. He was willing to try the CGM to allow him to see his blood glucose levels more easily throughout the day and perhaps motivate him to take the prescribed bolus insulin. He was referred to ambulatory diabetes education.

In March 2018, the patient met with the diabetes educator for his first formal visit. The patient reported the following 24-h diet history recall:

Breakfast:	bowl of cereal and granola and raisins, berries, and banana with 1/2 cup half and half (6 days a week = 102 g of carbohydrates)
Sundays:	2 eggs, 4 pieces of pork bacon, and a scoop of rice
Lunch:	6-inch tortilla with piece of Havarti cheese and 2 pieces of ham or bologna and yogurt
Dinner:	meat or fish or pork roast and 1 cup rice *or* roast chicken and baked potato *or* 2 chicken and bean burritos and beer
Snacks:	cheese and salami with toast
Beverages:	water, sparkling water, regular ginger ale (occasionally), glass of wine or beer (rarely)
Restaurant meals:	6 times per month

Table 9.1. Fasting Blood Glucose Report Provided by Patient

01/21/18	169	still treating sinus infection
01/22/18	178	
01/23/18	129	
01/24/18	210	
01/25/18	160	sinus infection over
01/26/18	157	Cat crisis
01/27/18	218	
01/28/18	170	
01/29/18	198	grant proposal due on 02/04; Tenure promotion report due 02/04
01/30/18	258	jury duty – get placed on jury for a criminal trial; 4 hours sleep
01/31/18	368	trial: 5 hours sleep
02/01/18	252	trial/conviction
02/02/18	313	catch up at work
02/03/18	336	
02/04/18	195	Super Bowl too many chips
02/05/18	260	

He reported taking glargine 54 units in the evening and 20 units every morning and insulin aspart 10 units with meals, with half a dose before a meal and half after a meal. Fasting glucose ranged from 69 to 219 mg/dL. He reported being too busy to take the time to test blood glucose at work. The patient was advised on carbohydrate sources and meal alternatives to cereal were discussed. He was counseled on following a low-fat diet.

The patient was shown available CGM options. He was interested in FreeStyle Libre CGM and was given a handout on Medicare requirements to qualify for the device. The diabetes education plan was to change the breakfast meal (include protein), aim for 45–60 g of carbohydrate per meal, and add 25% more insulin aspart when eating meals with 25 g of fat or more. He was instructed to SMBG 4 times a day so that Medicare Part B would pay for the personal CGM.

During the time between visits with the diabetes educators, he provided the following blood glucose logs of his fasting blood glucose (Table 9.2).

In May 2018, the patient was seen by his endocrinologist. His hemoglobin A_{1c} improved to 9.5% (from 12.3%) likely because he had lowered the carbohydrate content in his diet. He reported lowering carbohydrates at breakfast. He continued SMBG checking once daily and was not motivated to test differently or more often.

Table 9.2. Fasting Glucose Report

March 2018

03/10	118	03/11	115	03/12	87	03/13	105	03/14	114	03/15	72
03/16	108	03/17	107	03/18	185	03/19	145	03/20	155	03/21	225

--------Trip to New York ----

03/22	154	03/23	117	03/24	66	03/25	93	03/26	115	03/27	142
03/28	173	03/29	131	03/30	104	03/31	122				

Average for March – 138

April 2018

04/01	128	04/02	164	04/03	127	04/04	154	04/05	111	04/06	96
04/07	126	04/08	156	04/09	122	04/10	72	04/11	88	04/12	79
04/13	88	04/14	95	04/15	79	04/16	77	04/17	88	04/18	69
04/19	73	04/20	99	04/21	92	04/22	168	04/23	96	04/24	128
04/25	157	04/26	99	04/27	142	04/28	123*	04/29	262	04/30	159

*12:30 AM 4/29 54
Average for April – 104

May 2018

05/01	135	05/02	166	05/03	91	05/04	122	05/05	142	05/06	110
05/07	105	05/08	100	05/09	78	05/10	100	05/11	162	05/12	66
05/13	135	05/14	121	05/15	134	05/16	83	05/17	74	05/18	126
05/19	108	05/20	132	05/21	84	05/22	66	05/23	86	05/24	92
05/25	135	05/26	111	05/27	106	05/28	166	05/29	123	05/30	114

Average for May – 106

At the visit, the patient was fitted with a FreeStyle Libre personal sensor and reader (sample courtesy of Abbott) to assess glucose control. The patient was instructed on use of the device and reviewed Medicare requirements (SMBG 4 times daily) to get approval. He contacted the clinic a day later and requested a formal prescription for purchase as he was enjoying the data and its ease of use. The patient was scheduled for a follow-up appointment with a diabetes educator.

In July 2018, the patient met with the diabetes educator. He reported that he enjoyed the data the sensor provided (Figures 9.1 and 9.2). The CGM system report showed 4% of the readings were <70 mg/dL, 67% of the readings were in target range (70–180 mg/dL), and 29% of the readings were above target (>180 mg/dL). The average sensor glucose was 154 mg/dL with an estimated hemoglobin A_{1c} of 7.0%.

The patient reported the CGM system was especially helpful to use at work. He could use the system discretely and quickly to assess glucose control (Figure 9.3). Blood glucose meter results showed overall average glucose was 154 mg/dL with a range of 62–333 mg/dL. He was scanning the CGM 16–29 times/day as well as recording bolus doses in the reader. The patient was more engaged in managing his diabetes because of ease of use and the information provided. In a study of more than 800 patients using CGM, 96–100% of patients reported positive experiences, such as discreetness, convenience, increased quality of life, and more productive clinician-patients interaction facilitating better disease management.[2]

Before the visit, the patient adjusted the glargine 40–54 units in the evening and discontinued the morning dose of insulin glargine. He increased insulin aspart

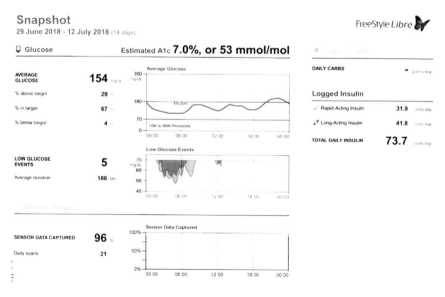

Figure 9.1. CGM snapshot report: June 29–July 12, 2018.

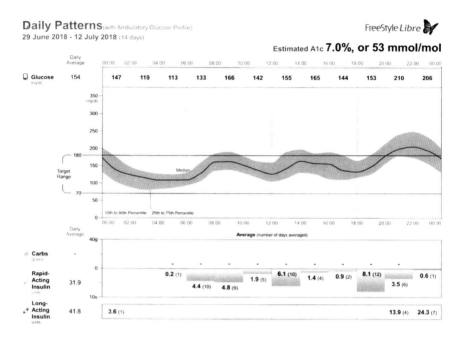

Figure 9.2. CGM daily patterns report: June 29–July 12, 2018.

to 10–12 units before meals and was no longer splitting the dose before and after the meal. The CGM daily pattern report showed a drop of ~97 mg/dL from bedtime to wakeup because of the basal insulin dose (Figure 9.4). He was counseled to decrease glargine but increase the insulin aspart at dinner to prevent postmeal hyperglycemia. He was advised to have a follow-up with the diabetes educator for meter download and to evaluate insulin changes.

In August 2018, the patient met with the diabetes educator. The patient further reduced insulin glargine to 32–40 units and reported using insulin aspart 8–10 units with meals. The CGM was downloaded and reviewed (Figure 9.4). The CGM report is a visual tool that shows patients the effects of insulin dosing and glucose and that helps explain why therapy changes are necessary. The drop in glucose overnight indicated too much basal insulin. The patient was instructed to continue to decrease insulin glargine and increase bolus insulin aspart, as needed.

The patient continued to record bolus doses in real time and scanned the CGM 14–16 times a day (Figure 9.5). The patient commented that his glycemic control improved greatly with FGM information and he reported feeling better and having more energy. On 31 August 2018, his hemoglobin A_{1c} was 7.3%.

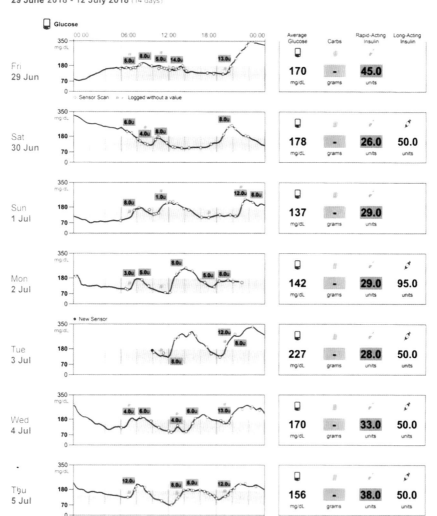

Figure 9.3. CGM weekly summary report: June 29–July 12, 2018.

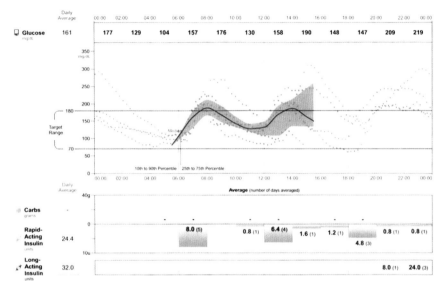

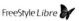

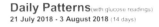

Figure 9.4. CGM daily patterns report: July 21–August 3, 2018.

CONCLUSION

This case study is a good example of how CGM technology can engage patients to improve glycemic control. The patient had averaged SMBG once daily, but with CGM, he was scanning the device an average of 15 scans/day. His hemoglobin A_{1c} dramatically improved over the 3-month period from 12% to 7.3% (Table 9.3). Patients with higher numbers of daily CGM scans show significantly improved levels of A1C, most likely because of better insulin adjustments for the consumed food and an improved ability to correct out-of-target glucose values in a timely fashion.[1]

The CGM was able to provide some context to his dietary pattern, stress, illness, and insulin dosing. Novel devices such as this can encourage a person with diabetes to reinvest in their management of diabetes and give them a new-found motivation for self-care. Note that the sample personal CGM was provided to the patient during a clinic visit. It is unclear whether he would have invested the time and cost for this device on his own.

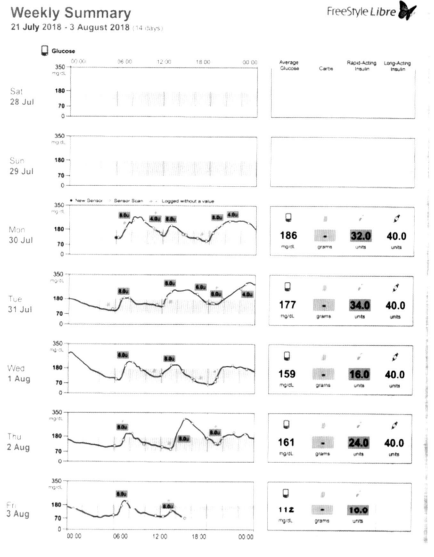

Figure 9.5. CGM weekly summary report: July 21–August 3, 2018.

Table 9.3. Hemoglobin A$_{1c}$ Trends

Date	08/25/16	02/27/17	08/31/17	02/23/18	05/17/18	08/31/18
Hemoglobin A$_{1c}$	12.5%	9.5%	12.0 %	11.7 %	9.5%	7.3%

REFERENCES

1. Hayek AA, Robert AA, Al Dawish MA. Evaluation of FreeStyle Libre flash glucose monitoring system on glycemic control, health-related quality of life, and fear of hypoglycemia in patients with type 1 diabetes. *Clin Med Insights: Endocr Diabetes* 2017;10:1–6

2. Kesavadev J, Shankar A, Ashok AD, Srinivas S, Ajai NA, Sanal G, Krishnan G, Ramachandran L, and Jothydev S. Our first 825 T2DM patients on 14-day factory-calibrated glucose monitoring system: clinical utility and challenges. *J Diabetes Sci Technol* 2017;12:230–231

Chapter 10

Practical Automated Insulin: Using a Hybrid Closed-Loop System in an Adolescent Boy with Type 1 Diabetes

Laurel H. Messer, RN, MPH, CDE;[1] Cari Berget, RN, MPH, CDE;[1] and Gregory P. Forlenza, MS, MD[1]

The utility of insulin pumps and continuous glucose monitors (CGMs) changed tremendously with the advent of automated insulin delivery. With automated insulin delivery systems, sensor glucose levels are used by the pump to calculate insulin delivery, instead of the user-programming fixed rates of insulin that are independent of glucose levels. Randomized controlled trials on automated insulin delivery systems have shown improved time in the target range of 70–180 mg/dL by 12–15% with their use when compared to sensor-augmented pump therapy.[1] To put this in concrete terms, individuals may spend almost 3–4 h/day more within the normal blood glucose range when using automated insulin delivery systems even when comparing to individuals who already are using pumps and sensors.

Currently, two commercial insulin delivery systems suspend insulin delivery when CGM glucose levels cross into the hypoglycemic range or are predicted to become hypoglycemic in the near future. One additional commercial system, the MiniMed 670G, automatically calculates basal insulin delivery based on sensor glucose readings and total daily insulin. This system is called a hybrid closed-loop (HCL) system, because the user still manually programs bolus insulin for food intake or correction doses. Other HCL systems likely will be approved commercially in the future.

The MiniMed 670G HCL system is unique in that it operates in 2 modes: open-loop mode (manual mode) and HCL mode (auto mode). In the open-loop mode, the system acts like a traditional insulin pump and all programmable dose parameters can be modified: basal doses, sensitivity or correction dose, insulin-to-carbohydrate ratios (ICRs), blood glucose targets, and insulin action time. All of these settings will affect insulin delivery in an open loop. When using the system in HCL mode, the pump controls the basal insulin delivery and sensitivities are determined automatically by the system to achieve a target glucose level of 120 mg/dL. The user or clinician is not able to modify these settings by changing programmed pump parameters. Bolus doses can be modified however, as the user or clinician must program the ICRs, and the insulin action time. Additionally, the user may set a "temp target"—that is, a temporary period of time in which the system automates to a glucose level of 150 mg/dL instead of 120 mg/dL. The system can be manually switched between open-loop and HCL

---

[1]Barbara Davis Center for Diabetes, University of Colorado School of Medicine, Aurora, CO.

mode but will also automatically exit HCL mode to open loop under a variety of conditions including lack of CGM data, persistent hyperglycemia, or system-driven insulin delivery constraints. Because the majority of adolescents using HCL systems spend roughly 70% time in HCL mode and 30% time in open-loop mode,[2-4] the clinician must consider how to optimize the pump settings for both open loop (i.e., evaluate all settings) and HCL (i.e., only evaluate ICR and insulin action time).

When evaluating automated insulin delivery, the acronym CARE provides a simple framework to employ when working with various systems.[5] Clinicians should consider how the system *calculates* insulin, what insulin dosing *adjustments* can be made, when to *revert* to open-loop delivery, and how to *educate* individuals. As discussed earlier, the MiniMed 670G system calculates insulin by automating basal dosing to achieve a target of 120 mg/dL, but it still requires the user to administer bolus doses for meals and corrections. The clinician and pump user can adjust the ICRs and insulin action time to modify insulin doses to account for times when the system is operating in HCL mode, and the rest of the insulin doses can be adjusted for use during open-loop mode. The user should revert to open loop if they have given an injection of insulin by syringe, if they have ketones that require extra insulin administration, or for periods of illness when temporary basal rates should be employed. Finally, clinicians should educate the patients on how to optimize time in HCL mode and glycemic range. As new systems come to market with new capabilities, the CARE model utility can be increased by adding S for *sensor* or *sharing* characteristics. The CARES framework will help distinguish whether individuals can use sensors non-adjunctively, and whether systems have access to remote monitoring and cloud-based data.

AIDEN THE BASEBALL PLAYER

Aiden is a 15-year-old adolescent boy with type 1 diabetes (T1D) for 2 years. He is a baseball player with practices twice per week and has games on the weekends. He is in 9th grade at a public school with a regular lunchtime and gym class in the afternoon. Aiden is allowed to test his blood glucose levels in the classroom and bolus independently. He can treat low glucose levels on his own, but also has the option of seeing the school nurse at any time if he wants assistance with diabetes management.

Aiden is seen every 3 months by an endocrinologist and certified diabetes educator at a specialty diabetes clinic. At his current appointment, he weighs 88.5 kg (a gain of 2.1 kg in the past 3 months) and is 68.5 inches tall (a gain of 0.5 inches in past 3 months). Aiden has used the MiniMed 670G HCL system for the past year. His HbA_{1c} at his current visit was 8.5%, above the Association target range of <7.5% for adolescents with T1D.[6] The goals of this visit were to optimize insulin doses and diabetes self-management behaviors to increase time in glycemic range 70–180 mg/dL and to lower his HbA_{1c}.

Assessment

Aiden says he likes using the MiniMed 670G and guesses that he tests blood glucose levels 4–6 times/day. He is less happy about wearing a sensor, stating "it is annoying to change, and sometimes I like to take a break because I get less alerts and alarms." He sometimes waits 1–2 days before changing the CGM sensor for this reason.

Aiden's glucose meter and insulin pump were downloaded and show the following (Figure 10.1):

For the past 2 weeks, Aiden has tested 5 times/day. He has averaged 71 units of insulin lispro (Humalog) per day (0.8 units/kg/day), with 58% administered via basal insulin and 42% by bolus insulin. He has been using the HCL mode (auto mode) 64% of the time and calibrates his sensor 2.8 times/day. Aiden is consuming an average of 387 carbohydrates/day. Sensor glucose levels are in target range (70–180 mg/dL) 60% of the time, >180 mg/dL 37% of the time, and <70 mg/dL 2% of the time.

Aiden's sensor overlay shows a consistent rise in glucose levels after breakfast that remain elevated until midday (Figure 10.2). The glucose levels decrease after 12 P.M., with some possible hypoglycemia in the afternoon. Glucose levels elevate again around 5 P.M. but return to euglycemia (<180 mg/dL) in the later evening. The overnight period is consistently within range.

When looking at the daily report, it appears Aiden oscillates between low and high glucose levels in the afternoon (Figure 10.3). Hypoglycemia in the afternoon appears to occur on weekdays but not on the weekends. When asked about his afternoons during weekdays, Aiden explains that he eats a "small to medium" lunch and then has gym in the afternoon. They usually run and play basketball. He notices that his glucose levels drop pretty quickly during gym, and he feels shaky and tired after it is over. This is when he states he is the hungriest as well, so he usually eats a large "snack" of 80–150 g of carbohydrate throughout the hour after gym and school. He starts with juice or a sports drink and then adds chips, frozen

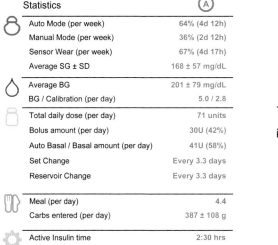
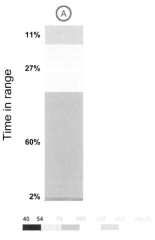

Statistics	Ⓐ
Auto Mode (per week)	64% (4d 12h)
Manual Mode (per week)	36% (2d 12h)
Sensor Wear (per week)	67% (4d 17h)
Average SG ± SD	168 ± 57 mg/dL
Average BG	201 ± 79 mg/dL
BG / Calibration (per day)	5.0 / 2.8
Total daily dose (per day)	71 units
Bolus amount (per day)	30U (42%)
Auto Basal / Basal amount (per day)	41U (58%)
Set Change	Every 3.3 days
Reservoir Change	Every 3.3 days
Meal (per day)	4.4
Carbs entered (per day)	387 ± 108 g
Active Insulin time	2:30 hrs

Figure 10.1. Patient device download: statistics.

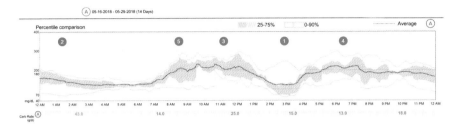

Figure 10.2. Percentile comparison report: May 16–May 29, 2018.

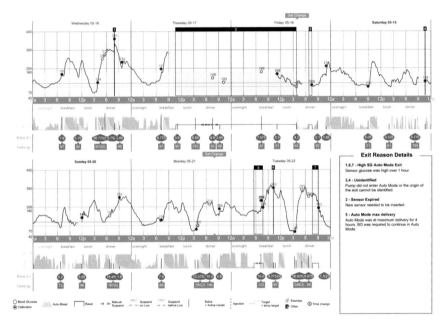

Figure 10.3. Daily report: May 16–May 22, 2018.

pizza, or a sandwich. He boluses for the carbohydrates after he is sure that his glucose levels have risen >70 mg/dL. He then eats dinner at home around 6 P.M.

Aiden's insulin dose settings have not been changed since his last clinic visit 3 months prior (Figure 10.4). His total daily basal dose is 31.2 units/day, his ICRs range from 1:13 (dinner) to 1:43 (overnight), and his sensitivities range from 90 to 125 mg/dL/unit.

Assessment and Plan

We discussed Aiden's HbA$_{1c}$ being above target of 7.5% and explained that our goal for today's visit was to make insulin dose adjustments and discuss ways that

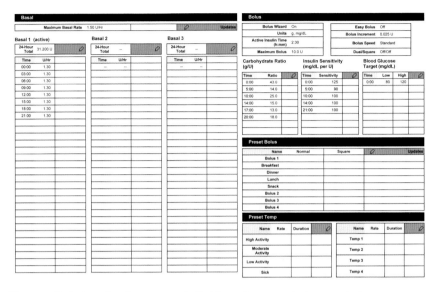

Figure 10.4. Insulin dose report. Settings have not changed since patient's last clinic visit.

Aiden can help increase his time in glycemic range of 70–180 mg/dL. We used the CARE model to discuss issues that are unique to automated insulin users.

Calculate. We reinforced with Aiden that in HCL, the only programmable settings used by the pump for insulin dosing are the ICR (for meal doses) and insulin action time (which will affect the amount of insulin-on-board subtracted for repeated correction boluses). We also noted, however, the importance of keeping his basal rates adjusted for the time he is in open-loop mode. Aiden is currently using the HCL mode 64% of the time. This means that the other 36% of the time, the pump is delivering his programmed basal rates.

Adjust. To optimize HCL mode, we suggested Aiden increase his breakfast ICR from 1:14 to 1:12 to contend with the midmorning hyperglycemia. We also increased his dinner ratio from 1:13 to 1:12 to help with evening hyperglycemia. The active insulin time (2.5 h) was not adjusted, because we found little evidence of correction doses being too strong or weak after previous correction doses. To optimize open-loop mode, we evaluated his basal rate settings. We identified a significant mismatch between his open-loop basal total (31.2 units) and his average daily basal using HCL (41 units). We therefore increased all of his basal rates by 0.25, increasing his 24-h basal total to 37.2 units. This is approximately a 20% increase to his basal rates and is closer to the HCL autobasal total of 41 units.

Revert. We reinforced education for Aiden that he should switch to open-loop mode if he requires a syringe injection of insulin or experiences illness in which temporary basal rates could better manage his glucose levels. We also suggested Aiden switch to open-loop mode if he has positive ketones in order to have better control over bolusing larger correction doses of insulin and no insulin suspensions.

Otherwise, Aiden should try to spend as much time as possible using the HCL mode. The low-threshold suspend feature should be activated each time the pump is switched to manual mode.

Educate.   The primary education focus was on treating hypoglycemia or pending hypoglycemia when using HCL. We showed Aiden how insulin had been suspended by the HCL for the period of time during gym class when glucose levels were falling rapidly. We also explained the importance of testing a glucose level, treating hypoglycemia with carbohydrates, and retesting 15 min later to ensure that glucose levels had risen. With HCL decreasing insulin before hypoglycemia events, we explained that Aiden may need only 10 g of carbohydrate for glucose levels >55 mg/dL. We also suggested that he could still eat a meal or more carbohydrates if he chose to, but it was better practice to wait until the glucose level was >70 mg/dL, and then to prebolus for the additional carbohydrates. The difficulty with this plan, however, is how hungry Aiden feels when glucose levels are falling rapidly, and he had just exercised for an hour.

In light of this, we also discussed using the temporary target feature for gym class. We explained that the temporary target feature of the HCL mode could be considered akin to a temporary basal rate, in that it reduced the amount of insulin for periods of high activity (by having the HCL system target a glucose level of 150 mg/dL instead of 120 mg/dL). We suggested he try this feature for a 2-h period of time, starting 30 min before gym and ending 30 min after gym. We discussed how this might reduce the rapid decrease in glucose levels during gym class and reduce the overtreatment of hypoglycemia afterward. Furthermore, Aiden could consider consuming 10–15 g carbohydrates in the middle of gym class to mitigate rapidly falling glucose levels before they occur.

To optimize time spent in HCL mode, we reinforced the importance of wearing the CGM sensor and responding to system alerts when they occur. Although Aiden stated that he did not like wearing the sensor, upon further discussion with him, it sounded like he was more irritated with the HCL alerts than with the actual sensor itself. We explained that with hyperglycemia, the system will exit HCL mode and require the user to restart HCL mode. We suggested that the insulin dose changes we made today, less carbohydrates for hypoglycemia treatment, and a temp target actually could prevent more hyperglycemia, thus reducing the burden of having to exit from HCL mode. He expressed relief at this proposal, as he stated the repeated exits were a cause of frustration. HCL can be considered a virtuous cycle, in which better glucose control leads to more time in HCL mode; and, likewise, HCL can lead to better glucose control. By motivating Aiden to continue to wear and respond to the CGM sensor, he may experience less frustration with the system overall.

Success with automated insulin relies both on strategic insulin dosing and reinforcing good diabetes self-management behaviors. Clinicians can help individuals using automated insulin by providing critical education on how the system works and how individuals can best work with the system. Systems that suspend with hypoglycemia, systems that provide HCL, and future systems will all work in fundamentally different ways, making targeted education essential for individual success.[5]

REFERENCES

1. Weisman A, Bai JW, Cardinez M, Kramer CK, Perkins BA. Effect of artificial pancreas systems on glycaemic control in patients with type 1 diabetes: a systematic review and meta-analysis of outpatient randomised controlled trials. *Lancet Diabetes Endocrinol* 2017;5:501–512

2. Garg SK, Weinzimer SA, Tamborlane WV, Buckingham BA, Bode BW, Bailey TS, Brazg RL, Ilany J, Slover RH, Anderson SM, Bergenstal RM, Grosman B, Roy A, Cordero TL, Shin J, Lee SW, Kaufman FR. Glucose outcomes with the in-home use of a hybrid closed-loop insulin delivery system in adolescents and adults with type 1 diabetes. *Diabetes Technol Ther* 2017;19(3):155–163

3. Berget C, Messer LH, Pyle L, Westfall E, Forlenza GP, Driscoll KA. Real-world use of hybrid closed-loop therapy in pediatric patients with type 1 diabetes [abstract]. *Diabetes* 2018;67(Suppl. 1)

4. Messer LH, Forlenza GP, Sherr JL, Wadwa RP, Buckingham BA, Weinzimer SA, Maahs DM, Slover RH. Optimizing hybrid closed-loop therapy in adolescents and emerging adults using the MiniMed 670G system. *Diabetes Care* 2018;41:789–796

5. Messer LH, Forlenza GP, Wadwa RP, Weinzimer SA, Sherr JL, Hood KK, Buckingham BA, Slover RH, Maahs DM: The dawn of automated insulin delivery: A new clinical framework to conceptualize insulin administration. *Pediatr Diabetes* 2018;19:14–17

6. American Diabetes Associates. Glycemic targets: standards of medical care in diabetes, 2018. *Diabetes Care* 2018;41:S55–S64

Chapter 11

Using Hybrid Closed-Loop Technology to Minimize Hypoglycemia in Type 1 Diabetes while Maintaining Excellent Diabetes Control

Elizabeth A. Doyle, DNP, APRN, CDE, BC-ADM,[1] and Beatrice C. Lupsa, MD[2]

INTRODUCTION

Since the results of the Diabetes Control and Complications Trial (DCCT) were released in 1993,[1] the goal of management in type 1 diabetes (T1D) has been to try to get the best diabetes control possible, with the hope of eliminating or at least minimizing long-term microvascular complications of the disease. Indeed, the American Diabetes Association, in its practice guidelines, suggests that a reasonable HbA_{1c} (A1C) goal for most nonpregnant adults with diabetes should be <7%.[2] For many patients, however, attempting to achieve this level of metabolic control has come at the cost of significant hypoglycemia, including in the DCCT study itself, where the incidence of severe hypoglycemia was 62 events per 100 patient years in the intensively treated cohort, who were able to achieve a mean A1C of 7.2%.[1]

Thankfully, diabetes technology has advanced over the years, and later multicenter studies have demonstrated that with improved technology the incidence of severe hypoglycemia can be decreased. For example, in a more recent study sponsored by the JDRF in which patients used insulin pumps and continuous subcutaneous glucose monitors, the adult subjects had an A1C of 7.1%, with a severe hypoglycemic rate of 20 events per 100 patient years.[3]

Technology has continued to advance, and in the fall of 2016, a hybrid closed-loop (HCL) system, manufactured by Medtronic MiniMed, was approved by the U.S. Food and Drug Administration (FDA). With this system, a subcutaneous insulin pump automatically delivers interprandial insulin based on data from a continuous glucose sensor [targeting a sensor glucose (SG) level of 120 mg/dL], and the user delivers premeal bolus doses based on the planned carbohydrate content in the meal.[4] Results of a relatively short (3-month) outpatient multicenter study demonstrated that adult subjects were able to achieve excellent diabetes control (mean A1C of 6.8%) with 0.0 severe hypoglycemic events per 100 patient years.[4,5] Although of a short duration, this study does suggest that with

[1]Assistant Professor, Yale School of Nursing, West Haven, CT; APRN/CDE, Yale Pediatric Endocrinology, Yale New Haven Hospital, New Haven, CT. [2]Assistant Professor of Medicine, Endocrinology, Yale School of Medicine, New Haven, CT.

the use of newer diabetes technologies, the ability to achieve excellent diabetes control while minimizing significant hypoglycemia indeed might be possible. The following case illustrates this fact and describes a 57-year-old man with T1D who has successfully used the HCL system in an outpatient setting.

CASE STUDY

Chief Complaint, History of Present Illness and Past Medical History

Bob was a 57-year-old man with a >35-year history of T1D, treated with basal-bolus multiple daily injections, who was referred to our office to learn about different diabetes technologies because of a history of severe hypoglycemia, with hypoglycemic unawareness. He reported having many minor hypoglycemic events and that he no longer experienced any adrenergic symptoms when his blood glucose (BG) levels were low. Bob did report "feeling different" when his BG levels were between 20 and 50 mg/dL. Within the past few years, he had experienced two severe hypoglycemic events, resulting in an unconscious state and necessitating treatment by emergency personnel.

Past Medical History

Bob's past medical history was significant for T1D for >35 years. He reported that his diabetes had been well controlled for at least the past 5 years, with A1C measurements always <6–7%. Since diagnosis, he had been treated with insulin injections, and he previously had not had any interest in using an insulin pump. As for microvascular complications, he had stable proliferative retinopathy, and chronic kidney disease (most recent eGFR was 43 ml/min/1.73m² and creatinine was 1.72 mg/dL). He denied any neuropathic symptoms. His additional comorbidities included well-managed hypertension and hyperlipidemia and depression and anxiety.

Current Diabetes Therapy

His insulin regimen consisted of 40 units of glargine daily. He took lispro before each of three main meals: 5 units for breakfast, 5 units for lunch, and 15 units for dinner. Bob additionally corrected his BG with lispro when it was >120 mg/dL, using a sensitivity factor of 1 unit of lispro insulin per 15 mg/dL. He admitted to taking many additional injections of lispro throughout the day if his BG was higher than his target glucose level, and the duration between lispro injections occasionally was <2 h.

Bob knew how to count carbohydrates, although did not use a ratio at meals, as he reported eating a consistent diet, to reduce glucose variations. If he ate something out of the ordinary, he would check his BG 2 h after the meal and take additional lispro insulin to bring it to target. At his initial visit, his weight was 97 kg (BMI = 33.5 kg/m²), which he reported was typical for him.

As for exercise, his full-time work was typically sedentary, but he walked his dogs 2 miles every evening with his wife.

Bob kept detailed written records, revealing that he checked his BG on average 10–11 times/day over the past few weeks, with a mean of 129.5 mg/dL and a range of 59–245 mg/dL. He reported treating at least one minor low BG level (either discovered when he checked his BG or because he had symptoms) every day. Bob checked his sugar at least twice during the night, reporting "not sleeping well anyhow." Only 7% of his routine readings were <70 mg/dL, although he reported that he typically did not have any obvious hypoglycemic symptoms unless the level was <50 mg/dL. He denied having any severe hypoglycemic events in the past month. Bob used Skittles to treat his low BG levels—as he has had the best success with this—and they were easy to carry in his pocket.

Current Labs

His HbA_{1c} at his initial visit was 6.2%. His lipid levels were at goal (LDL = 75 mg/dL). His measurements of kidney function were reportedly stable with an eGFR of 43 ml/min/1.73m², and creatinine of 1.72 mg/dL. All his other labs, including thyroid function tests and a comprehensive metabolic panel were otherwise within normal limits.

Assessment

Bob was a 57-year-old with a long-standing history of T1D, complicated by hypoglycemic unawareness, stable proliferative retinopathy, and stable chronic kidney disease. Although he had an A1C well below the goal for treatment, he had frequent, daily minor hypoglycemic events and a history of severe hypoglycemia. He admits to taking repeated correction doses of lispro by injection, which likely lead to insulin stacking and that may have contributed to his frequent hypoglycemia. He was somewhat anxious about his glucose levels, wanting them to be "perfect."

Management Plan

Our advanced practical registered nurse (APRN)/certified diabetes educator (CDE) had a long discussion with Bob about his diabetes treatment, particularly about the risks of hypoglycemia and hypoglycemic unawareness. He admitted that he "liked to feel low," that "it gave him a sense of euphoria," and that he "felt awful" if his BG was >180 mg/dL. The APRN/CDE again reiterated the risks of hypoglycemia, particularly given his long duration of T1D and other comorbidities. He agreed to try to minimize these events. He and his wife were taught how to use glucagon, and this was prescribed for him.

The APRN/CDE also discussed different technology available, which potentially could help him to minimize the hypoglycemia events he was experiencing. The current continuous glucose monitors (CGMs) that were available at the time were reviewed, and their pros and cons were discussed. All of the insulin pumps available were also discussed at length. In the end, Bob wanted to pursue the Medtronic 630G insulin pump, with an Enlite Sensor, knowing that he would be able to upgrade to the Medtronic HCL 670G system when it was available. The 630G has a "suspend on low" feature, in which the pump will suspend delivery for 2 h if the SG goes below the low limit that is set by the user. The hope was that this feature might decrease some of the hypoglycemia he was experiencing, while he awaited his transition to the HCL 670G system.

Follow-Up: Medtronic 630G with Enlite Sensor

Bob received our standard educational program for new pump patients and transitioned easily to the insulin pump. His initial pump doses were based on 80% of his injection total daily dose (TDD); however, he wound up taking a higher TDD on pump compared with his "usual" doses on injection (because he never provided us with the total amount he took for correction doses each day, his doses were based on his typical injection doses with meals and his basal insulin).

Table 11.1 gives some of the data collected at the visits. Bob initially struggled with "trusting the system," questioning whether or not it was turning off his basal rate appropriately. In fact, he decreased his "suspend on low" value from 80 mg/dL, which we had suggested (given his hypoglycemic unawareness) to 65 mg/dL on his own, so that the basal insulin delivery would suspend less frequently. Figure 11.1 shows some of the data downloaded through the CareLink software. This graph includes his insulin, CGM, and BG data after he had been on the pump and sensor for 12 months. At this time his basal rates were as follows:

12 A.M.	1.15 unit/h
3 A.M.	1.20 unit/h
10 A.M.	1.15 unit/h
3 P.M.	1.25 unit/h
9 P.M.	1.3 unit/h

His ICRs were as follows:

12 A.M.	10 g
6 A.M.	6 g
11 A.M.	7 g
3 P.M.	6 g
9:30 P.M.	8 g

His sensitivity was set at 1 unit per 15 mg/dL. Although his diabetes control remained excellent based on his A1C (see Table 11.1), as shown in Figure 11.1, he was taking many small bolus doses throughout the day (similar to what he did on injections), and likely still was "stacking" his insulin doses, trying to keep his BG constantly <120 mg/dL.

Bob admitted that he was still anxious about his BG levels remaining in range, but he was finding it easier to get them in range with the insulin pump. Of concern

Table 11.1. Data from Clinic Visits

	11/2016 Initial Visit	4/2017 3 mos 630G	1/2018 12 mos 630G	2/2018 1 mos 670G	5/2018 4 mos 670G
Weight (kg)	97.07	94.8	96.6	93.4	93
BMI	33.5	32.73	33.36	32.26	32.11
A1C (%)	6.2	5.9	6.0	—	6.3
TDD (units)	65 + corrections	67.5	81.6	74	78
% basal		37	36	39	31
# BG/per day	10.4	6.0	11.8	12.9	8.6

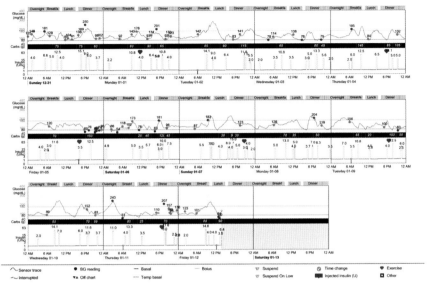

Figure 11.1. CGM, BG, and insulin doses data after 12 months of 630G pump and CGM use.

to his caregivers, during the 12 days that were downloaded from his pump at the follow-up visit (displayed in Figure 11.1), he had eight episodes where his SG was <60 mg/dL. Bob, however, thought that he was doing fantastic. He also continued to check his BG many times per day (see data in Table 11.1), and continued to eat Skittles whenever his sensor alarmed that he was <65 mg/dL. Thankfully, he did not experience any severe hypoglycemia. The APRN/CDE again expressed her concern about the hypoglycemia. The potential acute dangers of hypoglycemia related to operating a motor vehicle were discussed at length, although Bob assured the APRN/CDE that he made sure his SG was >90 mg/dL when he was driving.

Follow-Up: Medtronic HCL 670G

Bob transitioned from the 630G to the HCL 670G with ease. He returned to our office 1–4 months after beginning the 670G, and the APRN/CDE saw such a change in him personally. He was far less anxious and had "surrendered taking care of his BG levels to the pump." He remained diligent about his carbohydrate bolus doses, but he relied on the system to correct his BG between meals. He reported that he was still not sleeping through the night, but he was sleeping better than he had in years.

Figure 11.2 shows the data provided by the CareLink software at his 4-month visit. The APRN/CDE reviewed the graph in detail with Bob. The blue in the graph and the blue column A represents the current data. The APRN/CDE had Bob first look at the statistics in the right-hand column (marked with #1). He had remained in auto mode 92% of the time and had worn a sensor 94% of the previous

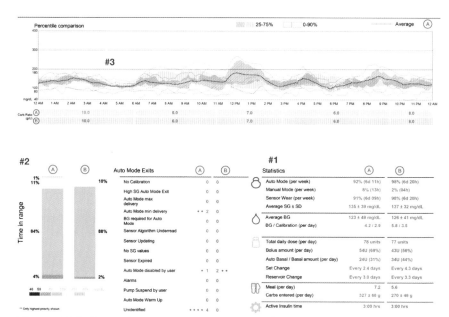

Figure 11.2. Data after 4 months on the 670G HCL.

2 weeks. He was praised for this excellent adherence to sensor wear. His average SG was 135 mg/dL with a standard deviation of only 39, representing little variability. The APRN/CDE examined the data on the left-hand side (marked with a #2) of the printout and showed him that his SG was within the target range 86% of the time. More important, only 2% of his SG were between 50 and 70 mg/dL and he did not experience any SG <50 mg/dL. His A1C at this visit was 6.3%, demonstrating persistent excellent diabetes control, despite the elimination of the majority of the hypoglycemia he previously was experiencing. Bob was quite surprised, but also extremely happy about this, as he had expected his A1C to be much higher because he thought his SGs were higher on the 670G system than on the 630G. Last, the APRN/CDE reviewed the SG graph (image #3 on Figure 11.2) with Bob, and pointed out that his SG did increase after his midday meal, so it was suggested that he change his 11 A.M. ICR from 7 to 6 g. The plan was for him to follow up in 3 months.

DISCUSSION

Attempting to achieve tight metabolic control in patients with T1D, per treatment guidelines from the American Diabetes Association,[2] can impose an increased risk of both minor and severe hypoglycemia. Additionally, despite education to the contrary, patients might be tempted to take frequent correction doses of fast-acting insulin to maintain glucose levels as close to the normal range as possible, which can further increase this risk of hypoglycemia. Diabetes technology is advancing at a rapid pace, and the combination of insulin pumps and CGMs can reduce the risk of hypoglycemia, while also improving overall glycemic control. This case serves as an example of how hypoglycemia can be nearly eliminated and excellent control can be maintained using the HCL 670G system. Although hypoglycemia persisted even with the use of CGM and an insulin pump with a suspend on low feature, the incidence of minor hypoglycemia was greatly reduced with use of the HCL 670G system. Clinicians should consider using this system in patients striving to achieve excellent metabolic control who are struggling with hypoglycemia.

REFERENCES

1. The Diabetes Control and Complications Trial Research Group. The effect of intensive treatment of diabetes on the development and progression of long-term complications in insulin-dependent diabetes mellitus. *N Engl J Med* 1993;329:977–986

2. American Diabetes Association. Glycemic targets: Standards of medical care in diabetes, 2018. *Diabetes Care* 2018;41(Suppl. 1):S55–S64

3. Juvenile Diabetes Research Foundation Continuous Glucose Monitoring Study Group; Tamborlane WV, Beck RW, Bode BW, Buckingham B, et al. Continuous glucose monitoring and intensive treatment of type 1 diabetes. *N Engl J Med* 2008;359:1464–1476

4. Bergenstal RM, Garg S, Weinzimer SA, et al. Safety of a hybrid closed-loop insulin delivery system in patients with type 1 diabetes. *JAMA* 2016;316:1407–1408

5. Garg, SK, Weinzimer, SA, Tamborlane, WV, et al. Glucose outcomes with the in-home use of a hybrid closed-loop insulin delivery system in adolescents and adults with type 1 diabetes. *Diabetes Technol Therap* 2017;19(3):155–163

Chapter 1
My 65 Years with Type 1 Diabetes

Robert H. Eckel, MD[1]

I don't recall what came first when I was 5 years old: being pushed down the steps by Ann Palmer, a daughter of one of my mother's friends, and landing on my head or being hospitalized at Cincinnati Children's Hospital with new onset type 1 diabetes (T1D) in February 1953 (Figure 1.1). Whichever came first that month, they were close enough to one another temporally that it has made me wonder whether the head injury perhaps precipitated the T1D. Could this be another environmental influence for new onset T1D? But I do remember a bout of mumps in the fall of 1952 when I was 4 years old, a more likely precursor to T1D, I think. Isn't it amazing that here we are 65 years later and we still have very little idea of what takes the genetically susceptible individual and brings on this life of T1D?

My remembrance of the initial hospital experience is nothing but a nightmare. Not only was I so sick and vomiting my guts out but also so frightened. What was this needle in my arm connected to a bag of water all about, all those urine samples I had to collect, and the finger-sticks with lancets as big as spears. Then they wouldn't let my mother stay. Can you believe this now? What was happening to me anyway, and there were so many tears, I'll never forget. After 3–4 days, I was homeward bound using Clinitest tablets with the following recipe: 5 drops urine plus 10 drops H_2O to evaluate levels of glycemia, ketone tabs for urine ketones, and of course insulin, ugh a shot, and every day. How long was this going to last anyway? I have no recollection of which insulin this was, but there weren't many options back then, so presumably NPH insulin or Lente? I remember so well that urine testing was a guess in the dark. Blue color meant no urine glucose and orange color meant tons of glucose in the urine, but then why was I hypoglycemic 30 min later?

The setting of my new onset T1D was not convenient. My father had already died when I was 10 months of age and my mother was working two jobs, as a 5th-grade school teacher and a church organist, to make ends meet for my older brother Ed and me. Moreover, I was in kindergarten at the time and arrangements for my care at home were needed with my mother and brother both at their respective schools; thank goodness for Mrs. Bonhaus. My diabetes care was in the

[1]Professor of Medicine, Division of Endocrinology, Metabolism and Diabetes, Division of Cardiology; Professor of Physiology and Biophysics, Charles A. Boettcher II Chair in Atherosclerosis; Vice Chancellor for Research, Interim, University of Colorado Denver Anschutz Medical Campus; Director Lipid Clinic, University of Colorado Hospital, Aurora, CO.

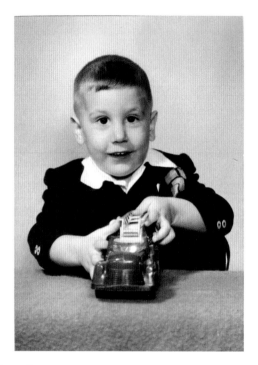

Figure 1.1. Robert Eckel, 5 years old.

hands of Dr. Clare Rittershofer, a pediatric diabetologist at Cincinnati Children's Hospital, who patterned his care of children after that of Dr. Harvey Knowles at the University of Cincinnati. Dr. Knowles was an early proponent of less rigorous approaches to glycemic control in adults and children with T1D and that suited my mother quite well in terms of avoiding hypoglycemia, an outcome that was occurring much more frequently than she liked at the time. To prevent episodes of severe hypoglycemia, Dr. Rittershofer put me on once-a-day pig globin insulin, which my mother injected every morning.

Now, my recollections of those early days of injections: Every morning, my mother would boil glass syringes and metal needles, that must have been gauge 21, and at times, this recipient unwelcomingly noted this large needle size. After a couple of years, my brother learned to substitute for my mom and then soon thereafter I would become both capable and willing. Then, there was changing the syringe or needle. For the syringe, it was done so only after it fell to the floor and broke, and with the needle, it was changed when pain occurred daily for a few days in a row on injection. Of course, my dose remained constant despite variable blue to orange Clinitest results. Then, I had one more hospitalization at Children's Hospital for diabetic ketoacidosis at age 7, but until the present, I experienced no further admissions for diabetes-related issues. Because of the complexities of diabetes management in those days, the only adventures out of the home until I was a teenager were to my grandparents in Van Wet, Ohio, and they became skilled at doing the glass needle thing.

Growing up with T1D affected my life. No Cub Scout or Boy Scout camping trips, and no overnight stays with friends, at least until plastic syringes became available and this wasn't until my high school years. However, because my mother wanted to avoid severe hypoglycemic events at all cost, I ate like any other normal kid. Thinking back, I had no restrictions, including simple or complex carbohydrates or in total or saturated fat. And I remember many trips walking to the nearby United Dairy Farmers for a chocolate malt with Mrs. Graf, my favorite babysitter. I must have had an HbA_{1c} of 12% in those days.

I did play sports, including knothole baseball, as a youngster, and pick-up football and church league basketball and softball throughout college and medical school, but growing up, I was small for my age and not good enough to make school teams. Then there were the lows that were sports related. My knothole baseball team was pretty good, and I was one of their two pitchers. We had a big game against one of our tougher opponents and I was on the mound. The strike zone seemed elusive, and then I realized it in part was because my vision was blurry. I remember stumbling and then being assisted by my brother and coach on the mound with a big glass of orange juice to follow. The game was halted for ~10 min and I resumed my role as the pitcher. But all I remember then was that I wasn't much better than before my hypoglycemic event.

Then I had another memorable hypoglycemic event during 6th grade of elementary school. I grew up in an all-white community, and such was the population of my elementary school. To gather some view of what the rest of the world was like, a trip was made downtown to an all-black school. I remember being a bit scared and standing in the lunchroom line. With details lacking, I had vomited and was confused, a sight that brought much attention, but was tomato soup the best remedy? Overall, these kinds of experiences were embarrassing, but in their absence, I recall feeling sorry for myself. Here I was, lacking a father, having T1D, and living a restricted life. Don't misinterpret this; I really did okay, it was just these occasional bouts of self-pity.

During junior high school, in those days that was grades 7–9, I found myself in a new school with some new kids, and I became somewhat nerdy. One example was the Arthur Ant Club, a small group of other nerdy guys who bonded to preserve the existence of small red-brown ants. So, how does this relate to T1D? It doesn't, but I found friends like me who accepted me without equivocation. Remember, I was small for my age and not good enough to make school teams. In junior high school as in elementary school, my mother always saw to it that the school and my teachers knew I had "brittle diabetes" and could demonstrate signs of hypoglycemia. Overall, my recollection of other T1D-related issues during these three years are minimal, but in 9th grade, I remember thinking girls were beginning to seem more interesting and particularly the good-looking ones. In fact, there was one, Sharon Cress, who caught my eye, but she seemed to be preoccupied and hanging out with another guy. Nevertheless, I had my eye on her and ultimately asked her to go on a church hayride. Of course, being 14 years old, I had to depend on my mother to pick her up and again, after the hayride, to pick us up and take her home. I'm sure my diabetes didn't come up on that first date, but it would. Initially, she had no feelings for me and her parents were restrictive.

Dates then were rare, but would become more frequent as years went by, and 8 years later, she would become my bride.

I began to play golf in high school but even today, I have a handicap that goes beyond the usual. I remember when my curiosity about the biology of T1D ensued, perhaps during my first year in medical school, I remember seeing an article by Dr. Arlen Rosenbloom from the University of Florida that demonstrated the impact of poorly controlled T1D during growth and development. These flexion contractures have impaired that straight left arm needed to consistently hit golf balls straight (Figure 1.2). Yes, this is an excuse but a good one for a handicap of 25 plus for a game I truly enjoy. I often walk, and that is part of living a diabetes-healthy lifestyle that's so important for all of us!

I started college at the University of Cincinnati (UC) immediately following high school. This was really my only choice because of convenience and cost. UC was an urban university at that time, and my mother and I lived within the city limits, so tuition was a great deal. Moreover, I was honored to receive a partial tuition savings by playing trombone in the college band— marching, basketball, and spring band. This required lots of practices, but I loved sports and UC had good football and great basketball teams in those years. I remember well my first band roadtrip to Memphis that fall. I had never had any alcoholic beverages in the past, I grew up in an alcohol-free home as did Sharon, but here I was away from home and nobody was watching. I got stone drunk and vomited throughout the night, and remember I had no glucose monitoring and short-acting insulin to correct an unknown but likely extremely high blood glucose level.

Apparently, my mother had already informed the band director, Dr. Hornyak, that I had T1D. He was quite concerned but didn't know quite what to do. Although I should have gone to the emergency room (ER), I somehow got through the day and marched with the band. From that point forward, I was the sober driver. The band included three other guys from my high school, and after most practices, a bar was the next stop, despite being late and on week nights. Remembering those nights and their level of sobriety, despite my T1D, for the most part, it was good that I often was one of the drivers.

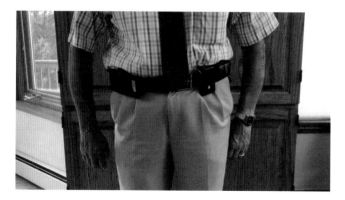

Figure 1.2. Flexion contractures.

During my last 2 years of high school and between my first year and sophomore year at UC, I worked on tennis courts for the City of Cincinnati. The first 2 years were hard work preparing clay courts for the evening visitors. This involved wetting down the courts, and then when they were somewhat dry, rolling them with a water-filled rotor and placing lines, soon to be eliminated once the evening tennis players arrived. I always made sure that sugar-containing beverages were within reach, and I clearly have survived to tell about it. During the last year of this summer work, a member of the School of Medicine faculty approached me, Dr. John Loper, and asked about my intentions. I told him that I wanted to go to medical school, and he offered me a part-time job washing dishes in his bacteriology laboratory. After 3 years working ~15 h a week, I was purifying an enzyme and doing chromatography.

The summer after completing my undergraduate education, with a major in bacteriology, Sharon and I married. I then entered medical school at the University of Cincinnati College of Medicine, again the only choice given that Sharon had a teaching job in Cincinnati and a tuition that didn't break the bank but was still enough to teach us financial management.

Now newly married, with limited resources and minimal furnishings, my own studying and my wife's making lesson plans until late at night created an entirely new agenda. As for many preceding years, a bedtime snack was routine to avoid nocturnal hypoglycemia and Sharon's cooking was outstanding. Over 4 years, I added another 12–15 lb. Then, there was pathology class during the second year. Despite biannual visits to an ophthalmologist while I was a child and a teenager, I really accepted this with little insight into why it was necessary. Now, the complications of T1D were front and center. Learning that my life expectancy would be shortened and perhaps so much so that my ability to see my children grow up and for my career in medicine be long lasting led to immediate concern. Moreover, I remember one of my instructors asking me why I wanted to be a physician with this expected scenario. Despite limited extra funds, Sharon and I anxiously sought term insurance policies that proved both costly but necessary. Then, the third year hit with a tough overnight call schedule for students including some rotations every other to every third night. We learned a lot of medicine, but the stress led to times of nausea after a late-night snack, likely unnecessary as some "lows" needed more immediate attention, mostly caused by yours truly. Remember, I did not have any glycemic determinants other than Clinitest and I don't recall that I ever took these with me to the hospital.

During late in my junior year of medical school, I decide that internal medicine would be the best choice to follow. My mother frequently told me of how good my father, a family physician, was in making correct diagnoses. Thus, internal medicine in those days was just that, and it provided much more in-depth detail than family medicine. To the disappointment to my mother, I would be leaving Cincinnati to train in Madison at the University of Wisconsin (UW) Hospitals. This was far from my first choice, but in retrospect, it proved beneficial in that it represented a somewhat less demanding schedule than many other house-staff training programs and that fit my T1D better.

Our family then began, with Kimberly being born 3 weeks after our arrival, and Kristin 2 years later. Memories of the impact of T1D on my life in general are few; however, I do remember a drive home from picking strawberries one hot

Sunday afternoon my mother-in-law and wife were screaming as my driving became erratic—and I was quite low. Thankfully, we arrived home safely and after some carbohydrate-containing beverage, Jeff Field and I played tennis. Sharon could not believe that my blood glucose could be so low and then I could go exercise.

Halfway through my house-staff training program, I had an experience that forever would change my career path. While rotating through a private hospital, where the best of private internists were our mentors, I realized that internal medicine was more than making a diagnosis and treating patients, and I became increasingly curious as to why people became ill and why the response to therapies was so inconsistent. With an undergraduate degree in bacteriology and an outstanding infectious disease faculty at UW, an infectious disease fellowship seemed natural. Having T1D, however, and the uncertainty as to whether the research experience would land me in academic medicine, I thought that endocrinology and metabolism made more sense. I didn't want to study my own disease but being preoccupied with my own complications of diabetes and the cholesterol–heart disease story momentum, I thought a fellowship focused on the interaction between lipids/lipoproteins, diabetes, and cardiovascular disease (CVD) would be my best choice. I applied to the University of Texas–Southwestern in Dallas, the University of California–San Francisco (UCSF), and the University of Washington, but I did not visit Dallas; Sharon didn't want to live in Texas. These were all metabolic-research intensive programs in this area of interest, and I would have been honored to be a fellow at any one of them. After visiting UCSF and University of Washington, whereat I was very conversant about how my T1D influenced my choice of fellowships, I became worried in late spring 1975 that I had not heard back from either UCSF or the University of Washington. I soon found out the UCSF didn't want me, but then in May, I was paged and notified that Dr. Ed Bierman from Seattle was on the phone. Although not known to me at the time, the rest of my academic and personal life with T1D was going to begin in Seattle.

I have trouble remembering the transition from globin to Lente insulin but believe it was during my residency in Madison. What I do remember well was at the terminus of my third year as a medical resident, and just following my mother's death from ALS (amyotrophic lateral sclerosis), I was making rounds on the cardiology service at the University of Wisconsin Hospital, and students and the intern on the service noticed I was "out to lunch" and making no sense in regard to current or historic information related to patient care. Somehow, someone obtained blood, and my glucose was 19 mg/dL. After orange juice, recovery was rapid; however, these episodes of severe hypoglycemia needing assistance are all memorable over the many years of this life called T1D.

With the help of my father-in-law, we moved ourselves to Seattle and an entirely new life began. We rented a house; I started on the endocrine consult service, in the clinic and in the lab. In those days, the American Board of Internal Medicine requirements for subspecialty certification were much less stringent than today. Although I was intent on not studying my own disease, I worked closely with Dr. Bierman on a clinical project that examined the relationship between plasma lipids, lipoproteins, and apolipoproteins to microvascular complications of T1D. In the laboratory, I worked under the mentorship of Dr. Wilfred Fujimoto and studied why fibroblasts obtained from patients with T2D had a reduced life span versus age-matched control subjects without diabetes. During the first 6 months, I became somewhat depressed about how slow research progressed. But then, using the tissue culture systems I learned in Dr. Fujimoto's lab and the lipoprotein lipase (LPL) assay from Dr. John Brunzell's lab, my LPL-focused career that continues today began.

Three additional memories related to this period of my life are worth noting, although there are many more, and two relate to T1D. The first is another one of those severe hypoglycemic events. While sitting in my very small office, and in no way isolated with three other fellow desks, I felt quite nauseated and became increasingly confused. Coincidentally, Dr. Bierman had stopped by, and the next thing I remember is being in the ER. Perhaps what makes this one so memorable is that the ER resident was Dr. George King, an esteemed physician scientist diabetologist at the Joslin Clinic. Every time I'm with George, this experience is relived.

The second is the birth of home blood glucose testing, initially with strips. Keep in mind now, I'd had T1D for 25 years and for the first time I could approximate my blood glucose by color matching with strips. The strips were expensive, and I could cut them into fourths and still be in the ballpark. Noting the importance of the postprandial period in overall glycemia, but no hemoglobin A_{1c} in those days, mealtime bolus insulin would ultimately follow. And there were no restroom visits when not at home, right through the shirt using the needle multiple times until dullness and pain ensued. Finally, I remember the many lessons of parenting, which at times were difficult lessons to learn. Within a year of Sharon's salvation, and despite my scientific mind-set, I became a born-again believer in the Lord Jesus Christ, an act of faith by God's grace that has permanently changed my life.

Following three wonderful years as an endocrine fellow at the University of Washington, I wondered, "now what?" I was fortunate to have five job opportunities and chose to come to the University of Colorado Medical School. The decision was based mostly on my division chair, Dr. Jerrold Olefsky. For a new tenure-track physician scientist, an active bench and clinical research was expected, and Jerry had both. But what I didn't know at the time I accepted the position is that he wanted me to have a First Award submitted 4 months before my arrival. Although I thought that I had submitted a First Award, by mistake, it was an R01, and to my surprise and Jerry's too, it was funded, and my career was jump-started. Over my nearly 40 years at the University of Colorado, so much has changed, including three more children, Elisabeth, Peter, and Clark, a move from the suburbs to the mountains, Sharon's death to breast cancer, 1.5 years as a single parent, my subsequent marriage to Margaret Scarborough, and then seeing child by child go on with their lives and be successful in their separate career paths. Now back to T1D.

Upon arrival to Denver, finger-stick glucose monitoring continued with sliced sticks, but soon thereafter, a meter was part of my armamentarium and assessment of more long-term glucose control began using A1C, was now approved by the U.S. Food and Drug Administration. I don't remember my first A1C, but I think it was somewhere in the low to mid 8.0%. Then in the late 1980s and early 1990s, when the Diabetes Control and Complications Trial data started to surface,[1] I finally was convinced that I needed pay more attention to my glycemic management. The overall environment I had in Seattle was that until proven otherwise, the avoidance of hypoglycemia was more important than maintaining tight control of glycemia. Many academic arguments would follow, but in 1988, major changes in lifestyle and improvement in glycemic control would ensue that have lasted.

For the first time, dietary simple sugars and saturated fat became important to limit. Although I had been seen by retina specialists when in Madison and Seattle, visits became regular. As glycemic control improved to A1Cs of ~7.0% my vision failed and my eye disease advanced from pre-proliferative to proliferative on the left and macular edema on the right. After panretinal laser treatment on the left and focal treatment on the right, my night vision began to fail and, ultimately, become so bad that in 2017 my license would be restricted to daytime only. In the mid-1990s, I traded in multiple daily injections for insulin infusion pump therapy and several years later continuous glucose monitoring (CGM) would begin. And another first, I went to see a diabetologist rather than myself, and I thank Dr. Michael McDermott for his remarkable and endless wisdom and care. I'm currently using the new Medtronic 670G and learning its many complex ways. This transition was a result of an increasing number of severe hypoglycemic events, one while in a swimming pool in Italy in 2017 that could have been fatal. All these events required assistance from others, many with glucagon administered by Margaret, and several with emergency calls.

Yes, I've had some other consequences of long-standing T1D, hypertension, including peripheral sensory neuropathy (numbness) and periodic angina with a coronary calcium score of over 3,000. The hypertension likely showed its ugly head when I was a medical student. I remember several systolic pressures in the 160 mm/Hg range under hospital-stressful situations; however, the first time an antihypertensive, diltiazem, was prescribed was after my first bout of angina driving home during a snowstorm in 1984. I reported this to no one. Then I had another bout of recurrent chest pain during an altitude climb, and a recently elevated coronary calcium score, with a coronary catherization to follow. My coronaries were not clean, but obstruction was not evident, so presumably my angina was microvascular. Of interest, despite my desire not to study my own disease (better called a life), with Merck support, I began a study of coronary heart disease in patients with T1D by obtaining coronary calcium scores using a new and popular technique, electron beam computerized tomography. Of course, I participated in my own study. Around this time, lisinopril would be added to my blood pressure regimen and my systolic pressure was now ~130 mm/Hg. Not mentioned was that while I was a resident and increasing data to support antiplatelet therapy to prevent CVD events, I began 325 mg of aspirin on Monday, Wednesday, and Friday that continues today.

Mild hypoglycemia in the workplace and beyond over the years has not been rare but easily managed. One such event, however, had unfortunate consequences. Just 5 min before a lecture in Denison Auditorium on the old School of Medicine campus, and before CGM was on board, I felt low and asked my administrative assistant to get me a soda. This followed promptly and per usual I was fine within 10 min. At some time subsequent to this event, not remembering the interval, I was sent a notice from the State of Colorado Medical Examiner's Office that a complaint had been issued by an outside party that my hypoglycemic events affected my performance as a clinical endocrinologist and put my patients at risk. What I would then discover was that this party was a friend of that same administrative assistant who had been fired months earlier for a substandard job performance. After meeting with an attorney at the CU campus and getting letters of reference from several colleagues, I was "acquitted" and deemed appropriate to continue as a clinician.

In summary, I've had T1D now for 65 years and feel fortunate to be alive. Despite aging and related stiffness, some *degenerative joint disease*, and a related right-knee replacement, I feel wonderful. My diet is heart healthy, I exercise 35–40 min 6 days/week with balanced routine of aerobic and resistance training, my A1C is 6.5% on an insulin dose of ~45 units daily. I thank my late wife Sharon, my five children, all my physicians, and particularly Margaret for their support over these many years (Figures 1.3–1.6). Moreover, the many advances in T1D-related science and medicine have given me a life far beyond that predicted by my pathology professor in 1970.

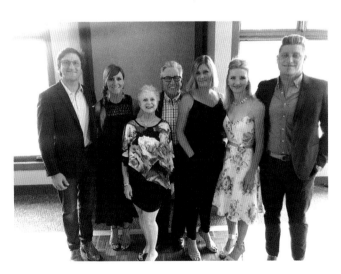

Figure 1.3. The Eckel family: Peter, Kristin, Margaret, Bob, Kimberly, Elisabeth, and Clark.

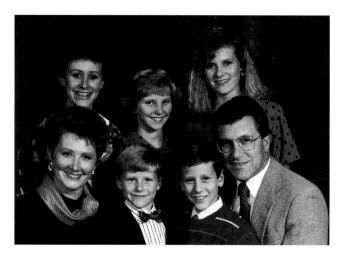

Figure 1.4. The Eckel family. Back row: Kristin, Elisabeth, and Kimberly. Front row: Sharon, Clark, Peter, and Bob.

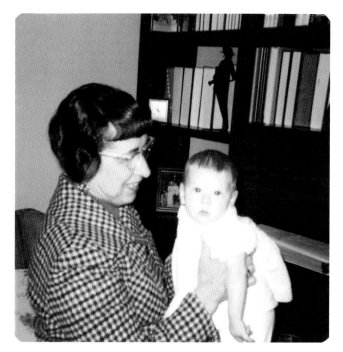

Figure 1.5. Ruth Eckel and Kimberly.

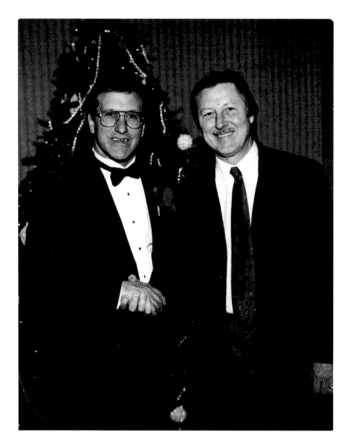

Figure 1.6. Bob and brother Ed.

REFERENCES

1. The Diabetes Control and Complications Trial Research Group. The effect of intensive therapy of diabetes on the development and progression of long-term complications in insulin-dependent diabetes mellitus. *N Engl J Med* 1993;329:977–986

Chapter 2
Resilience: How Technology Has Helped Me Flourish with Type 1 Diabetes

Elizabeth Stephens, MD[1]

My journey with diabetes is a bit atypical in that I was diagnosed when I was 24, while a 3rd-year medical student (Figure 2.1). I remember well during anatomy class joking with fellow classmates about which disease we thought we were more likely to get, as medical students can get quite hypochondriachal and anxious. Oddly enough, my chosen illness was diabetes. In retrospect, I am not really sure why I even considered that diagnosis for myself. I had no family history, no symptoms. Nevertheless, things changed in third year, and over ~6 months, I lost 20 pounds and couldn't go 30 min without having to stop to find a bathroom or slurp a jug of water.

Luckily, I was at a medical school that was quite advanced in terms of diabetes management. After my diagnosis, I was started on basal-bolus therapy using Ultralente and regular insulin. I received extraordinary amounts of diabetes education, taking in information about carbohydrate counting (or exchanges as they were called in that time) and from the get-go was adjusting insulin doses based on my food intake and glucose readings.

Now, those days are a bit of a blur. The stress of medical school was relentless, and adding on diet adjustments, insulin doses with meals, and unpredictable blood glucose levels while on my clinical rotations added to the complex challenges faced by a medical student. I remember vividly some of the intense hypoglycemic episodes I had on my surgical rotation when meals were delayed and my glucose would drop dramatically. My fellow students provided support, as I sat diaphoretic and shaky, shoveling in glucose tabs. In retrospect, I wonder why I didn't take some time off from school to adjust to this new life and develop better strategies for self-care. I think at the time, I couldn't possibly imagine prolonging my schooling and just took it all in stride, not realizing how diabetes had transformed my dream to become a doctor into a day-to-day struggle to survive.

Residency was also challenging, but luckily I made two friends in my residency class who also had diabetes and provided me with support and understanding. Because my diagnosis was relatively recent, I benefited from a "honeymoon phase" with my failing pancreas being able to release enough insulin on some days to keep my blood glucose levels marginally stable. On-call nights and long workdays,

[1]Clinic Medical Director, Providence Endocrinology East and West and Diabetes Education; Affiliate Associate Professor, Department of Internal Medicine, Oregon Health and Sciences University Endocrinology Faculty, Medical Education Department, Providence Portland Medical Center, Portland, OR.

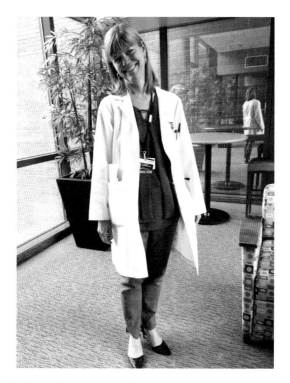

Figure 2.1. Elizabeth Stephens, MD.

however, disrupted my routines and shattered my glucose control. The unpredictable variability of my insulin needs and chaotic glucose patterns left me often utterly confused. I was fortunate during my residency to have wonderful mentors in endocrinology who helped me better understand diabetes and also sparked my interest in the hormonal feedback loops and diseases managed by specialists in this field. I eventually came to realize that my struggle to survive had become a way to thrive, and I wanted to share my unique perspective with patients with diabetes to help them live better and more fulfilling lives.

I began my endocrinology fellowship at the University of Colorado with these goals in mind and eventually chose to focus on innovative management strategies for diabetes self-care. But first I had to adjust to a new schedule plus a move to a new city, both of which challenged my glucose control. I covered three hospitals for inpatient consults, worked in a weekly clinic, and sacrificed a chunk of my time to create a social life in my new community. I didn't always get enough sleep or activity so my glucose levels suffered, and I had increasing difficulties with hypoglycemia that thankfully was not especially severe but just more frequent and annoying. I was under the care of a fantastic endocrinologist, the late Jan Perloff, who reviewed my glucose logs and encouraged me to consider an insulin pump. She explained that the device could provide a more flexible regimen given my demanding schedule and allow for lower insulin doses as I remained very insulin sensitive, requiring very small doses for meals and correction. I decided to move forward with the pump and had the good fortune to have access to a wonderful diabetes educator, Terri Ryan, who was also living with type 1 diabetes and could train me on the technology.

At the time, the most commonly used insulin pump was MiniMed (before they were owned by Medtronic), which was recommended by most diabetes experts in Denver. Being new to my endocrinology training, I was unfamiliar with the different pump options, so I elected to go with their suggestion.

There were a number of things that were helpful about pump therapy that remain so to this day. The ability to bolus as needed and use very small insulin doses; to adjust basal rates for activity or long spells of sitting; and to provide square-wave and dual-wave insulin delivery patterns for eating out or higher fat meals. All of these options allowed more flexibility with my busy life. In hindsight, I would have benefited from maintaining as much structure as possible because a daily routine with consistent insulin dosing would lead to more predictable glucose patterns. Being young, however, I valued the convenience of the pump to provide what I needed to match my hectic life of work and play.

I also had a great support system with my friend Terri Ryan, who had trained me in my pump. Over time she became a close friend and provided me with her expertise and emotional support during my transition to the pump. As a part of this experience, she opened my eyes to the value and importance to having a community of people with type 1 diabetes who can provide ideas for management, assist in coping with crises, and just acknowledge how difficult it is to live with a chronic disease. We ended up having an informal support group, including many of my colleagues in my department, as well as at the Barbara Davis Diabetes Center, where I ended up doing research in my second year of fellowship.

My endocrine training program also allowed me opportunities to experiment with different pump systems. I tried every pump on the market: Animas, Disetronic, Deltec Cozmo, and others. I have continued this first-hand experience with new technologies even today because I find that an intimate knowledge of the different devices helps me advise my patients about what system to consider based on their unique needs, resources, and skills. Trying out new pumps also keeps me engaged as a learner for my own self-care. Over the long years with a chronic disease, we all can slip into enduring without question mundane routines and numbing habits that may no longer represent state-of-the-art care. But more importantly, the moment I connect myself to a new technology, I feel a renewed sense of excitement, novelty, and, I should say, even hope akin to what I felt when I first learned as a medical student that I could not only survive but also flourish with diabetes. Each new device moves me closer toward a better understanding of my disease in its current state and wresting away its control of me.

Although the pump offered many advantages, other devices were becoming available that had great promise. My commitment to discovery expanded to my willingness to become a research subject. Colorado investigators enrolled me early in trials, such as the continuous glucose monitoring systems (CGMS). I was a study subject with Gluco-Watch, one of the first commercially available sensors worn on the wrist. It was hard to imagine this technology going very far, as it was quite uncomfortable with skin irritation and burning, as well as a short duration of use. These experiences, however, gave me a glimpse of what would be coming, and I felt the CGM would be a game-changer for those with type 1 diabetes. My glucose levels continued to be unpredictable during this period despite efforts to carbohydrate count and monitor. I found increasingly the number of variables that would affect my blood glucose levels was daunting: exercise, sleep, pump sites, stress, menstrual cycles. It was difficult to predict day to day what pattern would emerge. The CGM allowed for more continuous information, enabling the user to anticipate forthcoming trends in glucose levels. I tried using the Gluco-watch but found the skin issues too difficult to tolerate. But as other monitoring devices that were more comfortable and convenient came along, I became a regular user.

Today, I have become reliant on the CGM as my life continues to be full. Currently, I wear the Tandem t:slim X2, which integrates the t:slim pump and the Dexcom G6 CGM sensor. This system works for me as it is easy to access information from the pump and sensor, it is simple to dose and adjust, and the touch screen is user-friendly. I also like the small size. The recent addition of the threshold suspend feature with Basal IQ has made the device even more effective, reducing the frequency of hypoglycemia and the resultant swings in glucose levels that follow. It has reduced nocturnal lows for me as well as the amount of insulin that I need daily, while helping me shed a few extra pounds that were added by hypoglycemia treatment.

I feel fortunate that I have found a device that makes living with diabetes easier. But I have come to realize that there is no single answer for those living with type 1 diabetes in terms of management. We have many different options to choose from in deciding how we want to administer insulin. For me, the pump has been a great tool, with the ability to dose insulin on the fly, to take very small amounts and adjust the basal rate as needed for exercise or illness. The addition of the sensor has also been incredibly helpful in freeing me from finger-sticks, allowing me to set targets for my glucose levels so I can be alerted when I am going low or high, and alarming or adjusting insulin if I am distracted or sleeping but my glucose is dropping. Examples where the pump and sensor have been essential for my management include pregnancies and exercise. I have two boys, ages 11 and 13, and had them later in life with my last being born when I was 39. Both were uncomplicated pregnancies and deliveries, which I suspect was a result of my tight control using technology. Changes in insulin requirements as I moved through the trimesters were much easier to navigate with pump settings. The sensor was essential in the first trimester when hypoglycemia was more difficult to detect, and later, when I was really trying to tighten up my control postprandially.

I also find technology helpful for exercise. I am a regular bike commuter and also am very active in the day-to-day with my family. My insulin requirements vary quite a bit between work days and days at home, but they can become inconsistent at any time. The pump allows me to adjust insulin doses based on the patterns that I see, especially with temporary basal rate changes. I also tend to be very insulin-sensitive after exercise for hours, and a lower basal can help reduce my risk for low blood glucose.

Although the pump is definitely helpful, I would never say that this technology is easy. It takes a lot of time and attention to manage and is one more thing that can have issues and result in high or low blood glucose levels. A big challenge for me these days is finding sites for both my infusion sets and sensor. I am a lean person, and after my two pregnancies, my insulin absorption from my abdomen has never been the same. I have found alternative sites on my arms and legs for sensors, but I now have limited "terrain" for my infusion sets, which is concerning. I also get tired of the constant alarming, so I have been very mindful about only activating the alerts that I need. They are also a fashion challenge, as dresses or more fitted outfits just don't look the same with the lump of a sensor, or a pump under my waist or arm. Sleep is difficult with tubing and alarms. Finally, the technology is a constant reminder of my disease that can be fatiguing.

A few years ago, I decided to go on a "pump holiday" to give my skin a break and rid myself of diabetes reminders and devices. I did continue with my CGM. Being off the pump was a wonderful reprieve. I can imagine doing it again, especially for vacations where carrying all the pump gear and going through airports represent additional life burdens. At the end of my extensive pump holiday, however, I did find my blood glucose levels were more elevated as was my A1C, so I ended up going back to the pump.

The type 1 diabetes technology landscape continues to evolve with systems getting closer to the ultimate goal of the closed-loop or artificial pancreas. The currently available Medtronic 670G is the farthest along. Many patients who I have worked with have found this system to be incredibly helpful in reducing excursions and improving the frequency with which they wake up with glucose values at goal. For me, this system has been less useful likely because my life patterns and habits vary so much as I choose to live a rich, fulfilling, but often too busy personal and professional life. I still bike to work, see patients in clinic for 8 h straight, run to and from the hospital for consults, and often eat on the fly. Did I mention I have a family with two active and healthy kids (see Figure 2.2)? Every day is a new adventure. With this inconsistency, I find my own ability to

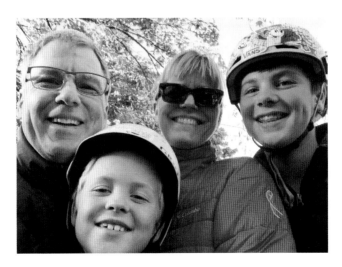

Figure 2.2. The Stephens family.

adjust my settings and targets more effective than asking the pump to do it all for me. I will say that the "suspend before low" pump feature has been very useful to reduce the frequency of hypoglycemia and need for treatment that inevitably results in rebound highs. I am eager for more of the systems to integrate that technology down the road.

In sum, I didn't invite diabetes into my life and I often wish for a day off, as its demands are relentless. I have many moments in which my sensor is alarming from hidden carbohydrates in a meal, or waking from sleep and having to eat, where I moan how I really don't feel like having diabetes right now. And yet, diabetes has given my life purpose and meaning, as well as an appreciation for health that I am not sure I otherwise would have had. It has also allowed me to meet and be a part of the care team for others struggling with the day-to-day management of glucose levels and to witness their determination, creativity, and bravery. Science and technology have enabled us to live better lives with diabetes and have helped to change the burden of living with this chronic disease. I am grateful to be inspired nearly every day.

Chapter 3
Personal Story with Type 1 Diabetes and Technology

Aaron Michels, MD[1]

I was diagnosed with type 1 diabetes (T1D) right before my 13th birthday (Figure 3.1). Like most people diagnosed with T1D, it changed my life. I have always said, "I was old enough to know that life is not fair, but not mature enough to cope with being diagnosed with T1D." My family and supportive medical team helped me through this difficult transition in life.

The diagnosis also helped define my career path at a young age. Living with diabetes introduced me to the medical system and the healthcare team that provided care to my family and me. Not only was the physician central to my managing diabetes, but also the diabetes educators, nurses, social workers, and dietitians were instrumental in helping us live with diabetes. From these experiences, I pursued a career in medicine. I graduated from Creighton University School of Medicine, completed residency, and then completed a fellowship in Diabetes and Endocrinology at the University of Colorado. I am currently a practicing diabetologist and physician scientist at the Barbara Davis Center for Diabetes, part of the University of Colorado Denver Anschutz Medical campus. It is an honor and a privilege to care for people who have the same disease as me. Having lived with T1D for more than 25 years, I was asked to reflect on the use of diabetes technology in my diabetes care and life.

When I was first diagnosed with diabetes, I was treated with multiple daily injections of insulin. As a teenager, this worked well for me and my psyche. I was a person with diabetes four times a day at breakfast, lunch, dinner, and bedtime, performing a finger-stick blood glucose and taking an injection. In between, I did not want to think or worry about diabetes. I experienced lows, however, especially overnight, and my diabetes care team encouraged the use of an insulin pump. As a teenager, I had no desire to have anything attached to me and be a constant reminder of having to live with diabetes. As time went on, I matured and was accepted to medical school. Still taking multiple injections of insulin each day, I began to consider the pros and cons of using an insulin pump.

At the age of 21 years, I eventually decided to use an insulin pump with the continued encouragement from my endocrinologist. During the summer before I began medical school, I was scheduled for an all-day insulin pump training class.

[1]Associate Professor of Pediatrics, Medicine, and Immunology and Microbiology, Frieda and George S. Eisenbarth Clinical Immunology Endowed Chair, University of Colorado Anschutz Medical Campus, Aurora, CO.

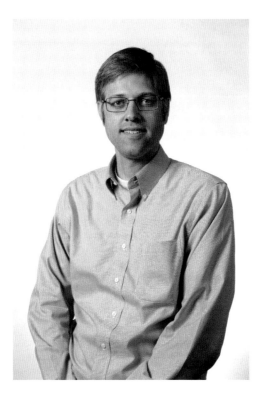

Figure 3.1. Aaron Michels, MD.

At that time, I received two insulin pumps: I was told I would have an extra one if one broke. With this, I briefly rethought my decision to use a pump but continued with the training. The first week involved a lot of blood glucose testing, including in the middle of the night to adjust basal rates. I remember one of the most challenging aspects of wearing an insulin pump for the first time was not programming settings, filling cartridges, or changing insertion sites: it was learning to sleep with the device, as it always seemed to be in the way. After ~3 months, all of the kinks were worked out in regard to basal rates along with showering and sleeping with an insulin pump. I felt quite positive about the ability to dose insulin more times a day and the ease of just pushing a button to bolus insulin. I wondered why I had not done this sooner. In terms of my overall blood glucose control, I experienced fewer lows during the night and my hemoglobin A_{1c} (A1C) decreased. I appreciated the ability to have more control over insulin dosing and learned to bolus for corrections before eating meals and to adjust basal rates during the day and night. I have been using an insulin pump now for 18 consecutive years and have never taken or considered taking a "pump break."

As I lived with diabetes going through medical school and residency, diabetes technology continued to advance. When I upgraded insulin pumps, I now received only one instead of two devices and minor changes were made such that even smaller fractions of a unit of insulin could be administered. The next big break-through came when I started using a continuous glucose monitor, that is, a sensor. I have been regularly using a sensor over the past 9 years with very little time off. I had tried sensors before this time; however, I was frustrated by the lack of accuracy and bulkiness of the sensors and devices during the early days of this technology. For a number of years, I found that more frequent finger-stick blood glucoses were better than using one of the available continuous glucose monitors.

All technology continues to advance, and in 2010, I tried using a sensor again and found it to be much more conducive to living life *with* diabetes and not *for* diabetes. When the sensor was accurate and transmitting a signal, this was one of the best learning tools I had come across for T1D. Being able to observe real-time responses to food and insulin action was eye opening. For the first couple of weeks, I had dozens of lows, as I was shocked by how high my blood glucose would increase after meals, and I tried to correct—it was easy to push a few buttons on my insulin pump. Quickly, I learned the importance of the old adage, "bolus before eating" and especially 10–15 min before eating. Having a functioning sensor reporting blood glucose levels every 5 min was indeed enlightening. Then it became a game to keep my blood glucose between 70 and 180 mg/dL. Using a sensor improved my overall blood glucose levels. For the first time in my life with diabetes, I was able to consistently keep my A1C <7.0%, and important, this was without a significant amount of hypoglycemia.

Sensor technology has continued to improve. It has now reached the point at which sensors are replacing finger-stick blood glucose checking and are being integrated with insulin pumps and algorithms to automatically adjust insulin delivery. These advances move use closer to a functional artificial pancreas and ultimately reduce the burden of managing diabetes.

I have experienced diabetes technology as a patient and as a physician, and recently as a parent. My oldest daughter also lives with T1D. We screened her for T1D-associated antibodies at the age of 2 years old and found that multiple antibodies were present. She started insulin at the age of 5 years. Within a week of starting insulin injections, she was also using a sensor. The ability to monitor blood glucose continually overnight greatly alleviates the parental fear of overnight hypoglycemia. Similar to myself, my daughter did not want to wear an insulin pump. Her reasons were much different than mine as a teenager—she thought my black insulin pump was ugly. Once she knew there were different colors and pink insertion sites, she was sold and has been wearing a pump for the past 4 years (even on our family vacations to the beach; see Figure 3.2). Insulin pumps and sensors have definitely made managing diabetes easier for our family.

I have experienced diabetes and diabetes technology in many facets of my life, as a patient, physician, and now as a father. I do hope to see a day when diabetes technology is no longer needed—that is, when T1D is prevented and cured. Living with diabetes and caring for patients with the same disease has also led me to conduct research to prevent and ultimately cure T1D. My research focuses on understanding the basic immunology of T1D to design safe, specific, and personalized therapies to prevent and stop the autoimmune destruction of insulin producing cells. One major focus is on the use of small "drug-like" molecules to inhibit the specific white blood cells involved in destroying insulin-producing

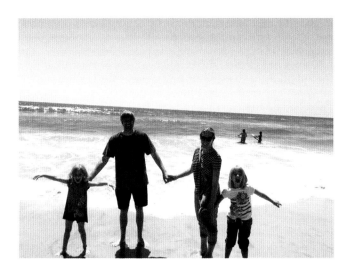

Figure 3.2. The Michels family.

β-cells. My laboratory has had success developing these therapies from bench to bedside, and clinical trials are now underway in children and adolescents at-risk for developing T1D. The ultimate goal is to stop the body's immune system from destroying insulin producing cells, making a cure for diabetes possible. Until that time, however, I remain connected to my diabetes technology.

Chapter 4
My Life with Diabetes and Technology

Justen Rudolph, MD[1]

My life with diabetes started in November 1994. I was a sophomore in college at the University of Montana in Missoula and was just getting used to living life off campus (Figure 4.1). I lived with two other roommates in a triplex learning to cook and clean for ourselves. I was taking pre-med classes, as I was planning on a future in medicine. My original goal was to become a family practice doctor and come back to the great state of Montana and care for the whole family.

Life was good at the time, and we had to make really hard decisions like, "are we going to go mountain biking after class today, or go hit the rivers and fly-fish the evening hatch?" I started to get terribly thirsty, however, from September through my diagnosis in November. On one weekend fishing trip to nearby Beaverhead River, I recall getting so thirsty over the day of fishing that I was "forced" to drink water from the river. I also had sprained my ankle that fall playing racquetball, and it just wouldn't heal. It was a nonbruising routine ankle sprain, similar to many others that I had had growing up playing basketball. This sprain lingered for months. After a month out of sheer frustration with the ankle, I tried to play racquetball again, but I just couldn't put much weight on in. As with most college kids, when there was a problem, I called my parents for advice. Complaining about the thirst, they thought perhaps it was due to the fact that I was cooking and making different foods now that I was living off campus and that maybe I was adding too much salt to my diet. Things progressed from there. I ended up needing to bring a 32-oz mug of Mountain Dew to each class, and at times, it was all I could do to get through a 1-h class without having to pee. I also had lost ~20 lb over this fall, but again, I thought maybe it was just how I was eating and trying to skimp by on a college kid's budget.

Finally, a week or two before Thanksgiving, I had another phone call to my parents, and they suggested I go to the student health center and get checked out—maybe it was diabetes or something else wrong. At the time, I had no idea what diabetes was. No one in my family had either type 1 diabetes (T1D) or type 2 diabetes (T2D), and I didn't know of any friends or classmates who had diabetes before this. I ended up going to the student health service for evaluation. They mentioned the possibility of T1D or T2D and needed to do some blood work.

---

[1]Director of St. Vincent Diabetes Center, Billings, MT.

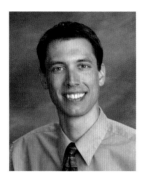

Figure 4.1. Justen Rudolph, MD.

I got a call the following day from the doctor saying, "It looks like you have diabetes."

My blood glucose level was 330 mg/dL. They recommended that I go see the diabetes educator at the local hospital in Missoula to get started on insulin shots, as the student health service wasn't equipped to teach me these skills.

I remember asking, "Are you sure it isn't type 2 that I can control with diet and exercise."

"No, I don't think so," was the response.

My next comment was, "Well, I'm really busy studying for my organic chemistry test. Can I go in next week?"

"No, you need to go today and get started on insulin," was the response.

Therefore, with fear, apprehension, and confusion, I started my journey with T1D.

I recall meeting with Judy, my diabetes educator. She gave me the crash course in diabetes. This was just before Thanksgiving, and I can specifically remember asking the question, "So, can I have mom's homemade apple pie?"

Judy's response was, "Well, pumpkin would be a better choice."

To that I lamented, "Well, I don't like pumpkin pie."

The other thing she told me was that I couldn't drink regular Mountain Dew. Given that I was drinking Mountain Dew at every class currently, this was going to be difficult. I refused to drink diet soda because it just tasted too bad, so I had to give up soda pop. However, over those first few weeks of life with diabetes, I also was grateful that at least I had a disease that I could manage. I was fearful of losing my vision over the course of my life, and I vowed to myself to keep my glucose levels controlled to prevent the long-term complications of diabetes. I could function in life if I had to lose my leg. I could continue living through dialysis or a kidney transplant if my kidneys failed. I didn't know, however, how I could function well without my sight. Judy mentioned an insulin pump during those first sessions with her and I told that I didn't think that was something I would need. I still had some denial that maybe the diagnosis was wrong and I could beat this thing somehow. Even back then, a cure was just around the corner, and I just needed to keep myself healthy until that cure was available. Nearly 25 years later, the cure is still just around the corner. Through technological advances with pumps, continuous glucose monitoring systems (CGMS), and now automated insulin delivery, however, treatment continues to improve and the burden of the disease continues to lessen.

I was started on N and R insulin for the first year and was taking two shots a day. I had to fix the amount of carbohydrates that I would eat for breakfast, lunch, and dinner and had to have a bedtime snack to avoid nighttime lows. I recall having to arrange my class schedule to make sure that I ate lunch before 12:30 or that NPH would peak and cause a low blood glucose level. That schedule and regimen continued for a year. I had a 1-year follow-up appointment with Judy, and she again talked to me about an insulin pump. Dr. Wilson was a local doctor who also had diabetes and who made it successfully through medical school with diabetes. He was wearing an insulin pump, was active, and was keeping his diabetes under good control. In my mind, if he was on a pump and successful, then maybe I should consider it.

I was getting sick of always eating the same amount of carbohydrates per meal and liked the idea of the freedom that an insulin pump provided. If I wanted to eat more for Thanksgiving this year than I did last year, a pump would allow me to adjust my insulin to match my food consumption. I also found that being an active college kid, I would need to snack and eat if I was going to exercise to prevent low blood glucose levels, and I had to make sure that candy or glucose tablets were with me at all times. It became somewhat of a joke in our house, that if you were going to eat my blood glucose candy that you also had to know how to give me a shot of glucagon and where it was kept. On the flip-side, it was the active lifestyle that raised concerns about me getting an insulin pump. I didn't want to have to be careful about my activity if I had a pump. If I was going to be mountain biking or whitewater kayaking, I didn't want to be concerned about the durability of the device.

So, despite me saying 1-year prior that I would not need an insulin pump, I ended up ordering and starting with a Medtronic 506 insulin pump. The factors involved were having a positive role model, wanting more flexibility in my diet, minimizing the risk of hypoglycemia, and having the durability to keep up with an active lifestyle.

When I started on an insulin pump, though, I wasn't sure if I was going to be successful. At that time, the bent needle cannula was still the standard. It was a steel-needle infusion set that would stay in place for a full 3 days. I remember as I put in my first infusion set nearly passing out from the pain and anxiety of putting that needle into my stomach. We had to pull out that set, and Judy had to place the first one for me. I wasn't sure I was going to be able to do this on my own going forward. Furthermore, you had these oh-so-desirable plastic shower bags that you had to place your pump in to keep water off it as there was no quick release mechanism on the bent needle sets at the time. We ended up trying a soft-set infusion set, which was still relatively new, and that was much more comfortable. Fortunately, around that time, the quick release mechanism also came out, and I was able to disconnect the pump to take a shower. Who knew how nice of a little perk that would be? That theme will continue throughout my life with diabetes and technology.

I greatly appreciated the ability to change my insulin doses based on how many carbohydrates I was eating. Certain foods continued to be problematic, however, such as pizza, and what college kid doesn't survive on a diet of pizza? The proverbial pizza effect (the exaggerated hyperglycemia that resulted after eating pizza) was in full effect. I learned to do things like dual-wave bolusing to try to compensate but always struggled. I did have a nice network of 6–10 people with T1D in the Missoula community who were on an insulin pump, led by Dr. Wilson, and we could learn from each other. About once a month, we would get together at the Mustard Seed (a local American Chinese restaurant) and we would each take our best guess method of carbohydrates counting for sweet and sour chicken or broccoli beef. We also would discuss how we each adjusted our insulin for exercise, or other challenges that came up living with diabetes and using an insulin pump.

I also appreciated the ability to reduce my insulin for exercise and activity as well. Hiking in the mountains, a day of walking and fishing in the river, or mountain biking became easier as I learned to use a temporary basal rate to reduce my insulin (Figures 4.2–4.7). It didn't eliminate the need to ensure that I always had glucose with me, but it did reduce my episodes of hypoglycemia. I remember thinking how difficult it would be if I was still on N and R insulin and couldn't really adjust my insulin to compensate for the activity level.

The pump held up to the rigors of a rough-and-tumble college life as well. It handled crashes over the top of my mountain bike. It handled water as well. MiniMed made a waterproof case back in those days that I could place my pump in and remain connected to the infusion set. Such was the case with whitewater kayaking. I would strap the case to my leg and as long as I stayed in the kayak with the skirt in place, things were just great. On one occasion, however, I flipped the boat and couldn't be turned back over. Now I was swimming down the river with my hands on the boat as I am kicking back to the bank. I could feel my insulin pump start to slide off my leg as I was kicking. This obviously would be a much worse

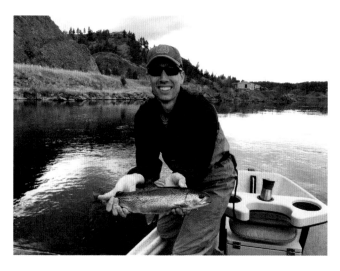

Figure 4.2. Rainbow Trout on Missouri River, MT.

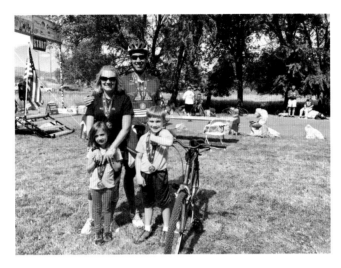

Figure 4.3. Red Rider at Montana Association Tour de Cure Event.

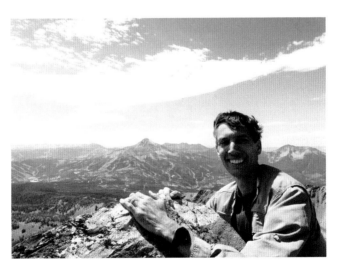

Figure 4.4. Climbing to the top of the Spanish Peaks with Lone Peak in the background, Big Sky, MT. Life with diabetes can be like climbing to the top of the mountain and then holding on for dear life.

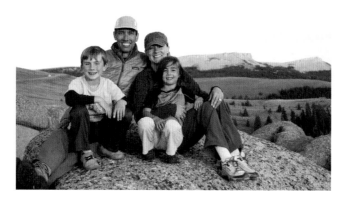

Figure 4.5. Family camping and exploring, Bighorn Mountains, WY.

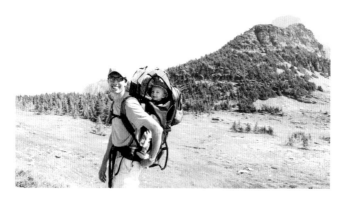

Figure 4.6. Hiking in Glacier National Park, MT.

situation to lose my pump in the bottom of the river. So I grabbed my pump strap, which was now around my ankle, with one hand, and kept the other hand on my kayak. I used one leg to kick myself back to shore. Each episode like this turned into a learning experience on how to live a little better with a pump; you learn from your mistakes. The next time I went out on the river, the pump went inside my wetsuit, and although it wasn't as comfortable, I didn't have an episode like that again.

Unfortunately, with diabetes technology, you have to learn to navigate the insurance system and the headaches involved with that. I find most patients end

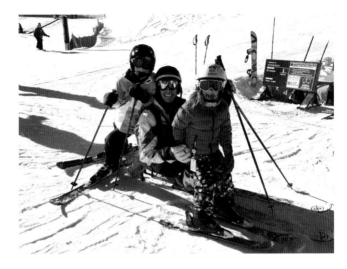

Figure 4.7. Skiing with the kids, Big Sky, MT.

up having a diabetes supplier or insurance nightmare. Mine occurred while I was in medical school. I upgraded my pump to the MiniMed 508 pump. This was also around the time that Medtronic bought out MiniMed and their billing department and customer service had changed. With my insurance during medical school, they essentially made me rent the pump while the insurance continued to pay Medtronic monthly. I certainly had to come up with the 20% copay, which I paid to Medtronic upfront. However, 2 years later, Medtronic sent me a bill for around $2,500 for the remainder of the pump cost. I was totally confused and livid that I had paid my portion and now they were billing me again. After multiple phone calls and hours on the phone, it turned out that Medtronic stopped billing my insurance the monthly rental charge to fully pay off the pump. This was certainly more money than a medical student living on loans was willing or able to spend. Medtronic maintained that it was ultimately my responsibility to pay for the pump. I continued to argue that it was not my responsibility that Medtronic stopped billing my insurance company. Ultimately, the situation got resolved, but not without excessive headaches and time trying to resolve it.

Recall one of my concerns when considering an insulin pump was the hardiness of the pump; I didn't want to have to be careful with it. I have been quite pleased with the durability of my insulin pumps over the years. While on vacation, I inadvertently dove into the ocean with my pump. I swam out ~50 yards before hitting my insulin pump with my arm and realizing my pump was still on. I thought for sure I had ruined my pump. After drying it out on the beach, however, it continued to function properly. The same thing occurred years later after diving into a freshwater lake. It has survived numerous wipeouts downhill skiing, mountain bike crashes, and pickup basketball games. It did meet its match versus the asphalt, however. I was a medical resident at the time. I was working the night shift on this particular night. There was a local teriyaki chicken restaurant close to the hospital

I was working at in Portland. I rode my bike to the restaurant to get dinner before I started my shift at 7 P.M. I had a plastic sack hanging off one handle bar and a backpack with my medical books on my back as I was riding to the hospital. I cut through a parking lot and thought I could weave in between the concrete parking blocks. As I weaved and tried to keep my dinner upright, however, I ended up sideswiping the parking block and went down. I landed on my right hip, which is where I typically carry my insulin pump. I brushed myself off, assessed whether my dinner survived, and then looked at my pump and saw instantly that I had a problem. The screen was completely shattered. The buttons for my pump seemed to work, but I just had no way to enter the blood glucose, carbohydrates, or dose my insulin accurately. It appeared to still be delivering basal insulin, so I thought I could at least get through my shift for that night.

Fortunately, I previously had enabled the "quick-bolus" feature on my pump at the time and because the buttons still worked, I could give boluses through audio queues. There was some anxiety involved wondering whether I could trust the pump to work properly after such a jarring event. I didn't feel like I had many options at this time, however, as I was the resident responsible for the night shift. It was these events over time that led me to my current backup plan. I keep a single insulin syringe with me in my glucose testing kit. If my pump were ever to suddenly fail, or have an infusion site problem, I could always get some insulin out of the reservoir of the pump and take a manual injection. This is why it is important to know your basal rates along with your carbohydrates and correction factor. Every person should have a pump failure backup plan. It certainly isn't going to be precise and blood glucose levels likely will not be optimal, but it will keep you out of the hospital and out of diabetic ketoacidosis (DKA).

This is one of the main concerns in using an insulin pump that every patient must take into account and plan for. As we have gotten shorter and quicker acting insulins (and more will be coming), the risk of going into DKA sooner than you would have otherwise on a long-acting basal insulin increases. For me, having a backup insulin syringe is the simplest and most portable way to have a backup plan available. I also recommend taking a picture of your insulin pump settings page from your pump download and keep that in your phone or in a cloud backup system so that you have the ability to reprogram your pump when you pump fails.

For 20 years, insulin pump technology was the most advanced mechanism for controlling glucose levels as we continue to try to mimic the fully functional pancreas. The next leap in technological advancement was CGM. It started with the professional Medtronic CGM Gold system when I was in clinical practice. A dedicated wired device connected to a separate pump-size box and gave you your glucose readings. You wore this for 1–3 days, at a maximum. Fortunately, the wired device quickly gave way to a wireless unit but had a "paddle" for a transmitter that you somehow had to tape to your body. The results were unreliable, and the sensor hurt quite a bit; it was about all I could do to leave it in for 3 days. The next step was miniaturizing the transmitter, making it much easier to keep in place. You still had to deal with the harpoon-style inserter and the pain involved in inserting that sensor and leaving it in place. I continued to try each iteration, hoping that it would help me identify the patterns to my blood glucose levels in response to different foods or activity levels. The sensor still could only be in place for 3 days, however, and it seemed that just about the time you got some good accuracy, it was time to pull out the sensor and replace it. For me, with this current generation of sensor, I could only psychologically manage about 2 weeks of using a sensor before I needed to take a break from it, mostly because of the pain and site irritation. It wasn't until the Dexcom CGM sensor came along that I started to be able to wear a sensor continuously, and I cannot fathom going back to managing my blood glucose levels without a sensor. The most obvious and clear advantage to CGM technology is being alerted to both low and high blood glucose levels in real time. It allows users to take an inventory of steps and actions that may have caused either the high or low blood glucose levels so you can make different decisions next time. I was able to get instant biofeedback.

I finally was able to closely follow my blood glucose levels after eating pizza and to follow my blood glucose levels to see how long the dual-wave bolus needed to be carried out. I recall thinking that managing blood glucose levels while eating pizza became "easy" over time, as I was able to see how much insulin was needed now and later, as long as I was eating the same amount of pizza. This was essentially impossible when I was on finger-stick blood glucose monitoring. I would eat pizza and could initially keep my blood glucose levels controlled until I went to bed and then the late effect of the pizza kicked in. I recall one Thanksgiving when I was in college before CGM. I was determined to keep my blood glucose levels controlled after that big meal, the largest of the year. I decided to check my blood glucose levels every hour for more than 12 h to see the pattern. Now, with CGM technology, this was possible to have a glucose reading every 5 min even if I chose to take a post-turkey nap.

Another more subtle benefit to using CGM technology was detection of nighttime lows. I think all people with diabetes have some underlying fear of nighttime lows, and either not waking up or waking up feeling so miserable from a low that you consciously or subconsciously do anything you can to avoid being low at night. But allowing your blood glucose levels to be high overnight means 6–8 h of high blood glucose levels, and this represents either a quarter to a third of your day spent high. If that amount of hyperglycemia persists, there is no way you have an A1C at goal or have a good time in range. For me, this really came into play with my dual-wave bolus again. Before CGM, I didn't want to go to bed with a normal blood glucose levels and have a lot of active insulin on board (i.e., insulin that is still actively working to bring down your blood glucose levels). Therefore, I would aim to keep my bedtime blood glucose a little higher. With CGM, over time, I became comfortable with the alarms and the detection of lows. I could confidently take enough insulin and keep a significantly higher percentage of insulin active in those first few hours of going to sleep and would know that if by chance I overshot my insulin bolus that I (or my wife) would wake up to the alarm and I could take corrective action. This really helped me to keep my overnight blood glucose levels at goal and wake up in the target range for glucose control.

CGM was also vital to keeping an active and variable lifestyle. I recall taking an overnight backpacking trip with a group of guys and how excited I was to have a CGM and that I could follow my blood glucose levels in real time. Of course, I had to plan where I was going to wear the sensor before the trip as I didn't want the hip strap or backpack to be rubbing on the sensor and forcing it out. A 6- to 8-h walk, with a 40- to 50-lb pack certainly is not part of my typical routine.

Clearly, I would need less insulin for this hike and for the subsequent trips to surrounding lakes. Using the pump's technology to reduce my insulin through a temporary basal rate and following how my blood glucose levels were responding was crucial. I initially used a temporary basal rate of 50%, which means I was getting 50% less insulin on an hour-to-hour basis. After 2 h of hiking, however, I could see on my CGM that my blood glucose was progressively dropping and ended up having a mild hypoglycemic reaction. I caught it early enough that I could correct it with glucose tabs, eat a granola bar to keep my blood glucose up, and then further reduce my basal rates. This allowed my blood glucose to stabilize, and I didn't need further adjustment to my basal rates. That evening, after setting up camp, I recall sitting back and wondering how I ever managed backpack trips without a CGM. Then, when the mountain goats woke us that night when they came into camp I was able to quickly check my blood glucose levels on my CGM, check out the goats, and safely return to sleep.

A similar process has evolved over the years when downhill skiing as well. To adjust my insulin and then periodically check my blood glucose on my CGM while on the chairlift has been invaluable. It helps me treat potential low blood glucose levels before they become problematic. This allows me to ski more freely knowing I'll be alerted if I start to drop low. Before CGM, I could not test my blood glucose while on the chairlift and I certainly didn't want to stop skiing to check it. Therefore, I would not test my blood glucose until lunchtime and treat for hypoglycemia if I felt low while skiing. Now that I am skiing more with my young kids, the intensity of my skiing has changed and I don't need to reduce my insulin as much as I once did. On adult ski days or days when hiking to the ridge is available, however, I can reduce my insulin further and follow my blood glucose levels in real time to keep me functioning at my peak.

The most recent data on CGM use in the population with T1D has come from the T1D Exchange, which our clinic has been fortunate to participate in. It states that even in the top diabetes centers in the country that only ~25% of patients are using CGM. My patients will often ask whether I use a sensor and I always respond with a "Yes, and I could never go back to life without a CGM." The value and benefit that it provides me outweighs the hassle of having another site, keeping it taped on, and dealing with the expense involved in paying for ongoing sensors. Insurance coverage continues to improve for CGM technology but the cost remains high. Unfortunately, even as sensor technology advances and doesn't require manual calibrations, the cost of strips doesn't offset the cost of sensors. The cost of sensors needs to come down at the same time as insurance coverage switches to a pharmacy benefit to allow patients better access to this life-changing technology.

AUTOMATED INSULIN DELIVERY

As the CGM technology has evolved and become accurate enough to dose insulin from, we now can consider automated insulin delivery. Simply put, this is using an insulin pump that is using CGM data to automatically adjust insulin to keep blood glucose levels at a target level through a computerized control algorithm. Medtronic entered into this space with their 670G insulin pump with automated insulin delivery in the spring of 2017. I had been holding onto my old 530 insulin pump for ~6 years prior and therefore my insurance company and I were ready to take the plunge when the 670 pump was available. My goals in pursuing the 670 pump were to wake up every morning with near-normal blood glucose levels and help control the highs late after dinner when the fat and protein are getting processed. I was using a dual-wave bolus for lunches and dinners the majority of the time. Dinner was especially tricky as my portion sizes were usually bigger and typically included home-cooked meals that were more difficult to guess the proper carbohydrates for. As I mentioned previously, I was able to do pretty well with pizza and adjusting that dual-wave, but other meals certainly provided many challenges. I would be apprehensive about going to bed with too much active insulin for fear of having a hypoglycemic event, which are never fun to wake up to. So, my hope was to have the 670 pump automatically adjust my insulin late at night to avoid the highs from the delayed processing of fat and protein; therefore, I could wake up with a normal blood glucose level rather than a blood glucose >200 mg/dL, which also doesn't feel great to wake up to.

I did have some reservations about the system, and specifically, it was around the accuracy and wearability of the sensor. When I had previously worn the sensor, I would frequently get dropped signals. I was told to put the pump on the same side of my body as my sensor. Frankly, I found this rather ridiculous. I just don't have that much body mass for a signal to go through, and I felt that shouldn't be part of the equation. I have my favorite spot to wear my pump, as all patients do. It's already a sacrifice to wear a pump 24/7 and then have a sensor with it, and the idea of having to wear it in a special spot just seemed too much.

Another problem I previously had with the wearability was keeping the clamshell transmitter adhered and in place. Inevitably, the back of the edges of the transmitter would catch on something, especially when I was wearing it on the back of my arm. One of my kids might accidentally grab it during a game of rough house. The act of swinging a golf club was just too much movement, and I couldn't keep it adhered. The tapes have evolved over the years; but, again, how much tape does one have to place to keep the transmitter in place? You also can't afford to lose too many sensors. A sensor is not cheap, and to lose a sensor prematurely because of normal life activities and the inability to keep it taped down becomes discouraging.

I also struggled with the accuracy of the Enlite Sensor in the past. I never got to the point of fully trusting the number I was getting without confirming a blood glucose level. Technically, this was how the original sensors were developed and marketed. It was adjunctive to blood glucose monitoring, which means you still had to test your blood glucose if you were going to dose your insulin from it. You could trust, however, the glucose trends, whether your blood glucose was climbing or falling, rather than the absolute number. This was especially true in the first 24–36 h of using a sensor when you are first getting it calibrated, the so-called wetting period, during which time the sensor is getting fully saturated with interstitial fluid and interstitial glucose (i.e., the glucose in the soft tissue rather than blood glucose).

So these were my goals, aspirations, and apprehensions in moving to the 670G pump. In terms of the sensor itself, there has been significant improvement. The reliability of the transmitter and the strength of the signal were resolved. I no longer had any dropped signals, and it didn't matter which side of my body I had the sensor on. I was getting consistent signals. The accuracy of the sensor was much improved but still not perfect. It certainly is good enough to adjust insulin and make treatment decisions. It still requires three or four blood glucose calibrations a day to achieve the best performance however. Now that sensors are factory calibrated and no longer require blood glucose calibrations, this feels extraordinarily frequent. For the benefit of automated insulin delivery, however, this is a reasonable trade-off.

The first month in auto mode can be arduous. I tell patients you have to agree to stick with it for at least a month before giving up and to expect frustrations with the alarms, and I had these same frustrations. You have to be at a place or time in your life that you can have and appropriately deal with a month of these frustrations. During this first 4–6 weeks of automated insulin delivery, expect that you will be checking your blood glucose levels more frequently and performing the "confirm BG" routine. This will get better over time, however, as one learns to trust the system and figures out what the system is trying to do. I also keep in mind that this is the first generation of automated insulin delivery. The goal from the perspective of the U.S. Food and Drug Administration was to have a system that was safe in terms of low blood glucose avoidance. To safely reduce or increase insulin, if the system detects something atypical, it will ask for a confirmatory blood glucose level to ensure that the system is getting accurate results and all parts of the pump are functioning correctly. Similarly, when blood glucose levels are high, if the pump has been giving you insulin through autobasal for a maximum period of time, it wants you to confirm that everything in the system is functioning. You need to be able to troubleshoot problems such as whether your infusion set is disconnected, whether the blood glucose value correct, and whether you need to check ketones.

The benefits of automated insulin delivery, however, are amazing when you have the system working as designed. Simply starting my day every morning with a blood glucose that is at goal is amazing. It means I'm not waking up cotton-mouthed from highs, I feel more refreshed and energized, and I feel like I can eat breakfast without the risk of worsening hyperglycemia if I was trying to eat on top of a high blood glucose. In addition, I can feel more confident with active insulin on board and not have to worry about hypoglycemia. I experienced this previously when first starting a CGM, but with automated insulin delivery, it takes it to the next level. So, having a system that can significantly reduce the risk of an overnight low, and the ability to trust that it will do that for me, is priceless.

Finally, there is the peace of mind knowing that I don't have to think about my blood glucose levels all the time. I don't have to constantly check what my blood glucose levels are doing and I know the system is working to get my blood glucose either up to 120 mg/dL or down to 120 mg/dL. I didn't recognize the amount of effort that was going into thinking about my blood glucose levels until I didn't have to any longer. I do wish that I could change that target to <100 mg/dL, but future advances in automated insulin delivery will get us there.

About 6 months into automated insulin delivery, I had clear validation of my trust in the pump's ability to avoid hypoglycemia. Before automated insulin delivery, I did not consider myself to be someone who had a lot of low blood glucose levels. Being a good planner with diabetes, however, I always tried to have glucose available in some fashion, just in case. Usually, it was packing some glucose tabs, jellybeans, or sweet tarts and having them stashed in my vehicle, desk at the office, workbag, or wife's purse. Traditionally, when we would pack for a trip, my school-age daughter was my official blood glucose candy packer. On this particular trip to the mountains, however, I had forgotten to pack any blood glucose candy. It was at this time, that I realized just how used to *not* having low blood glucose levels I had become. It didn't even cross my mind to pack glucose. I'm not advocating not having glucose with you and that you won't have lows with the automated insulin. It was certainly a mistake in planning, but it speaks to my peace of mind in knowing the system is working on my behalf to avoid lows, all without me having to think about it.

I continue, however, to look forward to an even brighter future. Diabetes technology has been advancing quicker than ever before and it is exciting to see and be a part of these advances. Until a few years ago, a 4-year warranty on a pump was adequate. Currently, that will leave you two generations behind in technology and having the ability to more safely and accurately control one's blood glucose levels. Of course, affordability continues to be a concern as these new technologies come to market. Ultimately, as these technologies advance, they continue to help me more safely and precisely control my blood glucose levels and enjoy life to the fullest while living with T1D.

Chapter 5
Staying in the Game with Continuous Glucose Monitoring Technology

David M. Tridgell, MD[1]

I was diagnosed with type 1 diabetes at the age of 15 years old in 1993. I was a responsible teenager. I tested my blood glucose levels at least 4 times/day and never missed an injection of R and N insulin. I majored in chemical engineering in collage and changed gears halfway through and decided to go to medical school.

Still, my journey to pumps and continuous glucose monitoring systems (CGMS) was slower than what one might expect. My endocrinologist would very gently encourage me to consider a pump, but I did not look forward to the thought of having something attached to me. I eventually decided that the prospect of greater flexibility and tighter control was worth it, and I got my first Animas insulin pump at the start of my third year of medical school. I haven't once looked back. Having been familiar with Animas, I decided to say with the pump each time I needed an upgrade, going to the Animas Ping and eventually the Animas Vibe. Now that Animas is no longer making pumps, I would like to remind the reader that the Animas Vibe was a sensor-augmented pump utilizing a Dexcom G4 CGM. I previously wore a loner Medtronic 530G insulin pump for a few weeks, which was kindly provided by our local Medtronic representative. I personally like the Medtronic and Animas insulin pumps the best, and I think that Medtronic has the best pump download of all the insulin pumps. My short-term experience with the Enlite Sensor was somewhat frustrating and mirrored what I witnessed in many of my patients, who also seemed to have much better experiences with the Dexcom. So, I was both intrigued but also hesitant about the 670G insulin pump. With such rapidly moving technology, I didn't want to commit to the 670G for 4 years, so I actually am now enrolled in a year-long 670G study. I've been in auto mode for a little over 2 weeks. My control has definitely improved, particularly overnight. The Guardian sensor is much improved over the Enlite, but I still think it has quite a ways to go to improve to the level of the Dexcom. I have had several Guardian sensors bleed extensively at insertion, I just removed them immediately and started over with a new sensor. The 670G often wants frequent and, what I consider unnecessary, repeat blood glucose confirmations on day one for a new sensor. To me, this clearly indicates there is more trauma with the sensor insertion than the Dexcom. Moreover, the insertion is not as simple as it is with Dexcom, and I've had reactions to the Medtronic tape a couple of times with some mild contact dermatitis, which is something I never

---

[1]Adult Endocrinology, Park Nicollet Clinic, St. Louis Park, MN.

experienced with Dexcom. I've noticed the same trend with my patients. Overall, I think the Medtronic 670G system is still the best system, but I think the Dexcom has by far the superior CGM, and I look forward to upcoming low-glucose suspend and hybrid closed-loop systems from the Tandem t:slim and Insulet Omnipod CGMs in cooperation with Dexcom. I also look forward to any improvements that Medtronic will make in their CGMSs.

I've never been an early adopter, I prefer to let other people work out the bugs. So, likewise, I was not an early adopter of a CGMS. You might think that a board-certified endocrinologist with type 1 diabetes such as myself would have been willing to jump at each new technology, but I never was. I didn't want more things attached to me, and more alarms going off. But, I must say, my diabetes control has improved with each new technology. Pumps gave me the flexibility to dose insulin without the hassle of injections. The ability to give fractions of a unit of insulin and to do the math for corrections and account for insulin "on board" to reduce hypoglycemia has been well worth it. Before using the 670G system, I previously would set a temporary basal rate or, on occasion, set to 0% basal rate for 30–90 min if exercising on short notice (life is unpredictable with three young children) or if my blood glucose level was dropping too rapidly during exercise, or if I my blood glucose level was falling too quickly from a correction. Also, given a nagging intermittent decade plus history of plantar fasciitis, I have taken to biking, and I particularly like having a pump and a CGM for my longer rides.

As a busy physician, married to a busy physician, with three young children at home, CGM technology has allowed me to minimize hypoglycemia so that I can be "in the game" as much as possible, and not have to take a 20 min time-out to treat as many lows. My sleep is disrupted enough though with my call schedule, my wife's call schedule, and my young children, so I set the high alert on my CGMS to 300 mg/dL so that it doesn't wake me up as much at night. I rarely get that high and watch it frequently enough during the day that I don't miss having a higher alarm for hyperglycemia. Personally, I'd rather wake up with a blood glucose level >200 mg/dL on occasion and have had a good night's sleep, than wake up high on occasion at 2 A.M. and then be stuck awake for 2–3 h. With the 670G, however, I really don't have to worry about that.

I admit that I've never really taken the time to download my devices at home. I know my habits, good and bad, and I can easily recognize if I'm having an increase in hypoglycemia—for example, due to an increase in exercise, such as occurs in the springs here in Minnesota—so that I can make adjustments on the fly, if needed. And if I need to adjust other things, I actually let my endocrinologist make adjustments as she is going to look at my data more objectively than I will.

I have had diabetes for 26 years with only some mild nonproliferative retinopathy, I've become much more relaxed regarding my control. I'm satisfied with an A1C of 6.8–7.2%, for example. My blood pressure runs in the 110s/60s mmHg, my total cholesterol is ~150 with LDLs in the 70s (without statins). Thus, targeting a lower A1C in my individual case won't really lower my risk of complications, but it would increase the risk of hypoglycemia, and that to me isn't worth it. I'm too busy living.

As for my patients, I encourage them to consider the technology, but I never push them. It took me time, and it will take many of them time, too. Some of them will never use a pump or CGM, and that's okay. It's their life. In general, I don't discuss my own diabetes much with my patients, but at times, I share my experience when I feel it is appropriate to do so. I think having firsthand knowledge of the technology really helps me to tailor my recommendations to each patient. My main concern is that this technology helps a fairly motivated patient improve their control, but it really doesn't help a patient who isn't motivated. I've certainly seen some exceptions. I can think of two patients who have pumps, and they seldom test their blood glucose levels unless they are wearing a CGM. When they wear the CGM, they generally test their blood glucose ≥4 times/ day. I have seen patients who have not been able to improve their control much at all with a CGM or a pump, but I have seen other patients who have lowered their A1C by 3% or 4% with a CGM alone. Recently I saw a patient with type 1 diabetes who had an A1C of 12.4% due to missed insulin injections. In just three to four months on a Dexcom G6 this patient brought his A1C down to 6.5% with amazing control and minimal hypoglycemia. CGM technology gave this patient enough feedback to help him remember to take his insulin consistently. This was by far the most draumatic improvement I have seen.

I am excited for where this technology is headed.

Chapter 6
Technophobe!

Mark R. Burge, MD[1,2]

INTRODUCTION

My name is Mark Burge (Figure 6.1). I am 58 years old and have had type 1 diabetes (T1D) for 39 years. Despite the fact that I have pursued a career as an academic endocrinologist and diabetologist (and have achieved some success in that arena), my relationship to diabetes technology has been somewhat conflicted. But before I tell that story, I need to provide some background about my crazy family. I come from a family that is thick with T1D; so much so that I had plans to become a diabetes doctor even before I was diagnosed with the disease myself.

My father was diagnosed with T1D in 1947 at the age of 19 years, and he was the only one on his side of the family who had the disease. On the other side of the family, my mother's older brother was diagnosed with T1D in 1932 at the age of 11 years. I also have two cousins on that side of the family with T1D, but it was my father and my uncle who shaped my earliest impressions of what it meant to live with diabetes. As such, I would like to relate a little bit of their histories, as well as to comment on their own contemporaneous struggles with diabetes technology.

DAVID E. PFUND, JR.

My mother's older brother, David Elmer Pfund, Jr., was born in the tiny Coast Range hamlet of Knappa, Oregon, on November 22, 1920. He was diagnosed with T1D in 1932 at the age of 11 years, <10 years after the initial commercial availability of insulin. His memories of the time of his diagnosis were dominated by "an extreme thirst" that was so severe that he had to drink out of mud puddles on the walk home from school. During the circuitous, 4.5-h car trip from the hospital in Astoria to a larger hospital in Portland, he went into a diabetic coma despite the fact that his physician had given him an injection of insulin in Astoria and had further insisted that they stop at another small town halfway through the journey to receive a second injection.

---

[1]Department of Internal Medicine/Endocrinology, University of New Mexico Health Sciences Center, Albuquerque, NM. [2]Dr. Burge's effort was partially supported by the UNM HSC, Clinical and Translational Science Center, NCATS grant # 8UL1TR000041.

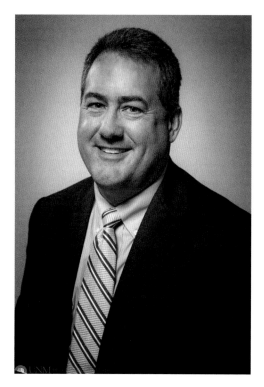

Figure 6.1. Mark R. Burge, MD.

Uncle David's initial insulin injections were strictly of the short-acting variety. A longer-acting (and notoriously unpredictable) insulin, protamine zinc insulin, became available in 1936. During those early years, urine glucose testing was performed using Benedict's Qualitative Test, which resulted in many family stories about boiling David's urine on the family's wood-burning stove in the kitchen. According to a description of the test by Free et al.,

> This time-honored test is based on the reduction of blue cupric ions to orange cuprous ions by sugar in the presence of heat and alkali. Five ml. of Benedict's qualitative reagent and eight drops of urine are mixed in a test tube and heated in a boiling water bath for five minutes. The mixture is cooled, the precipitate is re-suspended, and the colors are graded.[1]

The dietary recommendations that Uncle David received in those early years must have incorporated some high-fat, low-carbohydrate holdovers from the pre-insulin era, because even decades later he would routinely go around the holiday table at meals, asking, "Are you going to eat your fat?" As children, we gave up our turkey skin only reluctantly. But, indeed, the sixth edition of the *Joslin Diabetic*

Manual from 1937 recommends that 47% of daily calories be derived from the ingestion of fat, and it further provides the following dietary advice: "(A) Eat less, (B) Eat less sugar and starch, (C) Eat more vegetables, and (D) Don't lower the carbohydrate too much."[2]

Uncle David graduated from the University of Oregon and worked as a journeyman meat cutter from 1939 to 1942, a country-store owner from 1944 to 1978, a pig farmer from 1968 to 1971, a high school science teacher from 1955 to 1978, and a landlord from 1957 until his death in 2005. In 1942, David joined the U.S. Navy at the height of World War II, conveniently neglecting to inform them about his diabetes. He spent his war years working as a meat cutter in Ilwaco, Washington, and he was discharged in 1944 with full Veteran's benefits. He also taught science at an Air Force Base in Bermuda from 1961 to 1964.

Uncle David was famous in the family for his love of the wild Morel mushroom that grows abundantly in Oregon's temperate rain forests, and for his recurrent hypoglycemic events. In one legendary episode from 1965, he wandered into the woods near his home during an "insulin reaction," where he was discovered hours later by his family, unconscious but snoring. Another time, he was operating his tractor on the farm and fell off the tractor when he became hypoglycemic. The tractor kept going however, and rolled over his shoulder, shattering it. On another occasion, David spent the day cutting firewood on his farm. He had parked his truck inside the barn, so nobody knew he was there. When darkness fell, a neighbor called David's adult daughter and told her that they could hear some strange sounds coming from the woodshed. When she went down to check, she found a perfectly stacked row of firewood from floor to ceiling filling half of the woodshed from wall to wall, but she also heard bird sounds coming from behind the stacked rows of wood. After unstacking the wood, she found her hypoglycemic father sitting in a hidey-hole and making bird noises. The wonder is that if he had not been making any sounds, he may never have been found.

Uncle David was married to my Aunt Darlene for 62 years, and he died at the age of 84 years on October 13, 2005, after nearly 75 years of living with T1D. He lived his final few years without 80% of his gut after having it resected following a bowel infarction. He is remembered for his intelligence, his good humor, and for forgetting to pay me for pulling foxgloves (which are toxic to cattle) on his farm when I was 10 years old. But there are no hard feelings! Photos of David are shown in Figure 6.2.

ROBERT W. BURGE

My father, Robert William Burge, was born on October 28, 1929, in Klamath Falls, Oregon. He was raised in "Six Corners," near Sherwood, Oregon, and he grew up working in his father's berry fields and in the popular roadside "Burge's Store and Service Station" (featuring clean restrooms!) that also served as his home (Figure 6.3). Although Six Corners was located at the intersection of three popular highways, it was a decidedly rural locale. It is now a busy suburb of Portland.

Dad graduated from high school in 1947, and he joined the U.S. Navy shortly thereafter, during the brief interval between World War II and the Korean Conflict. During his period of "boot camp" training in San Diego, dad began to

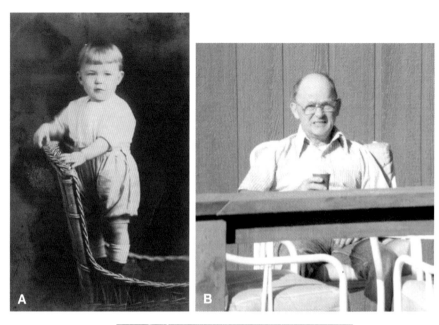

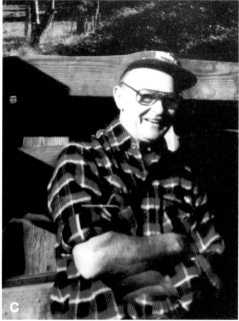

Figure 6.2. My uncle, David Pfund, Jr. **A:** Age 3. **B:** Relaxing circa 1984. **C:** At work on his farm.

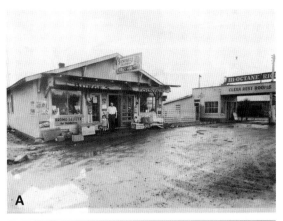

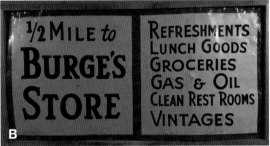

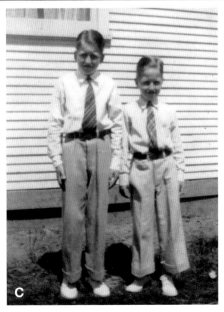

Figure 6.3. *(Continued on p. 354)*

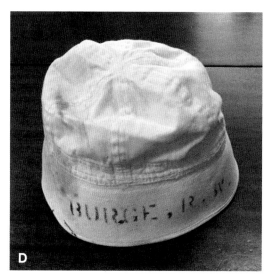

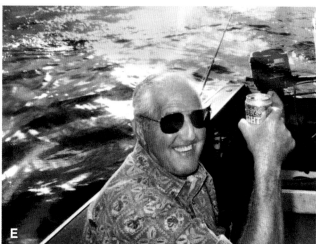

Figure 6.3. A: My grandfather, John M. Burge, and Aunt Beverly at Burge's Store and Service Station in Sherwood, Oregon, the place where my father grew up. **B:** Historic road sign from Highway 99E in Washington County, Oregon. The "clean restrooms" claim was a family joke because dad and his brother used to go in with a garden hose and blast them out. **C:** My father, Robert W. Burge (right) and his older brother Jerry (left), circa 1939, presumably shortly before going to clean the restrooms. **D:** Dad's hat from his short stint in the Navy, circa 1948. **E:** Dad on the Columbia River, circa 1998.

experience symptoms of fatigue and frequent urination. His symptoms became so severe that he frequently had to sneak out of marching formation to go urinate during the long training marches that were a part of the routine back then. He would occasionally get caught doing this, and as a result, he would be assigned additional guard duty at night as a punishment. When he reported to sick bay, the providers were suspicious that he was trying to wriggle out of these duties, and they sent him back out to work without evaluation. During leave for the Christmas holiday in 1947, dad remembered that his mouth was so dry on the train ride back home that he had to take a swig of soda just so that he would have enough moisture in his mouth to converse with his seatmate. By the time the train got to Portland, he was in a diabetic coma that lasted for 3 days. Dad received a medical discharge from the Navy shortly thereafter and was given full Veteran's benefits and a service-connected disability. Those disability checks came in especially handy when they helped put me through medical school. (Parenthetically, it is noteworthy that dad's disability designation was rescinded during the Reagan administration but reinstated during the Clinton administration, resulting in a windfall back payment!)

Dad subsequently graduated from the University of Oregon and worked for 22 years as an outgoing, personable, and effective sales representative for Monroe Industries selling office calculators. After Texas Instruments caused the bottom to drop out of that market in the mid-1970s, dad started another career with the National Park Service at Fort Vancouver, an outpost on the Columbia River that was established by the Hudson Bay Company in 1825. He worked there for another 20 years.

During my childhood, my dad cared for his diabetes by boiling his glass syringe every week or so to sterilize it and by injecting Lilly Iletin Regular and NPH insulin twice a day. I remember it was a big deal to him when the insulin changed from U40 (40 units/cc) to U80 (80 units/cc) and then to U100 in the late 1960s.[3] Those insulins were all derived from beef and pork by-products. He also assessed his glucose control by using Clinitest tablets to monitor his urine glucose levels. The test involved mixing 10 drops of water, 5 drops of urine, and a Clinitest tablet (which provided the heat and the alkali for the ensuing chemical reaction) together in a test tube.[4] After the violent, fizzing chemical reaction was complete, the color of the resulting liquid would reveal the result: blue meant there was no glucose in the urine, while red or orange meant that there was a little or a lot of glucose in the urine. When traveling, dad used Tes-Tape to assess his urine glucose, which was much more convenient but somewhat less accurate.[5]

Dad's first diabetes doctor was a former President of the American Diabetes Association, Dr. Blair Holcomb, from the well-respected Portland Diabetes Clinic, and dad admired Dr. Holcomb immensely. Like many diabetologists, Dr. Holcomb had self-published a series of diabetes self-help books that he would peddle to his patients, and these books featured a fictional character named Hezekiah Perkins, an ersatz diabetes patient who exemplified healthy, mindful living with diabetes (Figure 6.4).[6–8] Dad loved those books and would refer to them frequently, even occasionally verbalizing a rhetorical, "What would Hez do?" Seeing how dad idolized Dr. Blair Holcomb, and later Dr. John W. Stephens, from the Portland Diabetes Clinic made me want to become a diabetes doctor.

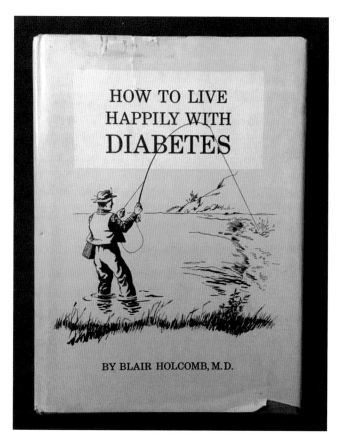

Figure 6.4. Blair Holcomb's Zen-like guide to how to keep a healthy attitude while living with type 1 diabetes.[7]

Shortly after he was diagnosed with diabetes, dad was told that exercise would be essential to his health and survival, and he took that advice to heart. He became an avid runner long before the University of Oregon track coach (and dad's hero), Bill Bowerman, published a book called *Jogging* that started a national craze.[9] Dad's typical routine would be to get up early and run 5 miles around the track of nearby James Madison High School, and he would do this ≥5 days/week. For variety, he would sometimes run to the top of Rocky Butte, a nearby county park. He even participated in one or two of the notorious "Hood to Coast" relay teams during the early years of that event.[10] In retrospect, all of this exercise explains dad's lifelong struggle with hypoglycemia, which was a recurring problem, especially in the days before home blood glucose monitoring. It was not uncommon for him to fall asleep on the couch and then to require a family-wide resuscitation effort that involved the force-feeding of orange juice and nasty, impossibly sticky glucose gel. Toward the end of his life, dad refused to drink any more orange juice, saying, "I've had enough orange juice in my life!"

During the 1970s, dad would be admitted every year or so to the "metabolic unit" of Portland's Good Samaritan Hospital for a week to "get regulated." This allowed his plasma glucose to be measured several times a day and his insulin doses to be adjusted accordingly. He was always scrupulous to follow his daily routine while he was in the hospital, including his daily running, so that the adjustments made to his regimen would reflect his real life. We would visit him in the hospital every night and watch him eat his bland supper. The food was always carefully weighed out so that every calorie of carbohydrate, protein, and fat was accounted for, and dad always wondered why they didn't let him eat like he ate at home. After he returned home, my mother would make a concerted effort for a few weeks to weigh out his food like they did at the hospital, but that laborious process would always eventually fall by the wayside.

One day when my father was 69 years old, he had just finished mowing the lawn and was speaking with his across-the-street neighbor about lawn fertilizer, when he suddenly fell to the ground. It turns out that the neighbor was Dr. Edward Hamel, a local physician with whom I had shared a house for a year during medical school while he was a pediatric intern. Recognizing cardiac arrest, Dr. Hamel performed cardiopulmonary resuscitation on my father for >11 min before an ambulance arrived, performed cardioversion, and resuscitated him. He subsequently underwent a five-vessel coronary artery bypass operation and lived for another 10 high-quality years. Thank you, Eddie!

Dad died on December 29, 2008, on the eve of Oregon's football victory over Oklahoma State in the Holiday Bowl. All told, he lived 79 years, and 60 of those with T1D. He always maintained that he lived a healthier life because of his diabetes, and I believed him. He also maintained that his decision to quit smoking in his 40s saved his life, and he was undoubtedly correct about that. But his decision to marry my mother, Barbara Rose Pfund, in 1959, was likely a more directly lifesaving decision, and they had nearly 50 years together. In many respects, mom disregarded her own dreams and desires out of deference to my father and his diabetes. And I feel that dad's life was necessarily defined by his diabetes in a way that I hope mine will not be, but he would probably disagree with that assessment. I miss him terribly. Photos of my father are shown in Figure 6.5.

MARK R. BURGE

During my second year of college, in December 1979, I returned home from the University of Oregon for the winter break full of pride because I had just received my first report card with straight As. And I was taking hard classes. Somewhat naively, I told my father that I was "working so hard that I was having trouble sleeping and losing a lot of weight." He asked if I was urinating much, and when I answered affirmatively, he marched me into the bathroom and had me go through the Clinitest routine. When the test came back bright orange, he said, "He's got diabetes!" and loaded me into the car. I was 19 years old. We drove to Good Samaritan Hospital, where my blood glucose was 649 mg/dL and my urine was strongly positive for ketones. I was admitted to the Diabetes Unit with diabetic

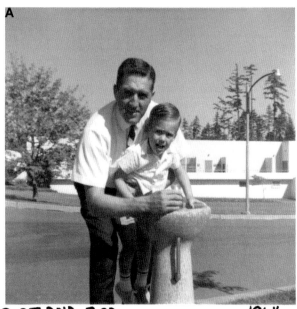

PORTLAND ZOO   1964

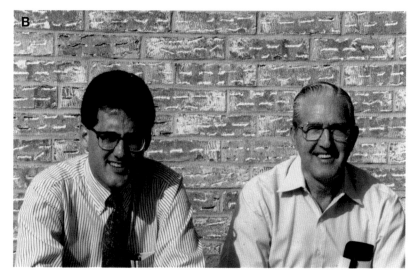

Figure 6.5. Dad and me. **A:** At the Portland Zoo in 1964. **B:** In Madison, Wisconsin, circa 1990.

ketoacidosis, and my family left me there to go to my aunt's Christmas party. Not that I hold a grudge or anything . . .

My father had specifically requested that I receive care from Joslin-trained Dr. John W. Stephens, and when Dr. Stephens came by to see me later that evening, we had a conversation that has stayed with me. He knew that I was familiar with the disease, and he said that the future did not look so bad for me. He said that he felt bad when small children were diagnosed with T1D, but he didn't feel too bad when adolescents were diagnosed with it because he felt that we currently possessed all of the tools necessary to live a healthy and rewarding life with diabetes. I then asked him whether or not a diagnosis of T1D would interfere with my plans to go to medical school, and he said, "Unfortunately, yes. While we have had patients who were diagnosed with diabetes during medical school, we have never successfully gotten a person with preexisting diabetes into the Oregon Health Sciences University (OHSU) School of Medicine."

I was crushed. And I was resentful of my family for leaving me alone while my hopes and dreams were dashed. (OK, maybe I do hold a grudge.) I subsequently switched my college major to "pre-law," but I was never really at peace with that decision, and after a year or so of adjusting to my new diabetes, I decided to risk it all and try for medical school. I matriculated to OHSU in 1983 as the first patient with T1D to be admitted to the School of Medicine, an achievement that I remain proud of.

Those first years with diabetes now seem like the dark ages to me. I initially used the Clinitest urine test to monitor my urine blood glucose and a glass syringe to inject my insulin, just like my dad did. I used regular and NPH insulin twice a day, and I frequently became hypoglycemic while walking around campus in Eugene. Even though I had little money, I became adept at slipping into the student union, a campus restaurant, or even the Faculty Club to grab a few sugar packets off of a nearby table to treat myself. I also remember the switch from beef and pork insulin to recombinant human insulin shortly after I was diagnosed, hoping that this would be a big deal, but ultimately discovering that it made little impact on my day-to-day routine.

In 1982, I got a summer job as a camp counselor working at Gales Creek Camp for children with T1D. The job lasted all summer long and turned out to be one of the most fortuitous opportunities of my life. Aside from making lifelong friends and confirming the career path that I aspired to, it was at Gales Creek Camp that I really figured out how to care for my diabetes. For the first time, I had ample access to Chemstrips capillary blood glucose strips, and with the help of the camp doctors (especially Neil Buist, MB ChB, FRCPE, DCH, and Dr. Kirk Jacobson), I learned how to incorporate self-management of blood glucose into my life. Another benefit of working at Gales Creek Camp was that I was able to procure a year's worth of diabetes supplies at a time. I kept that job for a three consecutive summers, and it instilled in me a true appreciation of the powerful impact that a diabetes camp can have on a young life. This July, I will serve my 29th year as either a camp physician or as the medical director at Camp 180, New Mexico's residential summer camp for children with T1D.

After I started medical school at OHSU in 1983, I met my future wife, classmate Sally Kroner. Sally feigned ignorance of diabetes while I patronizingly talked to her about it, and she enthusiastically helped me cut my Chemstrips lengthwise to make them last longer. And it was she who administered my first dose of gluca-gon during a severe hypoglycemic reaction. Sally eventually became a psychiatrist and enjoys telling people who ask her whether or not she psychoanalyzes me that she had me "figured out years ago." Sally went through medical school on a schol-arship from the U.S. Air Force, and I quickly learned that she owed the Air Force 4 years of service after her training was completed.

Upon the completion of internal medicine residency at the University of Wisconsin, Madison, in 1991, I had applied to all of the endocrinology fellowship programs that were located near an Air Force Base. I received several encouraging letters from people like Dr. Philip Cryer and Dr. Ralph DeFronzo, saying that if my wife were stationed nearby, they would make every effort to accommodate me into their fellowship program. Those letters felt like wonderful news to me. But Dr. David Schade, from the University of New Mexico Health Sciences Center, called me on the phone and asked me for "the name and phone number of the person responsible for making (Sally's) assignment." After providing him with the name and number of Major So-and-So, Dr. Schade flew me out to New Mexico for an interview, and we later learned from him (not the Air Force) the news that, "Your wife is coming to Albuquerque."

Once I started fellowship training, I began being exposed to patients who used "continuous subcutaneous insulin infusion" devices, or insulin pumps to manage their diabetes. When I asked Dr. Schade what he thought about the pump, he took the stance of a skeptical scientist and argued that the pumps were a racket (this is paraphrased) and that no degree of glucose control could be achieved with a pump that could not be achieved with a needle and syringe. As a result, I developed a somewhat distrustful view of my technophile patients. But I remained secretly curious.

Sally completed her Air Force commitment in 1995, and our plans were always for us to return home to Portland and for me to worm my way into the Portland Diabetes Clinic. But by the time she was free to go, I was a faculty member at the University of New Mexico Health Sciences Center with a brand-new grant from the National Institutes of Health and a coveted tenure-track position. Aside from that, we had jointly decided that Albuquerque was a pretty nice place to live and that housing prices were certainly more affordable than in Portland. Meanwhile, I managed my diabetes with Ultralente insulin (Eli Lilly & Co., Indianapolis, IN) injected twice a day, and I was thrilled when the rapid-acting insulin lispro (Humalog; Eli Lilly & Co., Indianapolis, IN) became available in 1996. The intro-duction of an improved basal insulin, insulin glargine (Lantus; Sanofi-Aventis, Bridgewater, NJ), in 2000 made my diabetes management even easier as long as I was willing to do four or five injections per day.

At some point around 2003, a sales representative from MiniMed (Northridge, CA) who had grown weary of hearing my tired argument against insulin pumps marched into my office and said, "Dr. Burge, I have a demo pump here, and I want you to agree to try it for six months." She had given me a MiniMed 508 pump, and I gradually learned to use it and accept it. I traded in the demo and got my own pump later that year, and I eagerly upgraded to the Medtronic Paradigm pump in 2006 (Medtronic PLC, Minneapolis, MN). As I adopted the insulin pump into my life, I was predictably irritated by the cost of the supplies and the inconvenience of kinked tubing, tubing that snagged on door handles, weird batteries, and bad infusion sets. But I continued to use the pump for two principal reasons: *1*) I was having much less hypoglycemia, and *2*) my morning blood glucose levels and A1C levels were undeniably improved by using the variable basal rates that the pump allowed. Conversely, I have had three insulin pumps ruined over the years when they inadvertently joined me in the swimming pool: once in Costa Rica, once at Diabetes Camp in New Mexico, and once in South Africa. Additionally, I gained weight as my glucose control improved, a consequence of wasting fewer ingested calories into my urine. My current pump is a Paradigm 772 pump, which I have used since 2009.

Around 2008, I procured a Dexcom 7 (San Diego, CA) continuous glucose monitor (CGM), and I was thrilled to see how much more stable my blood glucose levels became when I used this device. I was further delighted when, a few months later, I finally achieved an A1C <7% for the first time in decades. But I eventually grew weary of lugging all of the required gear in my pockets (an insulin pump and a CGM receiver in addition to a phone, a pager, my keys, a wallet, and loose change), and I stopped wearing my CGM.

I later started using the Medtronic CGM system because it was more completely integrated with my pump and required one less piece of gear to be carried around. My blood glucose control again improved considerably, and I again experienced the down side of wearing a CGM. Specifically, the Medtronic sensors did not last as long as the Dexcom sensors (3 days vs. 7 days), although I can usually squeeze 6–7 days out of them. More seriously, the low blood glucose alarm seems twitchy and is more likely to awaken Sally than myself during the night (much to her aggravation). And often these alarms are false alarms. Finally, I seem to have a special knack for discarding or losing the $300 sensor chips that are meant to be reutilized at every site change, and the expenses can mount up.

My current diabetes care routine is not unlike that of many of my patients. I have all of the CGM equipment that I need, but I do not use it regularly. My diabetes control is undoubtedly better when I do use it, however, and I experience less hypoglycemia when I am wearing my CGM. It is safe to say that my A1C runs <7.5% when I wear my CGM, and >7.5% when I don't use it. On the down side, I use more insulin when I am wearing my CGM, and I have gained a ton of weight over the past 10 years (~40 lb).

Another factor colors my opinion of current diabetes technology, and that is the aggressive corporate marketing of these products that is directed at both physicians and patients, as well as the large expense that state-of-the-art diabetes care entails. It has sadly become true that the cost of effective diabetes care can rival the cost of HIV or cancer therapy, if not curative hepatitis C therapy.[11] One cost analysis performed by Optum Inc. found that healthcare costs for their employees with diabetes cost 264% more than their employees without diabetes and averaged more than $16,000 per employee in 2016.[12] The absent or incomplete insurance coverage of the costs of insulin pumps and CGM present insurmountable obstacles for many of my patients. And I was particularly irritated when Medtronic's new 670G closed-loop insulin pump, the first to integrate CGM with insulin delivery, was initially made available only to those patients who were using the then-still-new Enlite 530G pump (with a threshold suspend feature). I have this vague, nagging, and only partially rational feeling that if I avail myself to all of the diabetes technology that is accessible to me merely because I can afford it, that I am somehow contributing to the growing divide in health disparity between rich and poor in America.

Conversely, my patients that have been rapid adopters of the technological advances in diabetes care are almost universally pleased with the results they have achieved. I have a half-dozen patients who are using commercially available closed-loop pump devices, and each of them has achieved normal or near-normal A1C levels. Even more inspiring, I have two or three patients who have jerry-rigged their own closed-loop pumps using salvaged hardware and open-source software. One of my patients describes his experience this way:

> In 2015, I became aware of OpenAPS, a group of people who were collaborating over the web to build their own "artificial pancreas system" (APS) using a Dexcom CGM and an old Medtronic pump. This was based on work previously done by the Nightscout Project, whose open source software allows Dexcom blood glucose information to be projected to just about any device, such as watches, phones, or clock radios. Using an obsolete Medtronic insulin pump, it is possible to use a computer to adjust the pump's basal rate over a radio link, and I bought an old $50 pump off Craigslist along with a very tiny pocket-size computer. The computer adjusts the pump using readings from my Dexcom CGM. I still manually control the boluses, but I can target any glucose level (even pre-meal) using my Apple iPhone. The OpenAPS algorithm continuously adjusts my blood glucose to my target, and turns the pump off if it predicts a low blood sugar. I get a lot more sleep, and my glucose curves are much smoother. For someone who has lived with type 1 diabetes for decades, it's heartening to know that there are patients all over the world whose lives are improved (or even saved) through the efforts of this extremely creative and motivated community. For decades, we have passively depended on the products brought to market by the world's pharmaceutical and medical device makers, but (to quote the motto of the Nightscout Project), "we are no longer waiting" (#WeAreNotWaiting).[13]

Progress sometimes seems inevitable, but that is not always the case. It is only through the persistent dedication of scientists, caregivers, educators, and entrepreneurs that advances in diabetes technology have been sustained over the past 100 years. The fact that these innovations are often expensive to the end-user is perhaps not surprising, but compared with other medical advances, the recent advances in technology that have revolutionized diabetes care have the potential to radically improve patient health and quality of life in ways that other medical advances do not. It is a continuing challenge for our society to find a way to offer these advances to all of the people who could benefit from them, just as it remains a challenge for diabetes educators and caregivers to discover ways of optimizing the adoption of these disruptive innovations by minimizing the inconvenience that they sometimes bring to the busy lives of our patients.

But as for me, I think it's time to stop whining and look into getting a closed-loop device . . .

REFERENCES

1. Free AH, Free HM. Urine sugar testing: state of the art. *Lab Med* 1975;6(2): 23–29

2. Joslin EP. Chapter IX: the diet of diabetic individuals. In *A Diabetic Manual.* Philadelphia, Lea & Febiger, 1937, p. 75–92

3. Sheldon J, Gurling KJ, Hill DM, et al. Insulin: U40, U80, or U100? *Br Med J* 1976;2(6047):1319

4. Anonymous. Clinitest Procedure. Available from www.pointofcare.net/ procedures/CLINITEST%20PROCEDURE.htm. Accessed 10 April 2018

5. Free AH, Free HM. Rapid convenience urine tests: their use and misuse. *Lab Med* 1978;9(12):9–18

6. Holcomb B. A study of blood sugar curves before and after thyroidectomy. *Endocrinology* 1929;13(5):467–476

7. Holcomb B. *How to Live Happily with Diabetes: Being the Chronicles of One Hezekiah Perkins, a Man Who Just Happened to Have Diabetes.* Portland, Barkerbrook Press, 1968

8. Holcomb B. *A Diabetic Notebook for Use of the Patient.* 4th ed. Portland, Arcady Press, 1946

9. Bowerman WJ, Harris WE. *Jogging: A Medically Approved Physical Fitness Program for All Ages.* New York, Grosset & Dunlap, 1975

10. Anonymous. Hood to coast relay. Available from https://hoodtocoastrelay. com/htc/relay-info. Accessed 23 April 2018

11. Riddle MC, Herman WH. The cost of diabetes care: an elephant in the room. *Diabetes Care* 2018;41(5):929–932

12. Anonymous. The rising cost of diabetes care. Available from www.optum. com/resources/library/rising-cost-diabetes-care.html. Accessed 26 April 2018

13. Klingler KD. Personal communication. 25 April 2018

Chapter 7
Ramblings on Type 1 Diabetes

JORDAN PERLMAN, MD[1]

I didn't make the decision to get an insulin pump so I thought I should ask the people who did—my parents:

> We were absolutely stunned at Jordan's diagnosis of type 1 diabetes (age 9). We assumed she just needed glasses. It was difficult to focus on management during her brief hospitalization. There was so much information and we were processing this tremendous loss. We wanted to be told what was best. As lawyers, we knew enough to seek expertise. The Chief of Pediatric Neurosurgery at Children's National Medical Center introduced us to Jordan's first diabetes doctor. This physician was enthusiastic about insulin pumps. She made the device seem like a reward for being responsible. The most appealing feature was that it would allow Jordan to be more spontaneous. As parents, we trusted Jordan's doctors to make good medical decisions. We focused on helping her find some semblance of normal. We insisted that Jordan have the latest technologies as a means of achieving this goal (no matter what they cost). Though we no longer manage blood glucose levels, we continue to provide financial support so Jordan can access any treatment she feels might make her life better.

As a physician, I wish I took better advantage of available pump technologies. I have a Medtronic 530G but I refuse to upgrade because I'm reluctant to forfeit control. I'm meticulous but not precise about blood glucose management. I don't use mathematical calculations to determine insulin doses so I haven't benefited from most of the existing pump features. I can't remember ever downloading pump data for review outside an endocrine office. I didn't choose to get an insulin pump, but I have occasional reservations about keeping it (not related to mechanics). I (sort of) blame the pump for some weight issues. It's much easier to binge, absent the need for extra shots. I realize this is a personal restraint problem, but shots provide an artificial barrier. I suppose a more tangible disadvantage is getting the tubing stuck on hooks and doorknobs (traumatic infusion set removal hurts). I've had great luck avoiding tubing occlusions and pump malfunctions— and continuous glucose monitoring (CGM) helps me detect these crises earlier. I do experience far less anxiety knowing the pump allows constant and immediate

[1]Internal Medicine Resident, University of Washington, Seattle, WA.

access to insulin. I'd argue that this is the adult version of freedom. I'm not aware of an alternative that can provide this same reassurance.

I believe CGM is the greatest diabetes advancement I've witnessed since diagnosis. This, however, is a more recent revelation. I had a disastrous introduction to CGM. I received the MiniMed RT-CGM system as part of a free pump (Paradigm) upgrade (2008). I don't think I ever got an accurate blood glucose reading from that sensor. I also recall seeing blood on the sheets following several (separate) barbaric insertions. I got burned on insulin doses because I was arrogant and stopped checking finger-sticks. I had so much hypoglycemia that I decided having no information was better than using CGM. I couldn't reconcile wearing an extra device just to detect trends, so I reverted to previous irresponsible practices. I was a college sophomore (I was 19 years old).

I went back to CGM because of peer pressure (plain and simple). I started medical school and met a much more responsible person with diabetes who wore a Dexcom Seven. I also wanted to impress my new endocrinologist. I was too embarrassed to admit I wasn't using CGM, so I lied and bought a Dexcom G4 (I was 24 years old). This purchase changed how I experience type 1 diabetes. It made management decisions more academic (and less emotional). The feelings of personal failure evaporated once I could demonstrate tangible causation. I have not had functional challenges using CGM. I do wish the Dexcom G5 would stop alarming high when I'm sick and want to sleep. There's so much available information that I sometimes struggle to reconcile the different metrics for blood glucose control. I'm no longer certain I understand what's most important for preventing complications. I sometimes wonder whether we need to give endocrinologists a few seconds to breathe.

I do have an incredible Dexcom experience to share (although it belongs mostly to someone else). This incident occurred soon after I graduated from medical school (I was 27 years old). I was an (inexperienced) emergency medicine intern covering overnight for the internal medicine teams. The schedule was brutal, and I was always exhausted. On this particular night, I had gone to a resident sleep room for a powernap. I hadn't been asleep for more than a few minutes when I heard a Dexcom alarm. I looked but it wasn't mine. I tried to go back to sleep, but the alarm persisted (and I had trained ears). I left the call room and wandered down the hall listening outside different doors. It took about 15 minutes but I found the source of the alarm and banged on the door. The room was locked and the (possible) occupant silent. I was joined by an orthopedics resident who (somehow) removed the doorknob. We entered the room to discover an unconscious male resident on the bed. His Dexcom receiver was on the table beside him. It was alarming low. I had a tube of decorative cake icing in my bag, and we managed to get most of it under the resident's tongue (I guess someone was also calling the emergency department). He awoke before the STAT nurses arrived but needed intravenous dextrose. I never saw him again but I'm guessing that Dexcom alarm saved his life.

Chapter 8

From Purified Pork to Pumps: How Technology Has Impacted My Life with Diabetes

JENNIFER SHERR, MD, PhD[1]

S itting on the exam table, at the age of 10 years, with the standard hospital-issued patient gown draped over me, I lowered my prop into place and waited for the door to open. My pediatric endocrinologist, Dr. Max Salas, knocked on the door and was greeted by the loudest snorting noise I could make. Grinning behind a plastic pig nose, I stated, "I think I may be on too much purified pork insulin."

Being diagnosed with type 1 diabetes (T1D) in 1987, I was keenly aware of how lucky I was. After all, the discovery of insulin meant my condition was not a death sentence and many reassured me that I would be cured in "the next 5 years." Although three decades have elapsed, I am hopeful for the day a cure will be found, but in the meantime, I am grateful for the technology that has revolutionized how I care for both myself and my patients.

A summertime diagnosis afforded me the time to adjust to this chronic medical condition for a few months before starting 4th grade. Recognizing the importance of testing my blood glucose, I knew I wanted to keep my glucometer with me at all times. I adopted the strategy of carrying a purse everywhere—not for the sake of fashion but merely in an attempt to be practical. I remember placing a drop of blood on my OneTouch and waiting the 45 sec (which felt like eons) when I knew I was hypoglycemic but needed to see the result before treating. There were meters that required blotting a drop of blood and used a colometric test, while others required cleaning the meter with a cotton swab. I tell patients about the lancet device that reminded me of a guillotine. Just remember to hold your hand steady as the needle whipped around to prick your finger.

At the start of the school year, I was determined to share with my classmates what had transpired over summer vacation. I stood at the front of the classroom and told them about my diagnosis and hospitalization. To assure them everything was okay, I tested my blood in front of them. I vividly recall watching a boy in my class become quite pale and require the nurse's attention after my demonstration. In fact, I was hyperglycemic, precipitating the teacher to buddy us up to walk to the nurse's office.

Although use of glucometer technology was a mainstay of my treatment plan since my diagnosis, I was leery to embrace continuous subcutaneous insulin pump therapy. As a teen, I could not reconcile having a piece of equipment that would

[1]Associate Professor, Pediatrics (Endocrinology), Yale University School of Medicine, New Haven, CT.

be constantly connected to me. While at Camp Nejeda, a New Jersey camp specifically designed for youth with diabetes, I recall that my aversion to pump therapy was further solidified by bunkmates when we headed to the showers. In separate stalls, I watched as one of my peers carefully hung a plastic bag holding her insulin pump onto the showerhead. The idea of the pump as a "constant companion" was the basis of my nightmares.

Yet, as high school wore on, my parents and Dr. Salas worked tirelessly to help me understand how a pump could improve my care. They discussed the flexibility it would afford me. I would no longer be tied to strict mealtimes because of my insulin regimen. With college on the horizon and an understanding that they all had my best interest at heart, I acquiesced to try this new insulin delivery modality. I did have one condition—the initiation of pump therapy had to be scheduled for the Monday *after* my senior prom. My concern about where to stash a piece of medical equipment in a gown was more than I could manage.

Transitioning to the pump was quite a production. My parents and I filed into my doctor's office to learn about how to fill the reservoir with insulin and insert a site, thankfully, one that could be disconnected. Our diabetes treatment vocabulary was expanded as we learned about basal rates and bolusing. Looking back, it strikes me that the MiniMed 506 required some extra effort. It was critical to prime the pump to ensure the pump motor driver arms were securely clasping the reservoir plunger and 357 batteries were required to make the machine work. My local pharmacy began stocking those batteries, and I paid close attention to that reservoir.

Despite the idiosyncrasies of pumping, it was evident from the start that I was reaping benefits. Testing my blood one day shortly after the transition, I was positive I would be hypoglycemic. Yet, the reading was well within targeted range. Thinking something was wrong with my meter, I repeated it two more times until I was convinced the result was true. Perplexed by the situation, I talked to my mom and realized that, for the first time, I could remember the sensation of hunger. I was no longer tied to a rigid eating schedule and instead I could let mealtimes become more fluid. Now my body was able to alert me to something that wasn't an urgent situation but rather a nuisance. I relished in the normality of it all.

I realized during the beginning of my freshman year at college that, just as I had done in grade school, I would just test and bolus as prescribed. This opened the door for me to begin sharing with a whole new group of peers that I had T1D. My diabetes technology provided me with a surefire way to break the news.

During my final year of medical school, a new feature for the pump was released—a bolus calculator. In considering whether I should pay out of pocket to upgrade to this new system and understanding that in residency erratic schedules would be my new norm, I made the leap. Although it seemed to some to be a small incremental step in pumping insulin, it made a difference for me. Before the use of a bolus calculator, all my boluses ended with a zero or a five after the decimal point. My reluctance to do math and my preference for rounding was evident. In the midst of my transition to pediatric residency, use of a smarter pump allowed me to let technology carry some of the burden of my chronic condition (Figure 8.1).

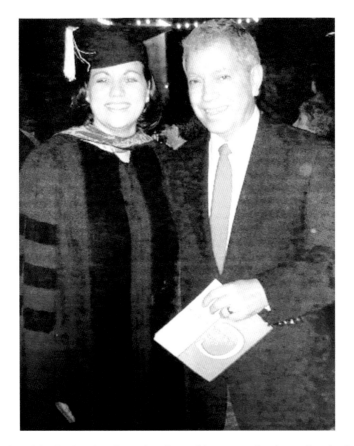

Figure 8.1. Medical school graduation with my pediatric endocrinologist, Dr. Max Salas.

With the advent of continuous glucose monitors (CGM), I was eager to visualize the degree of variability I was experiencing. Yale was one of the sites that was conducting the JDRF CGM trial, and as second-year fellow, I was so excited to sign the consent form. After going through the necessary blinded data collection phase, it came time for my randomization visit. As soon as I was placed in the sensor group, I had what I would consider to be a "The Price Is Right" moment. Just like someone in the audience who is chosen to play in the televised game show, I jumped out of my chair, waved my hands, cried, and called my mom. Needless to say, I was elated.

Beginning my sensor wear, I wanted to use the data to obtain perfection—that is, diabetes perfection. I set my low limit to 70 mg/dL and my high limit to 180 mg/dL. On the night after I started the sensor and it alarmed incessantly, my enthusiasm dwindled. In fact, over the next week, I distinctly remember ripping out the sensor in the middle of the night and throwing it across my bedroom. Clearly, I needed to evaluate my mind-set: what is perfection and is it attainable with this disease? So, I raised my upper limit to 300 mg/dL and then slowly lowered it step by step to 210 mg/dL, where it now remains. By allowing myself to set more realistic expectations, I was able to utilize the sensor effectively—learning how best to bolus for the pizza that has made New Haven famous. Exercise was more manageable as sensor glucose readings and trend arrows informed my decision to carbohydrate load and see how different activities impacted my glucose levels. Wearing a sensor was like being Dorothy in the Wizard of Oz, my world went from black-and-white Kansas, to the beautiful land of Oz that was drenched in Technicolor.

As I finished my fellowship, I met my soulmate. After years of focusing on medical school and training, I learned there was more to life. Like most brides, I dreamed of the perfect wedding dress. But, I wasn't looking for a certain cut or designer, I just wanted pockets. Why? How could I choose to be blind on my wedding day? Removing my pump and sensor would have been like taking away the blanket that Linus clings to in the Peanuts gang. Luckily, I found an amazing bridal shop that figured out how to create a pocket in the tuft of my dress, the tubing of my pump was strung through the layers of lace and provided me the opportunity to check my sensor glucose trend before I headed down the aisle (Figure 8.2).

After getting married, my mind and focus turned to my desire to have a child. Immediately following my wedding, I had the great fortune of joining a family, as my husband was part of a package deal with two children from his previous marriage. Yet, I yearned for one more child to complete our family (Figures 8.3 and 8.4).

Figure 8.2. Wedding day with Drs. Tamborlane, Weinzmer, and Ambrosino.

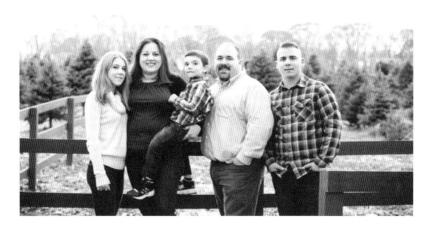

Figure 8.3. Family photo 2017.

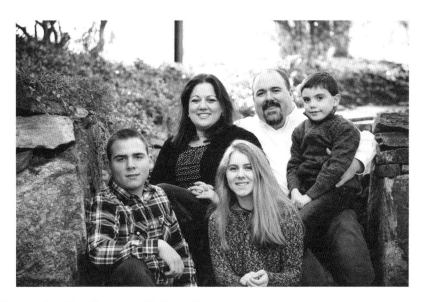

Figure 8.4. Family photo (Fall 2018).

Even before our marriage, we went for preconception counseling. In the preceding years, I had attended numerous sessions at conferences learning about neonatal complications secondary to diabetes. I was worried, fearful, and guilty knowing that despite my best efforts, my child would be exposed to a womb that was a little "too sweet." Here again, use of sensor-augmented pump therapy provided me a sense of control in what was an otherwise-daunting ordeal. I tightened my high alert, watched my sensor glucose constantly and bolused diligently.

When I went into labor, I advised the labor and delivery team that I would be managing my blood glucose levels with my pump during labor. Faced with a situation that felt entirely out of my control, I wanted to ensure I had control of my blood glucose levels. When it was decided that I needed a C-section, I remember being worried about whether I caused my child to be too large, precipitating the need for this intervention. The obstetrician on delivering my child remarked, "look at those shoulders, he is going to be a linebacker." My son's entry into the world was marked by the need to head to the neonatal intensive care unit because of some brief hypoglycemia and transient tachypnea of the newborn, a condition that can be seen in infants born via C-section (Figure 8.5). In my postpartum state, I struggled to cope with the fact that I had done the best I could to manage my glucose levels during pregnancy. The data downloads that I could review provided me with solace.

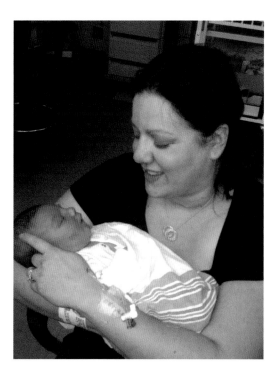

Figure 8.5. Birth of my son.

In summer 2015, our group at Yale was in the process of looking for participants for the Medtronic 670G pivotal trial. Having participated in numerous studies in the past, I was interested in enrolling. After discussing the situation with the ethics review board at Yale and assuring them I had not been coerced to participate, my desire to take part in the study was realized. Baseline data was collected from my usual pump settings programmed into the study equipment and, when the time came to transition to hybrid closed-loop insulin delivery, I was ripe with anticipation. But how would I, as someone whose strategy had been to constantly think about my sensor glucose levels and alter my insulin delivery with temporary basal rates and corrections, relinquish so much control to a device? It was very hard at first.

Despite working on closed-loop research endeavors for nearly a decade before starting in the study, I was leery to believe the system would work as intended. Was the autobasal suspending prior to a low, which at that point seemed inevitable based on my sensor glucose trend, adequate enough to avoid hypoglycemia? I obsessively counted up the micro-boluses delivered by autobasal and compared them to my pre-set open-loop basal rates questioning: did the units per hour make sense based on my sensor glucose values? I was quickly reminded about my aversion to math and realized that the system could be trusted. So, I sat back and watched it work. Yet, after working diligently to ensure that my fasting glucose was <100 mg/dL on most days, it was difficult to see it come in above this goal as I continued with system wear. I had been well within targeted control at the start of the study, and I wondered how it would pay off by the end of 3 months. To my surprise, my hemoglobin A_{1c} fell by 0.4%. I was astonished.

It was phenomenal to experience automation's success to better my painstakingly-achieved targeted glycemic control. Other outcomes, however, were the ones that truly made a difference to my life. In speaking to my kids at the end of the 3-month study period, I asked whether they noticed any difference (Figure 8.6). Without skipping a beat, my then 13-year old son responded, "Yeah, you are nicer." I was surprised by his judgment, but as we sat and pondered what that meant, it was evident that my nights were no longer interrupted by responding to sensor alarms or struggling to sleep with wide glycemic swings. Just as the pump had reintroduced me to the concept of hunger, the hybrid closed-loop system identified how chronically tiring living with T1D can be. This new system afforded me the opportunity to sleep and know that it would regulate things so each morning starts on the right foot.

From the time of my diagnosis, my goal was to enter the medical field. I emulated Dr. Salas in his support of my parents' contention that I was first and foremost a child; I just happened to be one who had diabetes. As I pursued a career in medicine my initial plan had been to be a clinician, more specifically, be Dr. Salas. I had wonderful role models, not just in my care team, but also in my family. Yet, I assured my mother, a clinical research nurse, that research was not for me. I went to the dual bachelor's and medical degree program at Rutgers College and the University of Medicine and Dentistry of New Jersey, Robert Wood Johnson Medical School. My path for residency took me to Yale, and there I met Dr. Bill Tamborlane. As I sat in his office soliciting advise on where I should apply to fellowship, he inquired about my career path. We knew each other from the wards, and as many are likely to attest, Dr. Tamborlane is quite a character.

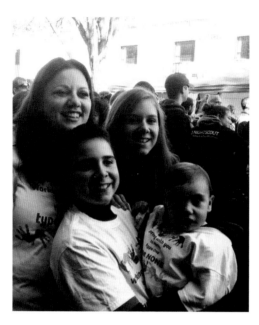

Figure 8.6. Walk with my three kids in 2014.

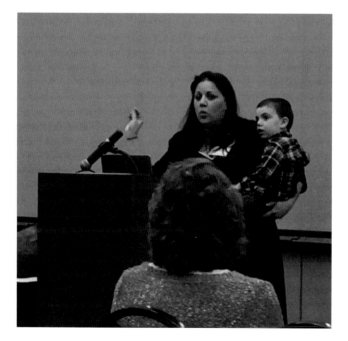

Figure 8.7. JDRF summit with my clingy son.

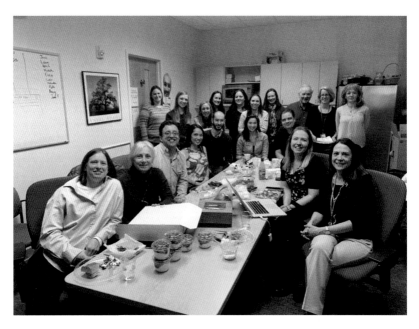

Figure 8.8. Yale pediatric diabetes research team.

He searched in his filing cabinet and pulled the *New England Journal of Medicine* paper describing the use of insulin pump therapy and wrote at the top of the paper "Jen, You're welcome for saving your life," —Bill. He took the time to explain to me that in clinical practice you will influence the patients you see, but in research your reach can be so much larger.

My course was altered. I set about my journey to become a physician scientist (Figure 8.7). Somehow despite my adamant stance as a young adult that research was not for me, with Dr. Tamborlane's suggestion, I found myself pursuing a doctoral degree in investigative medicine offered at the Yale Graduate School of Arts and Sciences (Figure 8.8). My ultimate goal was to help the many, who like me, are living with diabetes.

Looking back on the studies I have been a part of, both as a patient and as an investigator, I believe we are in the midst of a technological revolution. I am excited for what the future holds and I am grateful for my colleagues who continue to explore ways to prevent and cure T1D. Until that cure is found, I am hopeful that continued technological advances will allow all of us living with diabetes to minimize burdens of treatment and remain in targeted control; thus, increasing the likelihood we can be candidates for a cure when it is available.

Chapter 9

From Living in the Dark Ages to the Artificial Pancreas

Steven Edelman, MD[1]

L et me start from the very beginning. I was born on Labor Day, 6 September 1955. I was a typical kid until I was 15 years old, when I started to develop the classic symptoms of weight loss, excessive thirst, tiredness, and poor wound healing. I clearly remember at that time having a scab on my knee that just would not heal. In between my middle-school classes at Patrick Henry Junior High in the San Fernando Valley outside of Los Angeles, I would run to the restroom to urinate and relieve my distended aching bladder, and then slurp up as much water as possible at the drinking fountain. I just could not quench my thirst, and I remember all of the kids in line behind me yelling at me because I took so long. Then halfway through my next class, I would have to ask my teacher for a bathroom pass and urinate again and desperately seek out the nearest drinking fountain. My teachers were annoyed with me because I was the only kid to ask for the bathroom pass every single day. I was also reprimanded several times for falling asleep in class. I just could not keep my eyes open, and I had hardly any energy at all. By the time that class was over, my bladder was bursting again, and I would be dying of thirst. I would come home from school and go to bed at 3 p.m. and sleep until the next morning. I lost 20 lb, which I loved because I was always a little chunky. My nickname at school was "the stump." I also remember a family vacation in Mexico when I drank nothing but bottle after bottle of soft drinks, which were packed with sugar and, of course, made matters worse. Even if diet drinks had been available, I would not have ordered one, because I did not know I was developing diabetes, a condition I had never heard of before.

Finally, I realized something was wrong, and I asked my mother to take me to the doctor. We went to the urgent-care unit of my health maintenance organization and had my blood and urine collected for tests. The doctor spent a few minutes with me asking medical questions. After looking at the results of my tests, he called in an army of nurses who urgently wheel-chaired me off to the intensive care unit (ICU) to give me intravenous (IV) fluids and insulin. I was in the hospital for 1 week and during my stay, all kinds of people came to my bedside to tell me about diabetes. Several nurses kept telling me time and time again, "You can live a normal life"; I had no clue what they were talking about, but after a while, it started to make me nervous. When you are first diagnosed and in emotional shock,

[1]Professor of Medicine, University of California–San Diego, Veterans Affairs Medical Center, San Diego, CA; Founder and Director, Taking Control of Your Diabetes, Solana Beach, CA.

retaining information is pretty difficult. I do remember attending a diabetes class during the first week in the hospital. There I was, a newly diagnosed, young, naïve teenage boy with type 1 diabetes, sitting in a room with about 25 very obese, older people, all with type 2 diabetes. The single fact I remember from that class in 1970 was that ketchup has a lot of sugar in it. I kept thinking, "What am I going to dip my french fries in now?" I had lots of fun practicing how to give insulin injections into an orange, but the fun ended when it got to be my leg. Syringe technology at that time was just past the era of sharpening your old needles with an emery board. We have come a long way from 12-mm, 23-gauge needles to 4-mm, 32-gauge sharpened and lubricated syringes.

The other big fiasco that I remember at that time was the first injection I received from a new nurse after I was moved to a regular hospital room from the ICU. She came in with what looked like a horse syringe. It was huge and reminded me of a large supersoaker that I used for waterfights with the kids on my block. The nurse proceeded to inject me with this large syringe, which really hurt because of the large volume of insulin that was forced into my thigh. A short time later, the doctor who was assigned to take care of me, who was not a diabetes specialist, came in to see me. I asked him why the shot was so large, and he was also puzzled. To make a long story short, the nurse had misread the doctor's order. Instead of giving me 15 units of insulin (handwritten very sloppily as 15U), she gave me 150 units of insulin. Then all hell broke loose. They put me back in the ICU, stuck some more IV lines in me, made me drink very sweet fluids, and drew blood to test my blood glucose every 5 or 10 min for several hours. Talk about feeling like a pincushion. All hospitals now have a rule that the word "units" must be written out completely and not indicated by just a capital U. We now have electronic medical records, a technology that for sure has helped to avoid errors like this.

Even while attending the diabetes class that first week while in the hospital, my instincts told me that this was not the best learning environment for someone like me, and there had to be a better way. Eventually I was discharged to go home on only one shot a day in the morning of NPH and regular insulin, and I was given a strict diet using the old exchange system, by which I would weigh all of my portions of protein, carbohydrate, and fat on a little scale. What a pain! I was supposed to test my urine for glucose 4 times/day and keep records of everything. This was the state-of-the-art technology to follow how I was doing at home with my diabetes. At first, with the help of my mother, I did everything by the book, but eventually I lost interest. I did not realize why it was so important, and I certainly was not informed or motivated to take control of my diabetes. My father, who was not around very much, did not believe I had diabetes. That part of my family life deserves a separate book or television series; it would make *The Goldbergs* look normal.

I would see my doctor every 3 months, have my blood and urine collected in the morning, and then wait the usual 2–3 h for the results to come back from the lab. Remember that in 1970, there were no home glucose meters or A1C tests. My doctor would come into the room, look at the results, which was a single blood glucose level at one point in time from that morning, and say the same thing every time: "Steve, you are doing fine. I will see you next time." In addition, I never went to a camp for kids with diabetes or spent any time in support groups or classes for young people with diabetes. I was never educated about how to take an active role in my own diabetes care, and as a result, my control started to slip.

It took me several years before I realized that I should do something about the fact that I was probably not doing well, despite the repeated comments at every visit from my doctor that I was "doing fine." I truly did not know that I was doing harm to my body. I was not a rebellious teenager who purposely went out of control to gain attention. I simply was never told in a way that I understood what my goals of control should be and why it was so important.

On one occasion, I decided to test my doctor, because what he was saying to me at every visit did not make sense. On the morning of my next appointment, I went to Winchell's Donut Shop and ate five donuts, including two glazed, two chocolate cake, and one maple bar (my favorite!). I then proceeded to give my urine and blood samples at the office as usual. I remember using my own urine test strips in the hospital bathroom to test the sample I turned in for analysis. The strip turned black in ~3 sec, indicating that my urine was packed with sugar. I waited the usual 2–3 h, and finally, my doctor walked into the examination room holding his clipboard and studying the results of the blood and urine tests. He looked me straight in the eye and said, "Steve, you are doing fine. I will see you next time." From that point onward, I knew I could not trust him to take care of me, and I made a decision never to see that doctor again.

The bad news is that those early years of poor control contributed greatly to my development of several diabetic complications. I have proliferative diabetic retinopathy and macular edema, and I have received extensive laser surgery to both eyes to stabilize the problem. I was recently diagnosed with diabetic macular edema, which requires me to have intraocular injections every month. I have diabetic kidney disease, causing protein to spill into my urine and give me high blood pressure, for which I take three different medications to control the situation. I also have some manifestations of diabetic neuropathy (hypoglycemia unawareness and gastroparesis). The good news is that I sought out incredible diabetes specialists, such as Drs. Mayer Davidson and Richard Berkson, and started to receive the appropriate treatment to minimize and slow down the progression of these complications. I feel fortunate that I was able to improve my control at a time when my complications were not extremely advanced.

I was always interested in science and decided to go to medical school. At the University of California at Los Angeles (UCLA), where I did my undergraduate premedical studies, I became more interested in medicine and, specifically, diabetes. I worked in a diabetes research laboratory and observed patients in diabetes clinic. During that time, I also realized that one shot a day was totally inadequate, and I improved my regimen to allow for better control. Later, during my last year in medical school, I went on one of the first insulin pumps and became "fuel injected." Over the past several years, I have experimented with the new rapid-acting and long-acting designer insulin analogs, inhaled insulin, pramlintide (Symlin, an amylin analog), and continuous glucose monitoring (CGM) to try to find a regimen that fits my lifestyle the best. The advances in technology to manipulate the insulin structure made a huge difference for me and for millions of others taking insulin around the world.

I remember quite vividly when I studied physiology during my first year of medical school in 1978 at the University of California, Davis campus.

The professor was citing statistics from old textbooks about the high death rate in people with diabetes. He stated that 50% of people with diabetes die from diabetic kidney disease within 20 years after the initial diagnosis. During the lecture, my classmates were trying to avoid eye contact with me or attempted to give me some type of visual sympathy from across the lecture hall (both situations made me feel uncomfortable). That afternoon we had a physiology laboratory and had to dissect the cadaver of a 25-year-old male who had died of diabetic kidney disease. At the time, I was 23 years old with 8 years of diabetes behind me. My best friend, Ken Facter, always tried to comfort me by saying that at least I knew what I was going to die of. These early experiences motivated me to take better care of myself and to devote my career to helping people with diabetes. Tragically, Ken died suddenly of a heart attack at the age of 40 years. His death was a painful wake-up call to me that we must live every day to the fullest and not take one second of life for granted.

After my medical residency at UCLA, I did the first part of my diabetes specialty training (fellowship) at the Joslin Diabetes Clinic in Boston. I learned a great deal about all aspects of diabetes care and I also gave lectures to the patients admitted to the Joslin Clinic. I was always impressed by how thirsty the patients were for information about their condition. Those early interactions with patients had a profound impact on my career as a physician and educator.

I eventually ended up in San Diego, where I am a professor at the University of California San Diego School of Medicine and a staff member of the Veterans Affairs Medical Center for >31 years, if you can believe that! Here, I met two of my mentors and very close friends, Alain Baron and Bob Henry. They were two incredible role models who have selflessly supported the development of so many young people needing guidance in their careers. I now can say I have had the privilege of helping other younger doctors, such as Jeremy Pettus and Tricia Santos, in their career development. I also have had the honor and privilege of serving our country's veterans living with diabetes. This is such a special population of real heroes.

TAKING CONTROL OF YOUR DIABETES

Taking the Messages of Diabetes Care and Technology to "the People"

As a young faculty member, I spent a lot of time and energy after the results of the Diabetes Control and Complications Trial were released in 1993[1] trying to educate healthcare providers on how to take better care of their patients with diabetes. It was slow going, however, and diabetes care was not improving fast enough at the community level. I realized there were many barriers at that time that limited successful diabetes management. Here are a few:

- Managed care was beginning to hamper proper medical care in a major way.
- As a caregiver, I was fairly helpless in trying to fight the system.
- Very little education was directed toward people with diabetes.
- It took too long for information to filter down from the major research institutions to the specialists and then to the healthcare provider.

These specialists and healthcare providers, in turn, had to change their practice habits before their patients could be the recipients of a proven treatment strategy, new device, or medication. For these reasons, I decided to take the most important messages directly to those who were most affected by this condition.

In 1995, I had the idea of putting on a large conference for 1,000 people with diabetes called Taking Control of your Diabetes (TCOYD). I joined forces with my long-time colleague and friend, Sandy Bourdette, and we produced our first conference at the San Diego Convention Center, focusing on education, motivation, and self-advocacy. I realized early on that this approach could make a significant impact on diabetes care in this country, and it was a large piece of the diabetes-care puzzle that was missing.

Since the beginning of TCOYD in 1995, we have been pushing these three important themes and they have never lost their importance or magnitude:

1. *You have the main responsibility for taking control of your diabetes.* This is your life, and no one should be more interested in getting the best healthcare than you. The responsibility does not lie with your wife, husband, mother, father, sister, brother, or doctor. Your doctor does not bear the main responsibility for your health; that is your responsibility. It is you who will personally suffer if you develop blindness or kidney failure, not your physician.
2. *You are your own best advocate.* In these days of managed care and the shrinking healthcare dollar, it is becoming increasingly difficult to obtain the proper care you deserve and need to stay healthy. You must become knowledgeable about and get involved with the administrative aspects of your healthcare system so that you have timely access to the proper tests, most effective medications, and latest medical devices. This can be a frustrating and time-consuming process that can wear you down, but in the end, you will win if you are persistent.
3. *Be smart and be persistent.* Educate yourself about preventive measures, including advances in technology to avoid eye, kidney, nerve, and heart disease. Be knowledgeable about the screening tests used to diagnose diabetes-related problems early so that you can obtain proper treatment in time. Be current on all of the various treatment options available to aggressively treat any complication that you have so that its progression will be slowed or halted.

Simply stating these themes is one thing, but getting folks to take ownership of their health is another. That was the challenge. At that very first conference in 1995, I realized how thirsty people with diabetes were for information about their condition and how much more needed to be accomplished. Getting people to put diabetes high on their priority list is a key component for long-term success and depends so much on individualizing communication and education styles, as well as therapeutic strategies.

TCOYD became a not-for-profit organization and has grown steadily, while maintaining a high level of quality and impactful programs across the U.S.[2]

Several years ago, I realized there was another piece of the diabetes-care puzzle that was still missing. It was related to the communication and understanding between the caregiver and the person with diabetes.

A huge challenge is to improve the knowledge and attitudes of caregivers toward their patients struggling with diabetes and create an empathetic atmosphere with more open communication, avoiding the inappropriate labeling of patients as "noncompliant." I have never met a patient who did not want to live a long and healthy life, and the vast majority of healthcare providers went into the field of medicine to help people. Our unique Making the Connection initiative puts the doctor's learning environment smack in the middle of a TCOYD patient conference. For part of the day, they are in their own room receiving several cutting-edge lectures from experts in the field. They also join the people with diabetes attending the patient conference during several parts of the day. Keeping the healthcare professional up to date on the latest technology to help their patients is another huge challenge.

At the end of the day, the professionals have a better understanding of what it is like to live with diabetes on a day-to-day basis. In turn, the people with diabetes realize that our healthcare system is in need of repair and that the providers are under lots of different pressures. Most of all, the people with diabetes learn that their healthcare providers are on their side and need to be educated just as much as they do.

I believe that teaching institutions should educate both the professionals and patients together on a parallel track and encourage a bidirectional exchange of information between the caregivers and the people with diabetes. The key message for people with diabetes is to help your caregiver take better care of you. Our mission statement says it all:

> Guided by the belief that every person with diabetes has the right to live a healthy, happy, and productive life, TCOYD educates and motivates people with diabetes to take a more active role in their condition and provides innovative and integrative continuing diabetes education to medical professionals caring for people with diabetes.[3]

The main message I want to convey is that people can take control of their diabetes, even if they already have complications. It is never too late to get in control, both mentally and physically. The concept of TCOYD embodies the philosophy of self-help and self-advocacy.

Technology has made an incredible difference in my journey with diabetes. In the dark ages, it was basically urine testing and bamboo like insulin syringes. The following technology advances included the development of more physiologic insulins along with pumps and pens. The past 10 years has been the decade of CGM. Like many others, CGM has made a huge difference to me. To have a blood glucose value every 5 min with trend arrows, alerts, and alarms and the ability to share my information with loved ones in real time is nothing short of amazing. Using the advances in CGM technology, we now have advanced to pumps with predictive low-glucose suspend and hybrid closed-loop capabilities. Next the fully automatic artificial pancreas, which will be the bridge until a real cure comes around.

REFERENCES

1. The Diabetes Control and Complications Trial Research Group. The effect of intensive therapy of diabetes on the development and progression of long-term complications in insulin-dependent diabetes mellitus. *N Engl J Med* 1993;329:977–986

2. Taking Control of Your Diabetes. Available from https://www.tcoyd.org. Accessed 14 February 2018

3. Taking Control of Your Diabetes. Our mission. Available from https://tcoyd.org/mission. Accessed 14 February 2018

Chapter 10
My Story

Aaron Kowalski, PhD[1]

Type 1 diabetes (T1D) can be a death-defying disease. Hyperbole? For those living with T1D, it really isn't. A host of scenarios have to be avoided or carefully managed, including hypoglycemia (lows), severe lows, highs, seizures, emergency calls, car crashes, emergency room visits and the accompanying bills, and nerve-wracking glucagon injections. Many review articles describe hypoglycemia as the barrier to tight glycemic control. In the Kowalski family, this was acutely true. Diabetes technologies have changed this paradigm for our family. Although there remains the fear of hypoglycemia in the background, it is now dramatically reduced. Rather than being full of worry and obsessive management, life is instead full of successes and more easily overcoming the challenges of T1D. Life with T1D for the Kowalski's means marathons, 100-mile bike rides, career successes, and, most important, a happy and healthy family. Diabetes technologies are helping us live T1D without limits.

In 1977, my brother Stephen was diagnosed with T1D. It was, as it is for many families, an absolute shock. We had no other family members with the disease and knew nothing about it. It was a terrifying diagnosis for my parents. At the time, diabetes complications were common, and it was expected that diabetes would significantly cut Steve's normal life expectancy. The treatment then was crude: urine testing for the presence of glucose and two to three injections of animal insulin per day. My parents were highly engaged from the start. My father, a PhD microbiologist and my mother, a stay-at-home mom and later a teacher, worked tirelessly to manage Steve's diabetes. Interestingly, despite this being years before the publication of the Diabetes Control and Complications Trial,[1] their immediate focus was on "normalizing" glucose levels. The challenge, however, was obvious: the tools didn't allow for normalized glucose levels.

Imagine being the parent of a 3-year-old and knowing that high blood glucose was damaging his body. This fear was further exacerbated when we moved from Virginia to New Jersey and our new neighbor had been blinded by T1D in her early 20s. That reality was very upsetting. My parents worked incredibly hard to keep Steve's urine free from glucose, but they found it was a nearly impossible task. He was a toddler, his eating was finicky, he was active, and the tools were crude. It was around this time, probably 1978, that I remember Steve's first seizure. We were watching television with my father and Steve had fallen asleep on the couch, or so we thought. He then began moaning and screaming, yet still

---

[1]President and Chief Executive Officer, JDRF, New York, NY.

seemed to be asleep. Was it a nightmare? It became apparent very quickly that it wasn't. It was a severe low. I don't remember how my father treated Steve at the time, but I do know that in future events, we would use juice if we were lucky enough to be able to get him to drink from a straw or we would have to give him a glucagon injection. My main memory is that it was absolutely terrifying.

It was a few years later, in 1984, at the age of 13 years, that I, too, was diagnosed with T1D. I remember my father flying home early from a business trip and the sad look in his eyes. He knew he now had two children who would live with a chronic disease that put us at risk for devastating complications and significant daily risk. My memories of this time include the relief of the diagnosis, as I was losing weight, tired, had insatiable thirst, and was urinating multiple times a night and what felt like hourly during the day. The tools had improved slightly and I recall my first finger pokes and using colorimetric test strips and a crude lancet device that Steve and I called "the guillotine."

It was during this time that it became clear that my brother and I had very different phenotypes, and those phenotypes drove the challenges that we experienced in our lives with diabetes. Steve had, and still has, terrible hypoglycemia unawareness. We shared a bedroom until college, and I could be awakened from the deepest sleep simply by changes in his breathing. I would yell to my parents, "Steve is getting low." Most of the time, my mother and I would try to get him to drink juice, but often we needed glucagon and a subsequent trip to the emergency department. The worst event was my younger sister finding me at a summer job and screaming "Steve needs help!" He had been found passed out in his car on a near 100°F(38°C) day. His body was overheated, and he barely had a pulse. Had he been found any later he may have died.

My challenge was not low blood glucose; to this day, I have symptoms when my blood glucose is low. My problem was the deprioritization of diabetes versus school and sports through college. Fortunately, I believe thanks to dedication to exercise, I was able to maintain a good A1C during this time. This came with risks that I certainly underappreciated at the time. There were weeks at a time during college, which I would not test my blood glucose even once. I drank alcohol and didn't test before going to bed. In hindsight, I didn't always make the best diabetes decisions as a college student. Fortunately, I met my future wife, and it was at this time that I moved past a short-term focus to realizing that I had a long future ahead if I took good care of myself.

Diabetes technologies have changed my brother's and my life, as well as those of our loved ones and others close to us. It wasn't until I began as a scientist at JDRF that diabetes technologies truly entered our lives. My brother and I had different perspectives. I had contemplated getting a pump after graduating college and as I was beginning graduate school. Despite seeing an excellent doctor at a leading academic center, I was discouraged from adopting a pump. "You're doing great; you don't need a pump," I was told on more than one occasion. In hindsight, perhaps my clinical team didn't think I was a good candidate. That said, they certainly never conveyed their concerns to me if that was the case. My brother had a different school of thought. I've described him as "militantly anti-pump." He swore that he would never wear a device that would signal that he had diabetes, and that no one could convince him otherwise.

In October 2004, our world began to change in terms of diabetes technologies. In September of that year I'd taken a junior scientist role at JDRF. One of my first meetings was a Diabetes Technology Society (DTS) meeting in Philadelphia. My boss at the time asked that I participate in an National Institutes of Health–funded consortium meeting that was scheduled for the 2 days before the DTS meeting. The group was DirecNet and they were gearing up for a trial of a new, yet-to-be approved continuous glucose monitor (CGM)—the Abbott Navigator. I vividly remember attending breakfast of day two and a number of the clinicians who were testing the sensor were making comments like "This really works!" and "It's accurate!" I met some of the leaders in the field of diabetes technology, including Drs. Bill Tamborlane, Bruce Buckingham, Peter Chase, and Roy Beck. I remember talking T1D with Jen Block from Stanford (now at Bigfoot) and Laurel Messer at the Barbara Davis Center. It was a life-changing experience for me. I called my parents and my brother and told them that we were on the cusp of continuous glucose monitoring and our lives would very likely be changed for the better. Once I returned to JDRF, I argued that we should be investing in pushing diabetes devices to the market. The JDRF Artificial Pancreas Project was born.

In 2006, the Kowalski family's diabetes journey took a critical step in a positive direction when I put on a CGM for the first time. I was the first patient in my clinic, and I believe in New Jersey, to wear a Dexcom sensor. Although the Dexcom at that time was not very accurate, was difficult to use, and frequently had data dropouts, it was transformative to me. The glucose-trending information was game-changing. It was very shortly thereafter that my brother, convinced by my enthusiastic praise of it, put on his first CGM. Despite the challenges of the first-generation Dexcom, our lives were immediately improved. Not just Steve's and my life, but the lives of our loved ones.

When I speak about diabetes publicly, both to professional and lay audiences, I often ask two simple and seemingly silly questions: *1*) How many people in the audience don't have diabetes? and *2*) How many of those who don't have diabetes are wearing a diabetes device—a CGM or a pump? The punchline is that people without diabetes don't wear diabetes devices. I make this point because people with diabetes must make a decision to wear devices that they otherwise wouldn't wear; this is an investment. For investments, you expect a return. In diabetes, the return may come in different forms. There may be glycemic returns—for example, better A1C, less hypoglycemia, and less glycemic variability. There are also quality-of-life returns—for example, better sleep, less fear of hypoglycemia, less anxiety, and less poking. I believe that the reason many people opt not to wear devices is that for a long time the return on investment had not been large enough. How many more finger-sticks per day are worth doing for an incremental improvement in A1C? How much benefit drives pump adoption? These are individual questions and different outcomes drive these decisions. JDRF launched an initiative focused on outcomes beyond A1C. It's clear that diabetes technologies can improve A1C, but their true value is often found in other diabetes outcomes.

In the Kowalski family, the first and most important outcome that was significantly improved was reduction in hypoglycemia. CGM devices with glucose-trending information and threshold alarms were transformational, particularly for my brother with his hypoglycemia unawareness. That said, it was also important for me. Although I've never had a severe hypoglycemic event requiring hospitalization, I've certainly had lows that impaired my thinking and were very scary. As a frequent business traveler who is often sleeping in a hotel room by myself, having a CGM to alarm me of hypoglycemia has reduced anxiety and allowed for tighter glucose control.

After nearly 30 years of insulin injections, both my brother and I adopted insulin pumps in addition to CGM. The ability to modify basal rates further reduced hypoglycemia events and helped increase quality of life and, specifically, the ability to be active with our diabetes more successfully. There is ample evidence of the benefit of exercise for all people, but particularly for people with diabetes. These benefits are both physical and mental. My brother and I were always active, but sports exacerbated hypoglycemia risk and required significant effort and work. After adopting an insulin pump, I ran my first marathon. Today, I've run 20, including a 50K trailrun at altitude at Lake Tahoe and running a Boston Marathon–qualifying time. My brother has participated in multiple "century rides" (i.e., 100-mile cycling challenges). Steve is often among the first riders with T1D to finish and has been in the first group (with or without diabetes) at a ride.

The best advice that my parents gave my brother and me when we were younger was "you will do anything your friends do and more. It may take more work, but diabetes will not hold you back from your dreams!" That's easier said than done, but it rings true. Forty-one years later for Steve and 34 years later for me, I am happy to report that we are doing great. We are fortunate to have no diabetes complications. Steve is a successful architect running his own company. I've been lucky enough to work on the frontline of diabetes research. Diabetes isn't easy. There have been many highs and lows (pun intended!). Diabetes technologies have minimized both the literal and figurative lows. They have changed our lives. Both Steve and I are currently using the Loop app—a reverse-engineered hybrid closed-loop system. The results are amazing.

The future is bright. Diabetes outcomes of all forms will continue to improve until we find more advanced treatments, such as cell therapies. I'm proud of the role that JDRF has played in this process. I am also incredibly grateful to the diabetes technology community for the countless hours dedicated by so many incredible investigators, clinicians, and study participants to improve the lives of people with diabetes and their loved ones.

I'll end with my own loved ones. When I began in diabetes research, my motivation was the collective experience of my brother; myself; my siblings, who don't have diabetes yet but who have carried the tremendous weight of it; and my parents. Today, those are still top of mind, but even more so is the impact of T1D on my children. My wife has been a tremendous champion for me with my T1D and my work at JDRF, and it goes without saying that I want to be healthy for my children as they grow up. Diabetes impacts the entire family, and my family is my motivation. I wouldn't be here without them!

REFERENCES

1. The Diabetes Control and Complications Trial Research Group. The effect of intensive therapy of diabetes on the development and progression of long-term complications in insulin-dependent diabetes mellitus. *N Engl J Med* 1993;329:977–986

Chapter 11
My Own Story

Irl B. Hirsch, MD[1]

I developed diabetes in 1964. In those days, there was not much in the way of "diabetes technology," at least as we know it today. Disposable insulin syringes were still quite new, and I remember my parents having to boil the glass insulin syringes and using disposable, very painful insulin needles for my once- or twice-daily injections. These are not very good memories of diabetes in childhood. But at least everyone could afford insulin.

It is amazing to look at where we are today, and how we got here in a relatively short period of time. My personal change in technology came before starting medical school in 1980. I was fortunate enough to have met Dr. Julio Santiago at an Association meeting, and at that time, he was doing a study with insulin pump therapy. There would be no cost to me (which was quite important because I was a college student hoping to enter medical school that fall), but home blood glucose monitoring had not really started yet either. The plan was for me to stay in the hospital for a week to learn how to start checking blood glucose, while at the same time start an insulin pump. I wanted to wait until a smaller pump was developed, because the only insulin pumps available then were the so-called Blue Bricks (Figure 11.1). Fortunately, I was able to wait until the month before I started medical school, and I went on the smaller version of that pump from the same company (Figure 11.2). In those early days, we had to dilute the insulin (U40), and there was only one basal rate. We adjusted the basal rates by changing the dilution of the insulin with diluting fluid from Eli Lilly. I was told I was the first one in the U.S. on that pump. But what was equally important, as the result of that pump, was that I was also one of the first people in the U.S. to start home blood glucose monitoring.

It wasn't just the mechanics of these first pumps that were primitive. So too was the insulin. This was well before insulin lispro (Humalog) or insulin aspart (NovoLog), and even before human insulin. We used animal insulin. Although "purified insulin" was available, most of us didn't use that. And for the record, a vial of insulin in 1980 was at most about $10 per vial.

Over time, we eventually moved to human insulin and also "buffered insulin" that was developed specifically for insulin pump therapy. I really do believe as both a medical student and a resident training at the University of Miami, I could not have done as well as I did without pump therapy. The other options, I now realize, were scary.

---

[1]Professor of Medicine, University of Washington, Seattle, WA.

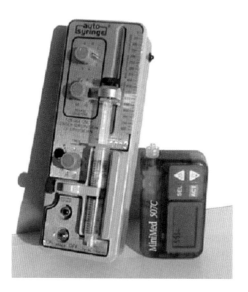

Figure 11.1. Auto-Syringe 2C insulin pump, also called the Blue Brick.

Source: Alsaleh FM, Smith FJ, Keady S, and Taylor KMG. Insulin pumps: from inception to the present and toward the future. *Journal of Clinical Pharmacy and Therapeutics* 2010; 35: 127–138. ©2009 The Authors. Journal compilation ©2009 Blackwell Publishing Ltd. Reprinted with permission from John Wiley & Sons.

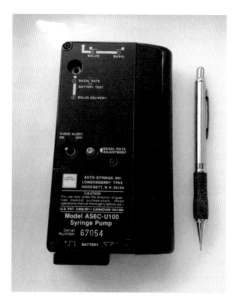

Figure 11.2. Auto-Syringe 6C: my first insulin pump.

Fast forward to 2006, and I think that as important technology as the pump was, continuous glucose monitoring (CGM) was maybe even more so. I recognized how important finger-stick blood glucose testing was at the time, but CGM was perhaps more important. That's because as we age, most of us lose the ability to feel hypoglycemia. Moreover, I discovered, in my case, that pumps cannot be used forever. I used those early animal insulins with straight-steel needles for so many years that I eventually ran out of infusion sites, and I had to give up the pump. The good news is that with the better basal insulins and, of course, with rapid-acting analogs and CGM, most of us do better now than we did with those initial pumps back in the early 1980s. In fact, for the current era, I'm not convinced pumps are any better than multiple injections for people like me as long as CGM is available and the person is intelligent about how to use insulin.

I have the advantage of historical perspective on diabetes technology. It is not something that I discuss much, but it is something that I think about often as I see young people who are doing so well but who don't really appreciate how the technology they are using has evolved so quickly. As we are now in the era of hybrid closed-loop systems and soon-to-be-completed closed-loop systems, I feel it is important that we recognize the many companies, foundations, and individuals who have allowed so many of us to lead productive lives. There are too many to acknowledge here, but I would be remiss if I did not mention the American Diabetes Association, the JDRF, the Helmsley Charitable Trust, Drs. Julio Santiago and Jay Skyler, and my parents, who raised more than $2 million to ensure improved care for all those with T1D, including their two sons and grandson.

Chapter 12

Continuous Glucose Monitoring and Insulin Pump Testimonial

Jeff Unger, MD, FAAFP, FACE[1]

M y wife, Lisa, thinks I'm crazy. "How many devices are you wearing today?" she asks with a puzzled face.

"As many as I need to eat, sleep, and exercise without fear of hypoglycemia," I opined.

I believe that God gave me type 1 diabetes so that I may help others not only achieve their metabolic targets, but to live life to the fullest. I often ask patients, "What are you most afraid of as a patient with diabetes?" There responses are universally similar. Each patient regardless of sex, race, and socioeconomic status tells me that they want to be able to watch their kids get married while maintaining all their birth-given body parts. Clinicians today have amazing pharmacologic tools as well as simple, yet advanced, technologies designed to make patients experts in diabetes self-management. When placed on the most appropriate medications and devices, patients can be "coached" to live their lives free of long- and short-term diabetes-related complications.

Patients now have access to a wide range of insulin pumps, continuous glucose monitors (CGM) and ultra-fast-acting insulin. Some closed-loop pumps allow patients to eat without calculating a mealtime bolus as insulin is delivered based on glucose excursions around mealtime. For the less technically astute patients, we can prescribe disposable patch pumps. These devices require <10 min of patient education time and deliver both basal and prandial boluses. Once used, the device can be discarded in the trash along with one's losing lottery ticket.

We have several approved CGM devices that provide patients with real-time glucose readings without the need for finger-stick calibration. These devices can be downloaded at one's home, at the office, or even into the cloud, which means that medical personnel no longer have to touch those bloody handwritten glucose log sheets. In fact, patients do not even have to lug their devices with them to an appointment as savvy medical assistants can download their data from "the cloud." Two CGM devices are able to audibly alert the user if their glucose levels are dropping too low or rising too high. Once the devices are downloaded, patients can be treated to a target based not just on A1C but toward "time in range." The

---

[1]Diplomate, American Board of Family Practice; Fellow, American Association of Clinical Endocrinologists; Assistant Clinical Professor of Family Medicine, University of California Riverside School of Medicine; Director, Unger Concierge Primary Care Medical Group; Director, Metabolic Studies; Catalina Research Institute, Rancho Cucamonga, CA.

Medtronic 630 G closed-loop pump and sensor data demonstrates that patients consistently spend >70% of their day within the range of 80–180 mg/dL while mitigating their chance of hypoglycemia.

The Abbott FreeStyle Libre sensor is factory calibrated and requires no finger-stick calibrations throughout its 10-day usage. The Dexcom 6 also allows patients to end finger-stick calibrations and turn off their tandem insulin pumps in response to a hypoglycemia event.

I've been known to go to extremes to successfully manage my diabetes. Years ago, I wore not one but two insulin pumps simultaneously. One pump delivered insulin while the second provided a continuous infusion of pramlitide (Symlin). One of my mentors, Steve Edelman, suggested that the use of pumped insulin and pramlitide might result in improvement in my overall glycemic control. It did not; however, this failed attempt at achieving physiologic glycemic control and blood glucose levels between 80–180 mg/dL demonstrates that it is as difficult as throwing a perfect game in professional baseball. One must remember that diabetes is a bihormonal disorder. We not only are insulinopenic, but also experience excessive and inappropriate glucagon production overnight and following each meal. Thus, targeting ideal glycemic control is a complex and frustrating process for all patients with diabetes.

Pumps and sensors make living with diabetes a "cake walk," yet I have experienced some moments of embarrassment. Last week, as I was getting behind the wheel of my truck, my daughter asked, "Daddy, what's your blood glucose?"

I replied, "62 mg/dL."

"Okay, give me your keys, NOW!"

"Wait a minute, you are just 14 years old," I argued. "Where are you taking me?"

I wonder what would happen to those of us with diabetes if we attended a "diabetes fantasy camp" for a weekend. For 48 h we could eat, drink, and exercise with no CGM, no insulin pumps, no noninsulin therapies, and no "food police" who are trying to tell us that they know how to count carbohydrates better than we do.

Over the past 2 weeks, I have been living with an integrated insulin pump and sensor. The sensor predicts when blood glucose levels are likely to drop and suspends the delivery of insulin until interstitial glucose levels stabilize. For many patients, the fear of experiencing treatment-emergent hypoglycemia results in nonadherence as well as more frequent office and ER visits. The goal of the sensor is to allow patients to spend more time within their prescribed treatment target and minimize the frequency of hypoglycemia.

For now, those patients with CGM and pumps have been deeply affected by these novel technologies and pharmacologic therapies. My patients with diabetes no longer fear this disease state. They accept diabetes as a chronic and progressive disease. With pumps and sensor technology, however, we all have the upper hand. We now control our diabetes to the absolute best of our ability. Diabetes no longer controls us.

Index